The Genetics of Aging

The Genetics of Aging

Edited by

Edward L. Schneider

Gerontology Research Center
National Institute on Aging
Baltimore, Maryland

PLENUM PRESS · NEW YORK AND LONDON

Library of Congress Cataloging in Publication Data

Main entry under title:

The Genetics of aging.

Includes bibliographies and index.
1. Aging – Genetic aspects. I. Schneider, Edward L.
QH529.G46   612.6'7'0157321   78-28
ISBN 0-306-31100-3

First Printing – May 1978
Second Printing – August 1979

© 1978 Plenum Press, New York
A Division of Plenum Publishing Corporation
227 West 17th Street, New York, N.Y. 10011

Printed in the United States of America

Contributors

Lew Bank • Department of Psychology, University of California at Los Angeles; Veterans Administration Hospital, Brentwood, Los Angeles, California

K. E. Cheney • Department of Pathology, University of California, Los Angeles, California

Samuel Goldstein • Departments of Medicine and Biochemistry, McMaster University, Hamilton, Ontario, Canada

Charles L. Goodrick • Laboratory of Behavioral Science, Gerontology Research Center, National Institute on Aging, National Institutes of Health, Public Health Service, U.S. Department of Health, Education and Welfare, Baltimore, Maryland

G. P. Hirsch • Division of Biology, Oak Ridge National Laboratory, Oak Ridge, Tennessee

Lissy F. Jarvik • Department of Psychiatry, University of California at Los Angeles; Veterans Administration Hospital, Brentwood, Los Angeles, California

David Kram • Laboratory of Cellular and Comparative Physiology, Gerontology Research Center, National Institute on Aging, National Institutes of Health, Public Health Service, U.S. Department of Health, Education and Welfare, Baltimore, Maryland

P. J. Meredith • Department of Pathology, University of California, Los Angeles, California

Edmond A. Murphy • Division of Medical Genetics, Department of Medicine, Johns Hopkins School of Medicine, Baltimore, Maryland

Thomas H. Norwood • Department of Pathology, University of Washington, Seattle, Washington

George A. Sacher • Division of Biological and Medical Research, Argonne National Laboratory, Argonne, Illinois

Harvey V. Samis • Veterans Administration Center, Bay Pines, Florida

Edward L. Schneider • Laboratory of Cellular and Comparative Physiology, Gerontology Research Center, National Institute on Aging, National Institutes of Health, Public Health Service, U.S. Department of Health, Education and Welfare, Baltimore, Maryland

G. S. Smith • Department of Pathology, University of California, Los Angeles, California

James R. Smith • W. Alton Jones Cell Science Center, Lake Placid, New York

Raymond R. Tice • Medical Department, Brookhaven National Laboratory, Upton, New York

R. L. Walford • Department of Pathology, University of California, Los Angeles, California

Preface

The Genetics of Aging is divided into several sections in an attempt to provide a logical progression from the level of the genome to the realm of human genetics. The relationship between the genetic material and aging will be thoroughly explored in the initial chapters. These chapters discuss in depth the various theories that have been proposed for the mechanisms of aging at the molecular level and present data which either support or contradict these hypotheses. Subsequent chapters will deal with the genetics of aging in organisms ranging from paramecium to mammals. The largest section of this volume will be devoted to several important areas in human genetics: human genetic disorders which feature premature aging, the effect of human parental aging on the production of genetically abnormal offspring, the genetics of human longevity, and a review of studies on aging human twins.

Over the last few decades genetic technology has provided enormous insight into a number of disciplines. Therefore, in the last few chapters, several genetic approaches to the study of aging are discussed: somatic cell genetics, immunogenetics, and behavioral genetics.

As the goal of this volume is to present a comprehensive examination of the genetics of aging, most chapters are oriented toward general review of their respective areas. It is my hope that this volume will encourage clinical, biological, and behavioral investigators to turn their attention to the genetic aspects of aging as well as to employ genetic technology to obtain further insight into aging processes.

Edward L. Schneider

Baltimore

Contents

Chapter 3
Aging and DNA-Repair Capability
Raymond R. Tice

Chapter 4
Somatic Mutations and Aging
G. P. Hirsch

PART II. ORGANISM LEVEL

Chapter 5
Genetics of Aging in Lower Organisms
James R. Smith

Chapter 6
Evolution of Longevity and Survival Characteristics in Mammals
George A. Sacher

PART III. HUMAN GENETICS

Chapter 7
Human Genetic Disorders That Feature Premature Onset and Accelerated Progression of Biological Aging
Samuel Goldstein

Chapter 8
Parental-Age Effects: Increased Frequencies of Genetically Abnormal Offspring
David Kram and Edward L. Schneider

Chapter 9
Genetics of Longevity in Man
Edmond A. Murphy

Chapter 10
A Longitudinal Study of Aging Human Twins
Lew Bank and Lissy F. Jarvik

PART IV. GENETIC APPROACHES TO AGING RESEARCH

Chapter 11

Somatic Cell Genetics in the Analysis of in Vitro Senescence
Thomas H. Norwood

Chapter 12

Immunogenetics of Aging
R. L. Walford, G. S. Smith, P. J. Meredith, and K. E. Cheney

Chapter 13
Behavior Genetics and Aging
Charles L. Goodrick

Introduction

Most biologic processes are the composite of both environmental and genetic determinants. Environmental influences on longevity range from the suddenness of an automobile accident to the subtle influences of cigarette smoking. In contrast to the relative clarity of some environmental factors, the genetic basis for aging is both complex and poorly understood. The existence of a genetic basis for aging and longevity, however, is incontrovertible.

The most convincing evidence for the genetic determination of longevity is the variation in life span among members of the animal kingdom. The mean life span of man is approximately seven hundred times longer than that of certain species of Drosophila. Even within superfamilies, considerable variation is observed: *Peromyscus leucopus,* the deer mouse, has a life span two to three times longer than the common laboratory mouse, *Mus musculus,* while the Philippine tree shrew, *Urogale everetti,* has a life span ten times shorter than that of its primate cousin, *Homo sapiens.* Finally, in regard to longevity variation within species, there are significant differences in life spans among inbred mouse strains.

The focus of this volume is on human longevity and aging. Therefore, it is particularly concerned with human studies. Evidence for a genetic component to longevity in man is somewhat less convincing than in lower organisms. Despite a wealth of anecdotal tales describing racial or geographic enclaves exhibiting longevity or families with unusual life spans, few studies have rigorously examined the genetic determination of human longevity. This important area will be reviewed by Dr. E. Murphy, who has reanalyzed one of the most extensive surveys of human longevity conducted by Dr. Raymond Pearl in the early part of this century.

Another approach to analyzing the genetic component to human aging and longevity is to examine the results of twin surveys. Individuals with the same genetic endowment—monozygous twins—should exhibit less variability in a particular function such as life span than dizygotic twins or siblings if the condition is genetically determined. This crucial area will be covered by Drs. Bank and Jarvik, who reviewed a number of studies of aging human monozygotic and dizygotic twins.

Finally, biologic studies have been greatly enhanced by the characterization of mutants which display variability in specific functions under scrutiny. Many biochemical pathways have been elucidated by research conducted on patients with inherited metabolic disorders. Therefore, human genetic disorders which display features of accelerated aging have drawn considerable interest. Although none of these conditions is a pure ''aging'' mutant, they do provide evidence for the genetic basis for many of the phenotypic alterations associated with aging.

How many genes are involved in regulating aging and/or controlling maximal life span? Some investigators, impressed by the increased life span that F1 hybrid laboratory animals exhibit over parental strains, have concluded that a single genetic locus may determine life span. However, despite the mathematical models which can be generated from such hybrid experiments, the overwhelming evidence derived from other sources points to longevity being controlled by a number of genetic loci. Evolutionary studies have indicated as many as 250 genes regulating maximal life span. Examination of human genetic disorders which have features of accelerated aging point toward an upper limit of 6900 genes related to aging. These numbers are certainly more realistic than a single genetic locus.

Several important questions need to be answered regarding the mechanisms for the genetic control of aging. Are there specific genes which code for senescence enzymes or hormones? Is there a gene or series of genes that programs the senescence and death of the organism? Are these genes quiescent during development and turned on only at maturity? Or, even more intriguing, could the same genes which regulate development also lead to senescence when development is completed? These questions have been raised by developmental biologists who feel that aging is just the terminal phase of the continuum of development. Of course, gerontologists can equally claim that development is merely the earliest stage of aging.

Another possible mechanism for the genetic regulation of aging is the gradual alteration of vital areas of the genome with aging. This could occur by several pathways: the genome could accumulate damage with time until a threshold is reached and cellular function is impaired to the point of senescence and cellular death. With sufficient cellular death in key organs, the entire organism could undergo senescence. This is the basis of somatic mutation theory. Alternatively, DNA damage could be occurring with an equal frequency throughout life, but the enzyme systems responsible for DNA repair may be altered with aging, leading to cellular malfunction and senescence. Finally, some organisms may have more efficient DNA repair systems. These organisms would therefore have longer life spans since their genetic material could be effectively protected. These possibilities will be further explored in the chapters on DNA repair and somatic mutations.

If aging and longevity are inherited traits, how did they evolve? Was there a gradual accumulation of senescent genes or alternatively, and more appealingly, has there been a selection toward genes which provide increasing longevity? Insight into the genetic regulation of aging may help to answer these intriguing questions.

The metabolic stability of the genetic material is unique. While most cellular macromolecules turn over with some degree of regularity in the various tissues of the body, DNA is not replaced and does not replicate new DNA. Thus the DNA in neurons, myocardial cells, muscle cells, and connective tissues fibroblasts of a 65-year-old individual is essentially the same macromolecule that was present at his or her birth. This stability of the genetic material, which is the basis for efficient conservation of phenotypic expression, is also a prime target for control of the aging process. Although it is possible to construct a model where the rate-limiting factor to aging is the alteration of a molecule such as an enzyme or ribonucleic acid, which is degraded within a period of hours or days, it is certainly easier to conceive of an accumulation of damage in a molecule such as DNA which has little, if any, turnover. In addition to this metabolic stability, DNA is also the key molecule in terms of cellular function. Almost all cell components are derived from the genome via transcription and translation of the genetic code. Thus alterations in the genome could lead to a multitude of effects which could be devastating, if not fatal, to the cell.

In this introductory chapter I have attempted to outline some of the important questions related to the role of genetics in human aging. These areas will be discussed in greater depth in the subsequent chapters.

Part I

Genome Level

Chapter 1

Molecular Genetics of Aging

Harvey V. Samis

1. Introduction

The mission of this chapter is to develop a background regarding molecular genetics and the place it holds and has held in experimental gerontology. My goal in writing this chapter is to point out fundamental questions that need serious and critical consideration before a "molecular genetics of aging" can take its place as a meaningful element in an understanding of aging phenomena. I do not intend an exhaustive review of the literature, and have therefore referred only to selected papers as examples of the kinds of thinking and the kinds of investigations that bear significantly on the arguments made.

One of the most prominent notions in experimental geronotology has been that organisms age because cells age. That is, deleterious changes that occur in individual cells seem to yield, up through the levels of biological organization, the deterioration of form and function which hallmarks senescence in the biome. It is a reasonable notion. Since 1665, when Robert Hooke drew attention to the cell as the basic biological unit, the cell has gradually become the reference unit, if not the prime focus, of biologists of most persuasions, from those concerned with matters of development to those interested in biological aging, working at all levels of biological organization from the province of anatomists to that of the biochemists.

Gerontologists have also been keenly aware that the patterns of senescent deterioration as well as life span are species-specific and appear to be inherited; i.e., there appears to be a "genetics of aging." The most compelling argument for a genetics of aging has been that each species has its own

Harvey V. Samis • Veterans Administration Center, Bay Pines, Florida 33504

characteristic life span, if normal environmental conditions are not drastically fouled (see Comfort, 1959, 1964). It is reasonable that genetics has played a predominant role in the thinking of gerontologists, as it has in all other facets of the life sciences. This is especially so, not because of the historically significant contributions of Mendel based on his studies of plant hybrids and their subsequent behavior, but because of the impact made by the elucidation of the structure of DNA and the success of investigators in unraveling the vagaries of the cellular information system.

Molecular genetics is the molecular biology of genetics, and it is defined by the sorts of things investigators working in the field do and have done. Molecular geneticists are concerned with such diverse areas of study as (1) unraveling the genetic code and understanding its ambiguities and subtleties as well as its evolution; (2) the translation of information stored in that code as DNA into protein; (3) the synthesis and chemistry of protein; (4) the synthesis of DNA and RNA; (5) the nature and cause of mutations; (6) the biochemistry of enzyme regulation; and (7) DNA repair. Certainly others would like to expand this list; some may wish to condense it. Nevertheless, the list does give some feeling for the kinds of phenomena that are considered to be components of molecular genetics.

Molecular biologists have addressed the problem of elucidating the structure and function of the gene. Their success is evidenced by the fact that their labors have led to certain dogmas that have stood the test of experimentation for approximately a quarter century. The first is that information flows from DNA to protein following a two-step sequence of events. The information coded in the linear sequences of deoxyribonucleotide residues in the DNA is first transcribed into sequences of ribonucleotides in RNA and then translated into linear sequences of the amino acids of proteins. The second is that the linear arrangement of the amino acid residues in the polypeptide chains of proteins is responsible for their three-dimensional form as well as for their specific functions. The third is that cellular components are constructed from macromolecular components synthesized either directly or indirectly under the direction of the information transmitted from generation to generation as nucleotide sequences of DNA and rendered functionally meaningful via the cellular information system. Simply stated, information for the development of an organism is transmitted from generation to generation coded in the linear sequence of nucleotide residues of which DNA is composed. Stored in the DNA, this information is of no use to the cell. The information becomes meaningful to the cell only when it is translated into protein, specifically enzymic protein. The flow of the cellular information system is from DNA and RNA to protein.

If organisms age because cells age, then it seems likely that cellular aging must be due to the occurrence of events that effect some sort of change in one or more of the cellular components. These alterations must accumulate in a component the altered state of which could functionally result in deleterious consequences. For these criteria to be met, the cellular component must be in a state of low flux relative to the rate at which the deleterious alterations take place. The genome seems a likely candidate when considered in the context of the other cellular components. It is relatively stable at least with respect to its information component, the DNA. Moreover, the accumulation of alterations in the DNA could be manifest functionally via the cellular information system as enzymic protein with diminished, lost, or otherwise altered function.

If these ideas prove correct, the site of the primary aging event would reside in the genome, with the gene-based information coded in the DNA suffering the primary degenerative alterations, ultimately effecting the deterioration of the host cell's function. Critical to these ideas regarding the cause of senescence is either (1) the accumulation of functionally altered proteins for which the alterations can be shown to be deleterious to the function of the affected cell or its fellows, or (2) a functionally significant change in the nature of the cell's complement of protein that can adversely affect its function. At the level of the cellular genetic information system, the genetic basis of aging could be subjected to the elegant methods and tools of molecular biologists and molecular geneticists.

Molecular genetics encompasses both the molecular basis of inheritance and the state and functional characteristics of the DNA-based cellular information system. It includes the molecular mechanisms of DNA replication, the transcription of DNA-based information into RNA, and the translation of that information into the functionally meaningful protein. In the broader sense, molecular genetics includes consideration of the regulation of these processes through the synthesis of protein and their sequencing and ordering in time and the fidelity that obtains throughout the information-flow system.

The molecular genetics of aging is usually interpreted as meaning the molecular genetic mechanisms of aging, with the implication that during adult life, changes occur in the central genetic information system that lead ultimately to a gradual deterioration of biological form and function. This bias has been translated intuitively into hypotheses, theories, and notions that propose that aging has its genesis in the central information system in the quantity or quality of the cellular protein population, especially among the many species of enzymic proteins.

It seems highly probable that changes of a degenerative sort do occur with aging in the system by means of which DNA-based information is ultimately translated into both structural and biochemically active protein. It is difficult to envision so complex a series of processes proceeding with absolute fidelity or an information store such as the genome existing, immutable, over long periods of time. The question is, however, does senescence, in the time frame that at present obtains for the various species, result from compromised fidelity in translation and transcription, or from the accumulation of degenerative changes in the genome? Alternatively, does senescence derive from some sort of genetically programmed sequence of events mechanistically analogous to the sort of programmed sequence that determines the characteristics of morphogenesis? Common to both these views is the notion that aging results from a change in the central information system. Consideration of the molecular genetic mechanisms resolves, therefore, into a consideration of the nature of the change or changes, on one hand, and their causes and consequences, on the other.

It is clear even to the most casual observer that longevity and the patterns of deterioration accompanying aging are genetically determined. The characteristics of senescence, as well as the rate of aging, life expectancy, and life span, are clearly fundamental characteristics of species and strains. How is a life span of 110 years genetically determined for humans and one of three years mandated for the rat or mouse? Even among rodents, what is the molecular basis for the difference in life span for the rat (3 years), the shrew (1 year), the guinea pig (7 years), and the rabbit (15 years) (Comfort, 1964). Even within the species, strains can exhibit marked differences. For example, the two different wild-type strains of *Drosophila melanogaster,* Oregon R and Swedish C, have mean life spans of 60 and 30 days, respectively, under identical environmental conditions (Clark and Gould, 1970).

The initial question is, are longevity and patterns of senescence inherited explicitly as positive events, or are they transmitted from generation to generation implicit in the physical and chemical composition and form of the organism? In 1928, Raymond Pearl (1928) juxtaposed these alternatives when he suggested that the "duration of life, considered of itself, is not a biologically separate characteristic of the organism, but instead, is simply the expression of the total functional–structural organization or pattern of the individual." These alternative means by which senescence and longevity may be initially determined will be the conceptual frame for this discussion of the molecular genetics of aging. It seems important that the ways by which aging is generated within an organism be compatible with the genetic means by which the patterns of senescent deterioration are inherited through generations.

The mechanisms postulated to explain aging in biological systems that invoke the DNA-based information system will therefore be discussed in terms of both the implicit and the explicit modes of inheritance. I hasten to point out that this approach is not a simple matter of semantics. To the contrary, it is a matter of imposing criteria for systematically considering the plethora of hypotheses and theories in order to judge their plausibility against the rather meager evidentiary background available at present. One goal of this approach is to obtain a clearer realization of the plausibility of the fundamental assertions of these hypotheses, theories, and notions.

I have chosen to exclude from these considerations matters of enzyme regulation. Although regulation of gene action, as expressed by enzyme activity, certainly does constitute a signal element in the molecular genetics of aging, it also involves extensive considerations of neurohumoral regulations and is a sufficiently discrete and important area of current endeavor to warrant separate treatment (see Adelman, 1972; Finch, 1976).

2. Mechanisms for the Inheritance of the Patterns of Senescence and Longevity

2.1. Explicit Inheritance

Mechanisms of senescence that could be reasonably inherited explicitly constitute those mechanisms grouped under programmed aging theories. Two general means by which aging can be programmed are readily apparent. The first may be considered to be analogous to the type of programming involved in morphogenesis (Wilson, D. L., 1974). Particular information blocks or segments of the genome would be repressed and others derepressed, thereby changing the biochemistry and the form and function of the cells involved. In this case, there would be a sequentially clocked series of events that would take place within the genome of an organism as it ages. These events would result in alterations that effect changes in the spectrum and level of gene products that are deleterious to the cell's normal function. In the case of morphogenesis, sequentially timed events result in the orderly growth and differentiation of the system. Viewed as a possible mechanism in aging, it is seen as a clocked destruction mechanism in which blocks of information are repressed or derepressed, resulting in alterations of the cell's biochemistry and changes in gene products that are detrimental to the cell, and ultimately to the entire organism. In this model, although the actual gene products become changed, the change is neither random nor accidental. The actual fidelity of the information flow is not impaired, nor is it the cause of loss or diminution of function for the affected cell. The gene products arise in the normal way from DNA to RNA to protein, but the products themselves are altered.

Contrasted with this model is one in which a finite amount of gene product is produced, and this product is not replaced when it is destroyed randomly by accidents or turned over as a function of use, thus leading to lost or decreased function or adaptive capacity. Conceptually tied to this idea is another programmed model that predicts that the products of metabolism in cells are not eliminated from the cell at a rate equal to that at which they are being produced and, consequently, accumulate as toxins. The rate at which they accumulate and poison the cell constitutes a genetic program for cell destruction. Another variation of this theme is that of programmed depletion. This variation encompasses the notions that the genetic information available in the genome can suffer destruction from use, and that the number of times a segment or block of information can be used before it is "used up" is genetically determined in terms of its inherent stability or resistance to "wear and tear." At this point, the distinction between aging as an active and possibly separate program and as merely the result of a morphogenic program running out is less than clear, and considerations of explicit inheritance seem to begin to merge with those of implicit inheritance.

Explicit inheritance of the patterns of senescence, however, implies a positive sequence of events. The senescence of an organism, if explicitly inherited, would be actively generated in much the same fashion that cell division, growth, and differentiation proceed according to a program that leads to the whole of morphogenesis. Clearly, programmed senescence need not be explicitly inherited. The program could reside in the characteristics of the biomolecules and the structural components of cells. Certainly, the susceptibility of biomolecules and the complexes of molecules and organelles to degenerative change is inherent in their chemical and physical characteristics, which are genetically determined. Under these circumstances, it would be the "chemical and physical nature of the organism" that would constitute the program for its patterns of senescence, which would be generated by means of stochastic accidents of one sort or another. Coupled with this tendency or susceptibility to change or damage would be the effectiveness of the pertinent repair systems or of those systems charged with the accurate renewal of the cellular as well as the extracellular components of the organism.

2.2. Implicit Inheritance

If patterns of senescence and longevity are implicitly inherited, the mechanism or mechanisms would be far more difficult to elucidate, greater in diversity and number, and far less amenable to manipulation.

Examples of implicitly inherited characteristics abound in the biome, since many of the characteristics of particular organisms are unique, species-specific, and genetically determined, yet are not explicitly inherited. For example, man cannot tolerate temperature beyond a certain limit, yet it would be patently absurd to suggest that such a limit is inherited by means of a "too-hot gene."

This absurdity is dramatically apparent when dealing with life span and life expectancy in poikilotherms. For example, life span and expectancy for the fruit fly *Drosophila* are markedly altered by changes in temperature (Loeb and Northrop, 1917; Pearl, 1928). That environmental temperature has a very real effect on the life expectancy of *Drosophila* is well known. How these effects are biologically determined and manifested is less clear-cut. For *Drosophila melanogaster,* Oregon R wild-type, survival at 36.1°C is (1) age-dependent and (2) dependent on the length of exposure at that temperature. Moreover, it is different for the two sexes. At all ages, the thermal sensitivity of males at 36.1°C, in terms of survival, is almost double that of females (Figs. 1 and 2). This characteristic of *Drosophila* implies a genetic basis for the sex difference in thermal sensitivity at 36.1°C. But it would be absurd to suggest that it is explicitly inherited in the form of a specific "thermal sensitivity" gene that switches on or off after a critical period of time at 36.1°C. It is more reasonable to think that this sensitivity is implicit in the uniqueness of the form and constitution of the two sexes of *Drosophila.*

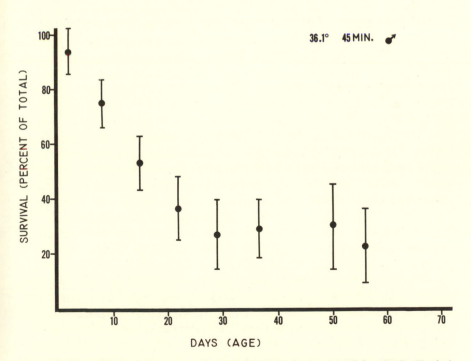

Fig. 1. Survival of *Drosophila melanogaster* males maintained at 36.1°C for 45 min. Vertical brackets denote standard deviations. In the experiment, 10 groups of 20 flies each of each sex (here, males; Fig. 2, females) were subjected to dry heat (36.1°C) in a water thermostat. Survivors were scored after being maintained at 25°C for 30 min following the heat treatment.

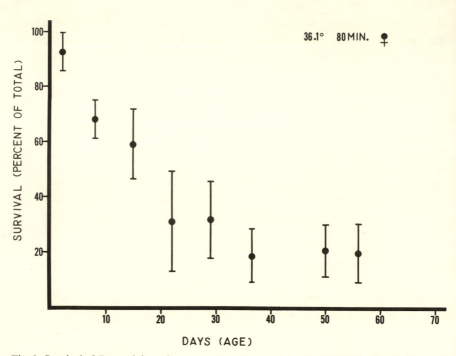

Fig. 2. Survival of *Drosophila melanogaster* females maintained at 36.1°C for 80 min. Vertical brackets denote standard deviations.

The notion that adaptability to temperature changes is genetically transmitted is plausibly compatible with the notion that the patterns of senescence, life span, and life expectancy may be implicitly inherited. They need not derive from some "happening" in the genetic store. The patterns of senescence and length of life can be viewed as implicit characteristics of the species not unlike those for the strength of skeletal musculature, fragility of bones, limits in height and weight, or the positions of and stimuli for copulation. All these are definite characteristics of an organism— unique and, in many cases, part of the description of the species.

The notion that senescent deterioration of form and function "must be due to some kind of occurrence, some kind of error, mutation or break-down in information flow or the fidelity of translation or transcription," though attractive, suffers from a paucity of data to support it (Finch, 1976; Baird *et al.*, 1975; Baird and Massie, 1975).

The sorts of models envisioned in this category are of two general types. The first type is formulated from those hypotheses that say that aging is due to stochastic accidents of one sort or another that occur in the DNA or the genome or in the system by means of which DNA-based information is translated into protein, resulting in an accumulation of aberrant proteins. The second type includes those hypotheses that suggest that aging is due to errors that occur in protein synthesis—errors that effect degenerative changes in the cellular information system itself, and in turn produce still other altered proteins (Orgel, 1973).

One can envision other types of events that would have little or no relationship to the genetic information system. Damage to membranes, decreased responsiveness of the endocrine system, and decreased sensitivity of target organs to neurohumoral control are a few examples of changes of this sort. Others would require no "primary cause" of the classic type, only the condition that biological repair systems and the systems responsible for the renewal of cellular and extracellular components and the removal of the products of their degradation be less than perfect, less than 100% efficient.

The clear fact is, rather, that such mechanisms are not required in order that there be a genetic basis for the uniqueness of the patterns of senescence and life span. These limits, like many others, may be viewed as implicit in the constitution of the organism, genetically transmitted, and established early on, during development; i.e., the genetically transmitted "cause" of senescence need not occur coincident with its manifestation.

3. Molecular-Genetic Mechanisms of Senescence

As has been stressed earlier, that there is a genetic basis for aging does not necessarily mean that senescence is generated through the cellular information system in terms of an unfolding genetic program for deterioration or as the result of stochastic accidents in the system that alter the basic store of genetic information in the genome or diminish the fidelity with which it is translated into functional protein. The genetic mechanisms that have been proposed to account for the apparent inheritance of the patterns of senescent change and longevity have nevertheless emphasized these sorts of changes. These ideas and proposals have consequently served as the hypothetical framework for much of the work in experimental gerontology. In consideration of the molecular genetic mechanisms of senescence, three views will be discussed. The first is the view that aging is due to stochastic accidents that occur somewhere in the cellular information system. The second is the view that aging may occur as a function of the nature of the organism and the uniqueness of its form and function. The third is the view that aging is an extension of development in that it is the result of a sequence of genetically programmed events that result in the gradual deterioration of form and function and thereby result in an exponentially increasing probability of death.

3.1. Altered Molecules

Errors here refer to stochastic accidents that occur in the cellular genetic information system. In this discussion, damage sustained outside the cellular genetic information, or not having a direct influence on the information flow in the system, will not be considered. For example, damage sustained by the oxidation of membranes or cross-linking populations of extracellular protein will not be discussed. The focus will be firmly on the cellular genetic information system by means of which DNA-based information is translated into protein.

3.1.1. Somatic Mutations

In 1939, Russ and Scott (1939) reported their observation that rats that had been subjected to ionizing radiation, though young chronologically, appeared old. Since that time, it has been repeatedly reported that exposure to ionizing radiation shortens life span (Curtis, 1961; Lindop and Rotblat, 1961). In addition, it has been shown that exposure to radiation can lead to the premature development of certain diseases and a reduced resistance to stress, usually associated with senescence (Curtis and Gebhard, 1960; Curtis, 1961; Upton *et al.*, 1963*a,b*). These observations naturally led many investigators to think that radiation, a known mutagen, might well be increasing the rate of aging in much the same way by which it was thought to increase the rate of mutation in germ cells. The reasoning was, of course, that like results derive from like causes—a highly questionable logical progression. The prerequisite had been met: radiation left the geometry of the survival curve unchanged, changing only the progression along the time axis (see Welch, 1967).

Szilard (1959) came directly and simply to the point. He proposed that somatic mutations accumulated in the genomes of somatic cells, gradually inactivating the "chromosome," until ultimately the functional capability of the chromosome was destroyed and finally the cell died. Szilard stated that his theory "assumes that the elementary step in the process of aging is an 'aging hit' which 'destroys' a chromosome of the somatic cell, in the sense that it renders all genes carried by that chromosome inactive."

This notion implies that genes of somatic cells are affected with time in a way analogous to radiation-induced mutations. According to Szilard, a mutant gene would be one not capable of producing a specific protein molecule in its chemically active form. Two alternatives arise from these notions. The first is that somatic mutations would result in the synthesis of altered protein, presumably altered in a way deleterious to the cell's function; i.e., the protein would be inactive, or would have a diminished activity, or would exhibit a degeneration in its specificity. The second is that the mutation would be of a sort that precludes transcription and ultimate translation into protein, with the result that the mutation would not be manifested as protein. If aging is due to the accumulation of somatic mutations, then it seems reasonable that cells would differ in the sort of mutations they sustain, and if cells with mutations do not die (Samis, 1966), a metazoic organism would become a mosaic of cells that are aging in different ways (Weismann, 1891), and even at different rates, depending on the functional significance of their particular array of somatic mutations. If, as Szilard has suggested, cell survival decreases as somatic mutations accumulate, then aging due to somatic mutations may be revealed, not through altered proteins, but through cellular attrition. If, in fact, cellular attrition is the "cause" or one of the "causes" of biological aging, then it is reasonable to think that aging does not occur in tissues and organs capable of undergoing mitosis, or that it occurs at a far lower rate. Aging would occur primarily through cell loss in tissues and organs incapable of cell division, the true post mitotics, and would result in a decreased functional capability in the affected organs and tissue, i.e., the CNS, skeletal muscle, and myocardium (Goss, 1966). If loss of cells is not the means by which organisms age, then one is confronted with determining how the random accumulation of altered proteins of vastly varying levels and assortments could be translated into the deterioration of functional capacity and form of an organism. Unique loss of function through mutations in one of the endocrine glands, if sufficiently widespread among the cells of the gland, could conceivably have widespread effects on the organism through loss of an element of humoral regulation. It would be difficult, however, to envision how a stochastic accident could generate mutations of such a specific sort.

Random somatic mutations have also been proposed as the bases of the age-related increase in autoimmune disease (Burnet, 1959, 1965, 1974). Burnet suggested that some of the immunologically competent cells may suffer mutations of a sort that cause a loss of tolerance for their host's proteins, and that the mutated cells may give rise to clones of cells that produce autoantibodies, leading to the damage of cells or their death. This variation on the error theme seems to have a basis in experimental evidence (Walford, 1967, 1969).

3.1.2. Error Catastrophe

It has been pointed out that it is not necessary to postulate somatic mutations to account for the accumulation of altered proteins in cells. Orgel (1963, 1970) suggested that there may well occur in the protein synthetic system errors that could lead to an accumulation of altered protein molecules.

In the process by means of which DNA-based information is translated into protein, there are three points at which the reading of the genetic code and the recognition and selection of particular molecules from others that are similar must take place. The amino-acid-activating enzymes must select a specific amino acid and couple it to the appropriate transfer RNA. The anti-codon of that particular transfer RNA charged with its amino acid must then pair with its messenger RNA codon. In addition, RNA polymerase must read the information coded in the DNA and select the appropriate ribonucleotide residues for the accurate transcription of the information into RNA. In each of these steps, errors could be introduced into protein. Orgel reasoned that since the protein-synthetic machinery is synthesized by that same machinery, errors in the enzymes involved in these steps could result in a progressively decreasing fidelity in translation or transcription or both. Errors of this sort could lead to an exponential increase in the level of altered proteins—an "error catastrophe."

That increasing amounts of altered proteins are generated that deleteriously affect the function of the cell is critical to this "error catastrophe" theory. In addition, if the accumulation of errors is a generalized phenomenon, not unique to a particular species of protein, it follows that with time, all protein species being synthesized should be represented by altered analogues, if these analogues are not selectively destroyed.

It is important to realize that errors in protein synthesis may also result in altered DNA polymerase, which would misreplicate DNA, thereby injecting errors into the genome that would lead to clones of abnormal cells (Orgel, 1973). In this way, errors in protein synthesis, whether at the transcriptional or the translational level, could also be considered as a mechanism for generating somatic mutations and initiating abnormal populations of cells.

3.1.3. Compensation and Repair

If it is accepted that somatic mutations and errors in the transcription of gene-based information into RNA and its translation into protein can and do occur, it seems reasonable to ask whether cells have any means by which they can recognize and compensate for the occurrence of errors or repair them.

In 1966, this author suggested mechanisms for the detection and repair of age-related alterations in DNA (Samis, 1966) as one process available to compensate for senescent change. There is no question that cells are capable of repairing damage to DNA; moreover, evidence is beginning to accumulate to suggest that this repair capability may decline with advancing age (Little, 1976). Yielding (1974) proposed that due to the differences in availability to repair enzymes of those DNA segments that are being actively transcribed, and those not involved in the renewal of cellular protein, errors may well accumulate preferentially in the inactive segments while being constantly repaired in those that are active. These errors in inactive segments of the genome would be of consequence in that they would be expected to affect cell replication deleteriously and thereby interfere with the replenishing of cells, rather than to affect postmitotic cellular function (Yielding, 1974), i.e., single- and double-strand scissions, cross-links, or even gross chromosomal lesions of the sort studied by Curtis and co-workers (Curtis and Gebhard, 1960; Curtis and Crowley, 1963). The relationship between DNA repair and aging is examined in detail in Chapter 3 of this volume.

In addition to the capacity to repair certain types of errors that arise in DNA, cells also possess a means by which they can selectively degrade proteins (Goldberg and Dice, 1974). Clearly, protein degradation is critical to the control of enzyme levels. Goldberg and Dice (1974) pointed out that protein degradation has been shown to follow first-order kinetics, i.e., that the probability of degradation is the same for both old and newly synthesized proteins. Furthermore, different protein species are degraded at vastly different rates (Fritz *et al.,* 1973; Russell *et al.,* 1970), and the rates vary widely and uniquely under different physiological conditions (Rechcigl, 1968; Millward, 1970; Goldberg, 1969) and for specific proteins (Schmike, 1964; Majerus and Kilburn, 1970). Rapid degradation allows for more efficient adjustment of the activity of enzymes to changing physiological demands. In addition, it appears that the differences in the role of degradation of the different proteins are dependent on the differences in their three-dimensional conformation. Differences in conformation induced by aberrance result in a higher rate of degradation for the altered molecule. It has been demonstrated that aberrant analogues of specific proteins are degraded at a far higher rate than their normal fellows (for review, see Goldberg and Dice, 1974; Goldberg and St. John, 1976).

3.2. Programmed Aging

Countering the argument that aging results from stochastic accidents is the position that senescence proceeds according to a genetically determined program, which is manifested as a gradual deterioration of the organism, in much the same way that growth and differentiation are programmed and become manifested during morphogenesis.

It has also been stated that aging is simply an expression of morphogenesis, and is generated by an active process requiring positive events (Woolhouse, 1967). It can certainly be stated that particular types or manifestations of aging are specific to particular species of animals and plants (Wilson, D. L., 1974). The argument being made is that this specificity derives from the species-unique genetic characteristics, thus constituting a particular "aging program" for each species. It has even been argued that the development of a directed senescence and consequent finite life span has evolved as a selective advantage for a species throughout the course of evolution (Guthrie, 1969). It is highly questionable that the hypotheses deduced from following this line of reasoning provide sufficient evidence for a general "genetic program" mechanism of aging.

One can see, for example, that a programmed shutdown of the production of enzymes involved in DNA repair could be a basis for the increase in the rate of accumulation of somatic mutations. Similarly, a gradual deterioration in the selectiveness of the cellular protein catabolic system could lead to an increased tolerance of, and therefore increasing levels of, altered proteins. Actual evidence for these two mechanisms, however, is lacking.

Barrows (1972) and Barrows and Kokkonen (1975) suggested that another sort of programmed senescence may occur in the bdelloid rotifer. They propose that the genetic material seems to be affected deleteriously, through usage, as these organisms age. The implication here is that if the use of this increasingly faulty information-flow system is decreased, the organism will age at a lower rate. This suggestion, however, is not based on a notion of positive or active programming, but rather on a theory of "wear and tear" similar to that enunciated by Pearl in 1928.

4. Conclusion

The acceptance of the existence of a genetic basis for senescence and life span is extremely widespread. Yet, with the exceptions of longevity and some unique pathologies that accompany advancing age, this notion is primarily intuitive. Actual experimental evidence for a genetic mechanism of aging has proved to be distressingly elusive, and the evidence that does exist is meager and often highly equivocal.

Data purported to show age-associated changes in enzyme activity are unimpressive. Those data that do exist suggest that if somatic mutations do occur, or protein synthesis does become faulty, the actual effect on the activity of the cell's enzyme complement is not serious and certainly not disastrous (Finch, 1972; Wilson, P. D., 1973). The lack of a conclusive change in enzyme activity with increasing age is not proof that these sorts of somatic mutations do not occur. Plausible explanations for this lack of net effect immediately come to mind. One possibility is that the mutations that do occur with age are of a type that preclude transcription of the affected site. This possibility is suggested by the work of von Hahn (1971) and O'Meara and Herrmann (1972), which shows an increasing tenacity in the binding of nucleoprotein with advancing age. A second explanation is that the loss of information potential of the genome, through the masking of segments of information, is compensated for by an increase in the synthesis of those proteins at other sites (Samis, 1966).

Support for an accumulation of altered or abnormal proteins with aging is derived from the work of Gershon and Gershon (1970, 1973*a,b*) and Zeelon *et al.* (1973), as well as from that of Holliday and his co-workers (Harrison and Holliday, 1967; Holliday and Tarrant, 1972; Holliday, 1975). The evidence from the Gershons' laboratory has shown that in *Turbatrix aceti,* there is a decrease in the specific activity of isocitrate lyase with advancing age (Gershon and Gershon, 1970). This decrease in enzyme activity was found to occur with a coincident increase in molecules immunochemically identical to those of the active enzyme. With Zeelon (Zeelon *et al.,* 1973), they were also able to show that fructose-1,6-diphosphate aldolase behaved in a similar fashion with advancing age. Their studies with fructose-1,6-diphosphate aldolase from mouse liver also showed an age-related decrease in specific activity and an increase in the amount of the inactive analogue (Gershon and Gershon, 1973*a*). Examination of mouse skeletal muscle aldolase by Gershon and Gershon (1973*b*) revealed no decrease in specific activity with age. These authors were able to show, however, that there was an accumulation of the inactive analogues of the aldolase.

In 1967, Harrison and Holliday (1967) reported that when larvae of *Drosophila* were fed amino acid analogues, a treatment that it was assumed would lead to the synthesis of abnormal proteins containing those analogues, the life span of the imagoes was decreased. As this author and co-workers have pointed out (Baird *et al.,* 1975), it is dangerous to reason from a study of this sort that since the introduction of amino acid analogues into protein leads to abnormal protein and this occurrence is coupled with a decreased life span, the accumulation of abnormal protein is the cause of aging. Such a conclusion assumes that like effects, of necessity, arise from like causes, which is clearly fallacious reasoning.

Thermostability determinations of glucose-6-phosphate dehydrogenase (G-6-PD) were carried out in cultures of fetal lung fibro-blasts by Holliday and Tarrant (1972). They were able to show that thermostability of a fraction of G-6-PD decreased with increasing *in vitro* culture age. These results have been questioned on the grounds that the cultures showing aberrant analogues of the dehydrogenase contained dying or dead cells, indicating that the accumulation of aberrant molecules may be a characteristic of dying or dead cells, rather than a function of senescence (Baird *et al.,* 1975).

The observations of many investigators that changes in enzyme activity with advancing age are rare and slight (see Finch, 1972; Wilson, P. D., 1973) lend little support to the arguments of Gershon and Gershon and those of Holliday and his co-workers. One could argue that the accumulation of nonfunctional enzymes or enzymes with diminished activity does occur, but that coincident with their generation, there is a compensatory increase in total number of molecules due to increased synthesis or decreased rate of degradation (Samis, 1966). If there were such an increase then one would expect to observe a gradual increase in total protein with advancing age. This, however, does not appear to be the case (Barrows *et al.*, 1960; Fonda *et al.*, 1973). There is also evidence of enzymes that do show a decrease in activity with age but without evidence of the accumulation of aberrant analogues, i.e., G-6-PD of rat liver (Grinna and Barber, 1972) and lactate dehydrogenase of mouse muscle (Oliveira and Pfuderer, 1973). In studies of catalase of rat liver, Zimmerman *et al.* (1975) showed that there is no age-associated change in either the thermostability of the enzyme or its immunochemistry, as evidenced by the almost identical immunoprecipitation curves for the enzymes from young and old rodents.

If the synthesis of altered molecules is to be taken seriously as a significant causative factor in aging, then one would expect that it would be the general case, i.e., that it would occur in all populations of protein. This is clearly not the case. One explanation for the lack of universality of evidence for aberrant analogues for all enzymes may be that in some cases the degradation of the altered forms is much greater than that of the normal form. This greatly increased degradation would maintain the altered form at a level too low to be detected. For other species of proteins, degradation of the aberrant molecule may closely approximate that of the normal form, and thereby maintain the altered form at a level close to that of the unaltered form.

Evidence to support the notions of a programmed genetic mechanism for aging is also very scarce. Some findings such as those of Barrows' group working with the bdelloid rotifer are amenable to interpretation within a variation of the programmed aging theme in the sense that the program "wears out" after a specific amount of use (Barrows, 1972).

It may well be that the question of Pearl (1928) regarding the genetic basis of longevity was prophetic. In most efforts to relate a genetics of aging to a genetic mechanism of aging, the tendency has been to assume that the mechanism is associated with some change in the cellular gene-based information system and coincident in time with the senescent deterioration. The genetic mechanism for senescence, however, may well be implicit in the inherited uniqueness of the organization and functional capacity of organisms, and not associated with deterioration or a programmed change in the information system.

Aging need not have a primary or single "cause" in the classic sense (Stewart, 1967; Samis, 1967). Most certainly, aging need not have its primary cause or causes in the genetic apparatus of somatic cells, as proposed by either the error theories or the programmed theories of aging.

It seems that it is more reasonable at this time to think that the genetics of aging resides in the genetic determination of the uniqueness of each organism's form and function, and that the basis for the uniqueness of patterns of senescent change and longevity are genetically transmitted implicit in the chemical and physical form of the organism.

ACKNOWLEDGMENT

The author's work is supported by the Medical Research Service of the Veterans Administration.

References

Adelman, R. C., 1972, Age-dependent control of enzyme adaption, in: *Advances in Gerontological Research,* Vol. 4 (B. L. Strehler, ed.), pp. 1–23, Academic Press, New York and London.

Baird, M. B., and Massie, H. R., 1975, A further note on the Orgel error hypothesis and senescence, *Gerontologia* **21**:240.

Baird, M. B., Samis, H. V., Massie, H. R., and Zimmerman, J. A., 1975, A brief argument in opposition to the Orgel hypothesis, *Gerontologia* **21**:57.

Barrows, C. H., 1972, Nutrition, aging and genetic program, *Am. J. Clin. Nutr.* **25**:829.

Barrows, C. H., and Kokkonen, G., 1975, Protein synthesis, development, growth and lifespan, *Growth* **39**:525.

Barrows, C. H., Falzone, J. A., and Shock, N. N., 1960, Age differences in the succinoxidase activity of homogenates and mitochondria from the liver and kidneys of rats, *J. Gerontol.* **15**:130.

Burnet, F. M., 1959, Autoimmune disease. II. Pathology of the immune response, *Br. Med. J.* **2**:645.

Burnet, F. M., 1965, Somatic mutation and chronic disease, *Br. Med. J.* **1**:338.

Burnet, F. M., 1974, Intrinsic mutagenesis: A genetic approach to aging, *Pathology* **6**:1.

Clark, A. M., and Gould, A. B., 1970, Genetic control of adult lifespan in *Drosophila melanogaster, Exp. Gerontol.* **5**:157.

Comfort, A., 1959, Studies on the longevity and mortality of English thoroughbred horses, in: *The Lifespan of Animals* (G. E. W. Wolstenhome and M. O'Conner, eds.), *Ciba Found. Colloq. Ageing* **5**:35–54.

Comfort, A., 1964, *Aging: The Biology of Senescence,* Holt, Rinehart, and Winston, New York.

Curtis, H. J., 1961, Radiation-induced aging in mice, in: *General Radiobiology* (P. L. T. Ilbery, ed.), pp. 114–128, Butterworths, London.

Curtis, H. J., and Crowley, C., 1963, Chromosome aberrations in liver cells in relation to the somatic mutation theory of aging, *Radiat. Res.* **19**:337.

Curtis, H. J., and Gebhard, K. L., 1960, Aging effect of toxic and radiation stresses, in: *The Biology of Aging* (B. L. Strehler, ed.), pp. 162–166, American Institute of Biological Science, Washington, D.C.

Finch, C. E., 1972, Enzyme activities, gene function and aging in mammals, *Exp. Gerontol.* **7**:53.

Finch, C. E., 1976, The regulation of physiological changes during mammalian aging, *Q. Rev. Biol.* **51**:49.

Fonda, M. L., Acree, D. W., and Auerbach, S. B., 1973, The relationship of α-aminobutyrate levels and its metabolism to age in brains of mice, *Arch. Biochem. Biophys.* **159:**622.

Fritz, P. J., White, E. L., Pruitt, K. M., and Vesell, E. S., 1973, Lactate dehydrogenase isoenzymes: Turnover in rat heart, skeletal muscle, and liver, *Biochemistry* **12:**4034.

Gershon, H., and Gershon, D., 1970, Detection of inactive enzyme molecules in aging organisms, *Nature (London)* **227:**1214.

Gershon, H., and Gershon, D., 1973*a,* Inactive enzyme molecules in aging mice: Liver aldolase, *Proc. Natl. Acad. Sci. U.S.A.* **70:**909.

Gershon, H., and Gershon, D., 1973*b,* Altered enzyme molecules in senescent organism: Mouse muscle aldolase, *Mech. Ageing Dev.* **2:**33.

Goldberg, A. L., 1969, Protein turnover in skeletal muscle. II. Effects of denervation and cortisone on protein catabolism in skeletal muscle, *J. Biol. Chem.* **244:**3223.

Goldberg, A. L., and Dice, J. F., 1974, Intracellular protein degradation in mammalian and bacterial cells, *Annu. Rev. Biochem.* **43:**835.

Goldberg, A. L., and St. John, A. C., 1976, Intracellular protein degradation in mammalian and bacterial cells, Part 2, *Annu. Rev. Biochem.* **45:**747.

Goss, R. J., 1966, Hypertrophy versus hyperplasia, *Science* **153:**1615.

Grinna, L. S., and Barber, A. A., 1972, Age-related changes in membrane lipid content and enzyme activities, *Biochim. Biophys. Acta* **288:**343.

Guthrie, R. D., 1969, Senescence as an adaptive trait, *Perspect. Biol. Med.* **12:**313.

Harrison, B. J., and Holliday, R., 1967, Senescence and the fidelity of protein synthesis in *Drosophila, Nature (London)* **213:**990.

Holliday, R., 1975, Testing the protein error theory of aging, *Gerontologia* **21:**64.

Holliday, R., and Tarrant, G. M., 1972, Altered enzymes in aging human fibroblasts, *Nature (London)* **238:**26.

Lindop, P. J., and Rotblat, J., 1961, Long-term effects of a single whole-body exposure of mice to ionizing radiations, *Proc. R. Soc. London* B154:332.

Little, J. B., 1976, Relationship between DNA repair capacity and cellular aging, *Gerontology* **22:**28.

Loeb, J., and Northrop, J. H., 1917, On the influence of food and temperature on the duration of life, *J. Biol. Chem.* **32:**103.

Majerus, P. W., and Kilburn, E., 1970, Acetyl coenzyme A carboxylase: The roles of synthesis and degradation of enzyme levels in rat liver, *J. Biol. Chem.* **244:**6254.

Millward, D. J., 1970, Protein turnover in skeletal muscle. II. The effect of starvation and a protein-free diet on the synthesis and catabolism of skeletal muscle proteins in comparison to liver, *Clin. Sci.* **39:**591.

Oliveira, R. J., and Pfuderer, P., 1973, Test for missynthesis of lactate dehydrogenase in aging mice by use of a monospecific antibody, *Exp. Gerontol.* **8:**193.

O'Meara, A. R., and Herrmann, R. L., 1972, A modified mouse liver chromatin preparation displaying age-related differences in salt dissociation and template ability, *Biochim. Biophys. Acta* **269:**419.

Orgel, L. E., 1963, The maintenance of accuracy of protein synthesis and its relevance to aging, *Proc. Natl. Acad. Sci. U.S.A.* **49:**517.

Orgel, L. E., 1970, Maintenance of the accuracy of protein synthesis and its relation to aging, *Proc. Natl. Acad. Sci. U.S.A.* **67:**1476.

Orgel, L. E., 1973, Aging of clones of mammalian cells, *Nature (London)* **243:**441.

Pearl, R., 1928, Evolution and mortality, *Q. Rev. Biol.* **3:**391.

Rechcigl, M., Jr., 1968, *In vivo* turnover and its role in the metabolic regulation of enzyme levels, *Enzymologia* **34:**23.

Russ, S., and Scott, G. M., 1939, Biological effects of gamma irradiation, *Br. J. Radiol.* **12:**440.

Russell, D. H., Medina, V. J., and Snyder, S. H., 1970, The dynamics of synthesis and degradation of polyamines in normal and regenerating rat liver and brain, *J. Biol. Chem.* **245**:6732.

Samis, H. V., 1966, A concept of biological aging: The role of compensatory processes, *J. Theor. Biol.* **13**:236.

Samis, H. V., 1967, Epilogue, in: *A Symposium on the Role of Biological Information Systems in Development and Aging* (H. V. Samis, ed.), *J. Gerontol. (Part II)* **22**:58.

Schimke, R. T., 1964, The importance of both synthesis and degradation in the control of arginase levels in rat liver, *J. Biol. Chem.* **239**:3808.

Stewart, P. A., 1967, Cybernetics and aging, in: *A Symposium on the Role of Biological Information Systems in Development and Aging* (H. V. Samis, ed.), *J. Gerontol. (Part II)* **22**:1.

Szilard, L., 1959, On the nature of the aging process, *Proc. Natl. Acad. Sci. U.S.A.* **45**:30.

Upton, A. C., Conklin, J. W., McDonald, J. P., and Christenberry, K. W., 1963*a*, Preliminary studies on late somatic effects of radiomimetic chemicals, in: *Cellular Basis and Aetiology of Late Effects of Ionizing Radiation* (R. J. C. Harris, ed.), pp. 171–175, Academic Press, New York.

Upton, A. C., Kastenbaum, M. A., and Conklin, J. W., 1963*b*, Age-specific death rates of mice exposed to ionizing radiation and radiomimetic agents, in: *Cellular Basis and Aetiology of Late Effects of Ionizing Radiation* (R. J. C. Harris, ed.), pp. 285–297, Academic Press, New York.

von Hahn, H. P., 1971, Failures of regulation mechanisms as causes of cellular aging, in: *Advances in Gerontological Research,* Vol. 3 (B. L. Strehler, ed.), pp. 1–33, Academic Press, New York.

Walford, R. L., 1967, The general immunology of aging, in: *Advances in Gerontological Research,* Vol. 2 (B. L. Strehler, ed.), pp. 159–204, Academic Press, New York and London.

Walford, R. L., 1969, *The Immunologic Theory of Aging,* Williams and Wilkins, Baltimore.

Weismann, A., 1891, The duration of life, in: *Essays Upon Heredity and Kindred Biological Problems,* Vol. 1 (E. B. Poulton, S. Schonland, and A. E. Shipley, eds.), pp. 1–66, Clarendon Press, Oxford.

Welch, J. P., 1967, Somatic mutations and the aging process, in: *Advances in Gerontological Research,* Vol. 2 (B. L. Strehler, ed.), pp. 1–30, Academic Press, New York and London.

Wilson, D. L., 1974, The programmed theory of aging, in: *Theoretical Aspects of Aging* (M. Rochstein, ed.), pp. 11–21, Academic Press, New York.

Wilson, P. D., 1973, Enzyme changes in aging mammals, *Gerontologia* **19**:79.

Woolhouse, H. W., 1967, The nature of senescence in plants, in: *Aspects of the Biology of Aging* (H. W. Woolhouse, ed.), p. 179, Academic Press, New York.

Yielding, K. L., 1974, A model for aging based on differential repair of somatic mutational damage, *Perspect. Biol. Med. Winter* **1974**:201.

Zeelon, P., Gershon, H., and Gershon, D., 1973, Inactive enzyme molecules in aging organisms: Nematode fructose-1,6-disphosphate aldolase, *Biochemistry* **12**:1743.

Zimmerman, J. A., Samis, H. V., Baird, M. B., and Massie, H. R., 1975, Properties of catalase molecules in rats of different ages in: *Explorations in Aging* (V. J. Cristofalo, J. Roberts, and R. C. Adelman, eds.), *Advances in Experimental Biology and Medicine,* Vol. 61, p. 291, Plenum Press, New York.

Chapter 2

Cytogenetics of Aging

Edward L. Schneider

1. Introduction

An analysis of the effects of aging on the genetic endowment of organisms would not be complete without an examination of cytogenetics. Early cytogenetic studies were focused on the chromosomal constitution of lower organisms such as *Drosophila,* since chromosomal preparations in these species were technically simple and chromosomal number was small. It was not until 1956 that the technology was finally developed to examine the human chromosome complement accurately. Until that date, the human chromosomal number was thought to be 48. The studies of Tijo and Levan (1956) demonstrated clearly, however, that human cells possess 22 pairs of autosomal chromosomes plus either an X and Y chromosome in the male or two X chromosomes in the female.

Once the normal human chromosome complement was defined, a search was undertaken to find abnormal chromosome complements. The observation by Lejeune *et al.* (1959) that children with the Down syndrome (mongolism) possess an extra chromosome was quickly followed by similar findings in the Patau (Patau *et al.,* 1960), Edwards (Edwards *et al.,* 1960), and Klinefelter (Zuppinger *et al.,* 1967) syndromes. A typical human karyotype prepared during this early period of human cytogenetics is shown in Fig. 1.

The human chromosome complement is comprised of three types of chromosomes, designated by the position of the centromere: (1) *acrocen-*

Edward L. Schneider ● Laboratory of Cellular and Comparative Physiology, Gerontology Research Center, National Institute on Aging, National Institutes of Health, Public Health Service, U.S. Department of Health, Education and Welfare, Baltimore, Maryland 21224

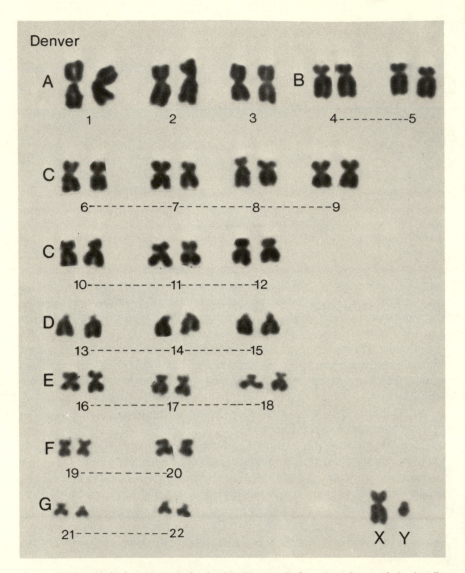

Fig. 1. Human male karyotype stained with Giemsa. Before the advent of the banding technique, it was possible only to assign chromosomes into groups on the basis of size and centromeric position.

tric chromosomes, in which the centromere is located near the end of the chromosome; (2) *metacentric* chromosomes, in which the centromere is at the center of the chromosome; and (3) *submetacentric* chromosomes in which the centromere is near but not at the center of the chromosome. The centromere is located at the end of *telocentric* chromosomes, which do not exist in man but are found in other species.

Although certain chromosomes (the 1, 2, and 3 chromosome pairs) could be identified by their size and centromeric position, most chromosomes could only be assigned to chromosomal groups (Fig. 1). Seven chromosomal groups were formalized by the Denver Conference on the Human Karyotype (1960): groups A–G. Unfortunately, it was impossible to accurately distinguish the X from the other C-group metacentric chromosomes and the Y from the other G-group acrocentrics.

The recent advent of the specialized chromosome banding techniques has greatly facilitated the study of human cytogenetics. Caspersson *et al.* (1970) made the initial discovery that chromosomes stained with the drug guinacrine mustard produced specific banding patterns on fluorescent microscopy. After the rush to buy fluorescent microscopes abated, a number of non-fluorescent-staining techniques were developed (Arrighi and Hsu, 1971; Dutrillaux and Lejeune, 1971; Pardue and Gall, 1970; Sumner *et al.*, 1971) that produced characteristic banding patterns. In the banded karyotypes seen in Figs. 2 and 3, all the autosomal chromosomes, as well as the X and Y chromosomes, can be easily identified by their distinctive banding patterns. In many cases, positive bands with one technique would produce negative bands with another. The important finding, however, was that consistent banding of human chromosomes was indeed possible, and that every chromosome in the human chromosome complement could be identified. These observations were formalized at the Paris Conference on the Human Karyotype (1971).

Following the development of these banding techniques, major advances in the field of somatic cell genetics have led to the assignment of over 100 genetic loci to specific chromosomes (Fig. 4) (McKusick, 1976*a*).

Cytogenetic techniques continue to evolve, and the recent report by Yunis (1976) suggests that it may be possible in the future to obtain the level of band resolution in human chromosomes that can be presently obtained in chromosomes from *Drosophila* and other lower organisms. The banding patterns of chromosomes obtained by Yunis in human prophase cells are shown in Fig. 5.

In this chapter, attention will be directed to examining changes in chromosomal number as a function of both *in vivo* and *in vitro* aging. Since the frequencies of chromosome aberrations such as breaks and rearrangements are discussed in depth in Chapters 3 and 4, they will not be considered in this chapter.

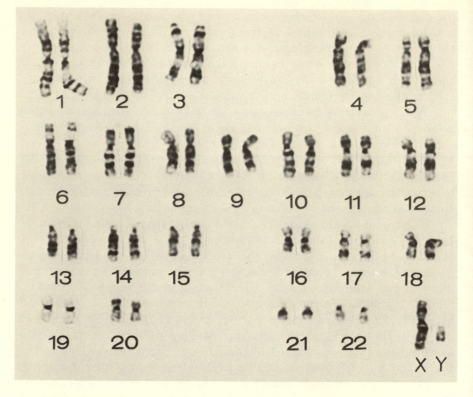

Fig. 2. Human male karyotype prepared by trypsin–Giemsa treatment to obtain chromosomal banding. With this technique, each chromosomal pair can be identified by their characteristic banding patterns. Note that the male possesses 22 pairs of autosomal chromosomes plus X and Y sex chromosomes. Karyotype courtesy of Helen Lawce, San Francisco, California.

2. Alterations in Lymphocyte Chromosome Complement with Human Aging

The initial investigation of the effect of human aging on chromosomal number was performed by P. A. Jacobs *et al.* (1961). They established peripheral leukocyte cultures from 97 individuals, aged 1–82 years, and examined approximately 36 metaphase cells from each culture. These investigators found significant increases in both hypodiploidy ($N < 46$) and hyperdiploidy ($N > 46$) as a function of human aging. The altered frequency of hypodiploid cells was the more impressive, with the percentage of hypodiploid cells increasing from 3.02% in the 5–14 age range to 9.54% in the 65-and-over group. A second part of this study was an examination of the frequency of hypomodal cells in subjects with abnormal chromosome

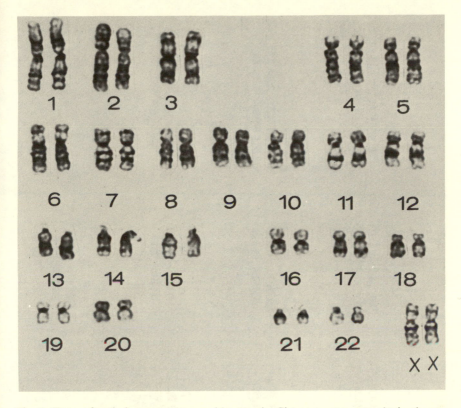

Fig. 3. Human female karyotype prepared by trypsin–Giemsa treatment to obtain chromosomal banding. Note that the female possesses 22 pairs of autosomal chromosomes plus two X chromosomes. Karyotype courtesy of Helen Lawce.

complements, patients with the Down syndrome (47, trisomy 21) and the Klinefelter syndrome (47, XXY). Once again, an increased frequency of hypomodal cells (in this case, $N < 41$) was observed as a function of aging.

These authors followed this important observation with an examination of the effect of sex on the increased frequency of chromosomal aneuploidy observed as a function of aging (Jacobs, P. A., et al., 1963). They found that while the frequency of hypodiploid cells increased in both males and females with normal aging, the pattern of increase was quite different. Until age 45, there is a gradual increase in the frequency of hypodiploid cells in both sexes. After 45, however, the frequency of hypodiploidy increases more sharply in females and then plateaus, while the frequency of hypodiploid cells in males continues to increase gradually up through the oldest age ranges.

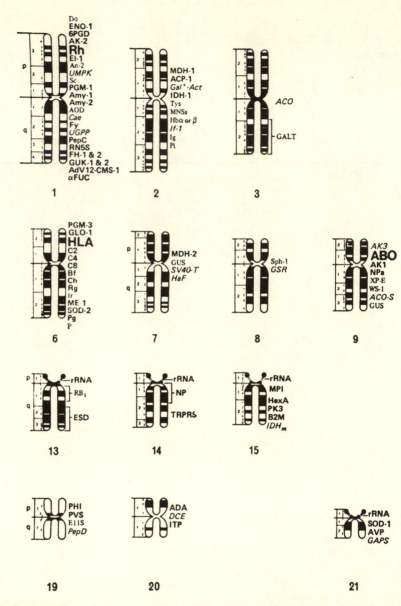

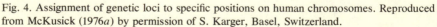

Fig. 4. Assignment of genetic loci to specific positions on human chromosomes. Reproduced from McKusick (1976*a*) by permission of S. Karger, Basel, Switzerland.

A confirmed assignment............ENO-1
A provisional assignment...........*UMPK*
An inconsistent assignment
or assignment in limbo...............Do
Particularly noteworthy assignments.. **ABO, Rh, HLA**

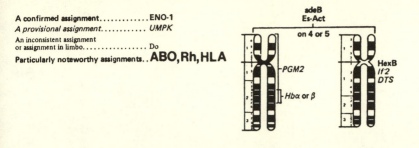

adeB
Es-Act
on 4 or 5

PGM2

Hbα or β

HexB
If2
DTS

4   5

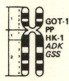

GOT-1
PP
HK-1
ADK
GSS

10

ACP-2
LDH-A
EsA4
AL

11

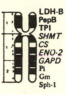

LDH-B
PepB
TPI
SHMT
CS
ENO-2
GAPD
Pi
Gm
Sph-1

12

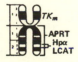

TK_m

APRT
Hpα
LCAT

16

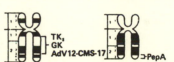

TK_s
GK
AdV12-CMS-17

17

⊐PepA

18

rRNA

22

TDF
H-Y

Y

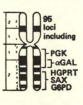

95
loci
including

PGK
αGAL
HGPRT
SAX
G6PD

X

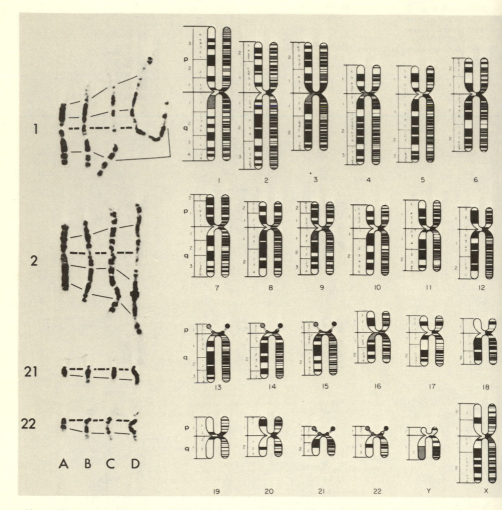

Fig. 5. Chromosomal banding obtained in human prophase cells. *Left:* The two largest (1 and 2) and two smallest (21 and 22) human chromosomes at midmetaphase (A), early metaphase (B), early prometaphase (C), and late prophase (D). *Right:* For each chromosome in this schema, the left chromatid represents the banding pattern observed in midmetaphase and the right chromatid represents the pattern observed in late prophase. Note the greatly increased resolution of chromosomal banding in late prophase. Reproduced from Yunis (1976) by permission of the American Association for the Advancement of Science, Washington, D.C.

An attempt was also made to identify the missing chromosome in the hypodiploid cells. Since these studies were performed before the current chromosomal banding techniques, no specific chromosome could be identified, and the closest approximation that could be achieved was the identification of the chromosomal group to which the missing chromosome belonged. In males, the missing chromosome appeared to come from the G group (21, 22, and the Y) while in females, the missing chromosome was from the C group (6–12 and the X). These studies from the Edinburgh group led a number of other laboratories to investigate this intriguing relationship between aging and chromosomal aneuploidy.

DeGalen (1966) was the first to challenge this reported increase in lymphocyte chromosomal aneuploidy as a function of aging. Subsequently, a number of other laboratories have produced both negative and positive findings. The results of 13 of these studies are summarized in Table I. In the majority (10/13) of these studies, a significant elevation in hypodiploidy was observed in females with increasing age, and the most frequently lost chromosome appeared to belong to the C + X group. There were three reports, however, in which no significant increase in hypodiploidy was observed in aged females (Bloom *et al.,* 1967; Kadontani *et al.,* 1971; Neurath *et al.,* 1970). The results in regard to hyperdiploidy and to hypodiploidy in males are largely negative. Interestingly enough, in several studies in which no age-related significant elevation in hypodiploidy was observed in males, analysis of the missing chromosome in both young and old cells revealed that the G + Y chromosomes were the most frequently lost.

Mattevi and Salzano (1975) summarized the results of nine of these studies plus their own experience (see Table II). Between 8900 and 14,200 cells were examined in both males and females in young (20–45) and old (60+) groups. Analysis of these pooled data reveals a significant increase in hypodiploidy in both male and female groups as a function of age. Once again, however, the increased hypodiploidy in females was significantly greater than that observed in males. There was no significant increase in hyperdiploidy with aging in either males or females.

3. Population Studies

The initial studies by P. A. Jacobs *et al.* (1961) were performed on a mixture of volunteers, hospitalized patients, and parents of patients with chromosomal disorders. Since this was far from a random population, there was much subsequent criticism of these results. This criticism led Jacobs and her group to confirm their results on a random population selected from the lists of general practitioners in Edinburgh (Jacobs, P. A., and Court Brown, 1966).

Table I. Summary of Several Studies of the Frequency of Aneuploidy as a Function of Aging[a]

Study	Females[b]			Males[b]		
	Hypodiploidy	Hyperdiploidy	C + X group lost	Hypodiploidy	Hyperdiploidy	G + Y group lost
Hamerton et al. (1965)	+	+	+	+	–	–
Sandberg et al. (1967)	+	–	NE	–	–	NE
Bloom et al. (1967)	–	–	–		–	+
Nielsen (1968)	+	–	+	NE	NE	NE
Goodman et al. (1969)	+	–	+	NE	NE	NE
Jarvik and Kato (1969)	+	–	NE	–	–	NE
Neurath et al. (1970)	–	–	–	–	–	+
Jarvik and Kato (1970)	+	–	–	–	–	+
Nielsen (1970)	+	+	+	–	–	–
Cadotte and Fraser (1970)	+	–	–	+	–	–
Kadontani et al. (1971)	–	–	NE	–	–	NE
Demoise and Conard (1972)	+	–	+	–	–	+
Mattevi and Salzano (1975)	+	+	+	+	–	±

[a]Following the initial studies by P. A. Jacobs et al. (1961, 1963).
[b](NE) Not examined.

Table II. Frequency of Hypodiploidy in Old and Young Males and Females: Combined Data from 10 Series[a]

Group	Age	Number of subjects	Number of cells examined	Hypodiploidy (%)	Hyperdiploidy (%)
Males	20–45	547	8,993	6.1	0.8
	60+	1034	11,395	9.1	0.9
Females	20–45	612	10,594	5.4	1.0
	60+	1601	12,470	11.2	1.2

[a]Data of P. A. Jacobs et al. (1961), Hamerton et al. (1965), Bloom et al. (1967), Sandberg et al. (1967), Cadotte and Fraser (1970), Jarvik and Kato (1970), Neurath et al. (1970), Nielsen (1970), Kadontani et al. (1971), and Mattevi and Salzano (1975).

Hamerton et al. (1965) were able to cytogenetically examine an entire isolated population, the people of Tristan da Cunha. Their results were similar to those of Jacobs in that the observed hypodiploidy was greater in females than in males, and the increase fit a cubic curve rather than the linear regression seen in males. Once again, the missing chromosome appeared to belong to the C group in female cells and to the G group in male cells. In this study, exclusion of cells with fewer than 44 chromosomes and those containing chromosomal aberrations, such as dicentrics, resulted in the elimination of the observed increase in hypodiploidy in male cells. The increase in hyperdiploidy with age was much less pronounced, and was seen only in the oldest age groups.

Another population that has been surveyed is in the Buffalo, New York, metropolitan area, which was examined by Sandberg et al. (1967). These authors confirmed the increased frequency of hypodiploid cells in female lymphocytes as a function of age. The remainder of their findings, however, were not in agreement with the observations of Jacobs and Hamerton. These authors did not find increased hypodiploidy in male cells or hyperdiploidy in either male or female cells with aging.

Two studies involved populations that were exposed to significant levels of radiation. Bloom et al. (1967) examined a population of Japanese survivors of the atomic blast at Hiroshima and found no significant increase in either hypo- or hyperdiploidy as a function of aging.

The other study involved a Marshall Island population that had been accidentally exposed to radioactive fallout (Demoise and Conard, 1972). This population comprised both exposed and unexposed persons. In the unexposed group, increased hypodiploidy was found as a function of age in the female group only, while in the exposed group, significant hypodiploidy was observed in both sexes. No hyperdiploidy was observed in any group. When cells from the unexposed persons were cultured in the presence of sera from the exposed group, no increase in hypodiploidy was observed.

In summary, the majority of these population surveys have clearly indicated that increased hypodiploidy does appear to occur in lymphocytes as a function of aging in females and to a lesser extent in males.

4. Aneuploidy, Aging, and Organic Brain Disease

Several laboratories turned their attention to the question whether chromosomal aneuploidy may be related to the development of accelerated mental deterioration. Nielsen *et al.* (1968) first examined the frequency of chromosomal aneuploidy in blood cultures derived from an older population of patients with senile dementia as well as from young and old control populations. All groups were comprised entirely of females. While the frequency of hypodiploid cells increased as a function of normal aging, the highest levels of hypodiploidy were observed in the senile dementia group. Examination of the missing chromosome revealed that the C + X was lost more frequently in the senile dementia population than in the control old normal population.

Studies of the relationship between chromosomal alterations and specific tests of mental functioning revealed a significant correlation between the Graham–Kendall Memory-for-Designs Test and hypodiploidy (Jarvik and Kato, 1969) and the Stroop Color-Word Test and hypodiploidy (Bettner and Jarvik, 1971).

These results were recently been challenged by Cohen (1976), who concludes that chromosome loss may not be related to organic brain disease. Further studies, particularly longitudinal studies, are indicated to assess this potentially important relationship.

5. Effect of Genotype on Aneuploidy

In certain lower organisms, it has been shown that specific gene mutations can lead to chromosomal nondisjunction and aneuploidy. It is therefore not surprising that the relationship between genotype and aneuploidy might be examined in man. One approach is to examine the frequency of aneuploidy in monozygotic twins, dizygotic twins, and unrelated age-matched subjects. If genotype played a major role in the production of aneuploidy, one might expect decreased intrapair differences in the frequency of aneuploidy in monozygotic twins in comparison with the other groups. In the study of Jarvik and Kato (1970), in which a small number of subjects were examined, intrapair differences between monozygotic twins were not significantly smaller than in dizygotic twins or unrelated subjects.

Although these results are preliminary, they do suggest that genotype may not play an important role in age-related aneuploidy. Further studies are indicated, however, to confirm these findings.

6. Specific vs. Nonspecific Chromosome Loss

Although the initial reports suggested that the C-group chromosomes were specifically lost in the female and the G + Y group in the male, subsequent reports suggested that chromosomal size may play the major role in determining chromosomal loss. Of particular interest was the report by Neurath *et al.* (1970), which demonstrated that chromosomal loss appeared to be inversely related to chromosomal size.

Fitzgerald *et al.* (1975) utilized the new banding techniques to demonstrate that the most frequent missing chromosome in cultured female leukocytes was the X chromosome. Unfortunately, these banding techniques have not yet been applied to studies of peripheral blood cells obtained from male donors. The results obtained from bone marrow studies (Pierre, 1974; Pierre and Hoagland, 1971, 1972) would suggest, however, that the Y chromosome is the most frequently lost chromosome in male cells.

7. Polyploidy

Tetraploidy ($N = 92$) is not uncommon in certain human cell populations (Falzone *et al.*, 1959; Epstein, 1967). Few studies, however, have been addressed to examining the frequency of polyploid cells as a function of human aging. The results of three studies of cultured human leukocytes that did measure polyploidy were conflicting. Goodman *et al.* (1969) found a significant increase in polyploid cells, from 0.3% in college females 19–21 years old to 0.7% in older "churchgoing" women aged 67–93. Sandberg *et al.* (1967), in their study of a more random population in Buffalo, found no increase in polyploidy, while Demoise and Conard (1972), in their study of Marshall Islanders, found decreased polyploidy with aging. The differences among these studies may be due to the different diets, drug habits, and radiation exposure of these three populations.

Studies of rat hepatic cells revealed no increased frequency of polyploidy with aging (Falzone *et al.*, 1959). Only with *in vitro* passage of human diploid fibroblasts is a consistent increase in polyploidy observed (Benn, 1976; Kadanka *et al.*, 1973; Saksela and Moorhead, 1963; Thompson and Holliday, 1975).

8. Cross-Sectional vs. Longitudinal Studies

All the studies described above were cross-sectional; i.e., old and young subjects were surveyed at the same time. There are many difficulties inherent in any cross-sectional study of human aging. Some of the questions that might be raised by cross-sectional studies of chromosomal aneuploidy with aging include: (1) Is the observed aneuploidy in the older population due to the selective survival of those subjects with increased frequencies of aneuploidy? (2) Are we observing the effect of certain chemicals or drugs that were prevalent 40–70 years ago and are not currently in use: (3) Is the increase in aneuploidy a gradual process, or does it accelerate in the last decades?

To assess the relationship between aneuploidy and aging most accurately, one should examine the same population of subjects as they age. Unfortunately, longitudinal studies of this nature are extremely difficult or almost impossible to conduct. Chromosomal techniques have been available for only a short time, and even during this brief period, there have been considerable improvements and expansions in cytogenetic technology; therefore, the longitudinal study commenced today may be obsolete tomorrow. The longest possible longitudinal study would have been a mere 17 years from Jacob's observation to the publication date of this volume.

One brave group, however, has performed a brief but important longitudinal study. Jarvik *et al.* (1976) conducted this study on 11 female and 6 male subjects over a 6-year period and found a significant increase in hyper- and hypodiploidy in female subjects, but not in males. The most frequently lost chromosome in the hypodiploid cells appeared to belong to the C group (6–12 + X).

It is to be hoped that further longitudinal studies will be pursued to help gain a better understanding of the increase in aneuploidy with aging.

9. Chromosomal Alterations with Aging in Tissues Other than Lymphocytes

Fang *et al.* (1975) established short-term cultures from human ovarian tissue derived from women aged 24–75 and examined the chromosome complements of these cells. They found no significant increase in aneuploidy with age. Examination of chromosomal loss in hypodiploid cells, however, revealed a correlation with chromosomal size. The authors also claimed a specific loss of the X chromosome with aging. They do not explain how the X was identified, and since these authors do not describe any banding techniques for chromosomal identification, one finds it difficult to accept their conclusions regarding loss of the X chromosome.

10. Effect of Experimental Conditions on Chromosome Number

Since direct chromosomal examination of human lymphocytes is impossible, phytohemagglutinin (PHA) is added to blood-cell cultures to stimulate lymphocyte proliferation. Cell division usually commences 24–48 hr after PHA stimulation and remains rapid for another 48 hr (Tice *et al.,* 1976). Cell cultures are usually harvested during this 48- to 96-hr period after PHA stimulation to obtain sufficient metaphase cells for chromosomal analyses. At 48 hr, most cells are undergoing their first *in vitro* division, and are thus closest to the *in vivo* state. In contrast, at 72 or 96 hr, cells have replicated 2–5 times (Tice *et al.,* 1976). If chromosome loss were purely an *in vitro* phenomena and were unrelated to *in vivo* chromosomal alterations, one might expect an increased frequency of aneuploidy to occur as a function of *in vitro* culture time.

While most studies of chromosomal number have involved 72-hr harvesting of lymphocyte cultures, several studies have examined the frequencies of aneuploidy at 48 as well as 72 hr after PHA stimulation. Unfortunately, these studies have produced somewhat conflicting results: two showed increased hypodiploidy in 72-hr cultures in comparison with 48-hr cultures (Court Brown *et al.,* 1966; Honda *et al.,* 1969), one showed no difference between 48- and 72-hr cultures (Jacobs, P. A., and Court Brown, 1966), and one revealed increased aneuploidy in the 48-hr cultures (Mattevi and Salzano, 1975). That significant hypodiploidy is seen in 48-hr cultures and that there is no clear trend toward increased hypodiploidy with lengthened *in vitro* culture indicates that the observed hypodiploidy in cultured human lymphocytes probably does reflect *in vivo* aneuploidy and is not an artifact of *in vitro* culture.

11. In Vivo Examination of Aneuploidy

Few investigators would contest that *in vitro* tissue culture conditions are not the ideal method for examining the loss of chromosomes as a function of *in vivo* human aging. Unfortunately, direct examination of chromosomes without tissue culture has been extremely difficult and has led to the *in vitro* studies that have been described.

Cadotte and Fraser (1970) were the first investigators to examine the chromosome complement of bone marrow cells as a function of aging. Although they found increased aneuploidy in cultured peripheral leukocyte cultures, their direct analysis of bone marrow cells did not reveal any significant aneuploidy as a function of aging. In contrast to these studies, Pierre and Hoagland (1971), in an extensive survey of males, found a markedly increased frequency of older males possessing 45,XO cell lines in their bone marrow. In a subsequent study of females by these authors, no loss of X chromosomes was found with increasing age (Pierre and Hoagland, 1972). Although the frequency of males with missing Y chromosomes increased with aging in their study, no correlation was observed between the degree of chromosome loss and the age of the donor.

Unfortunately, population studies of bone marrow cells are extremely difficult, since the procedure employed to obtain these cells is much more complicated than the venipuncture employed to obtain blood samples. Of necessity, these studies involve subjects being screened for hematological or malignant conditions or relatives of such subjects. Conclusions based on these studies must therefore be limited. They do suggest, however, that caution should be exercised in interpreting the chromosome aneuploidy found in peripheral blood cultures.

12. Studies of the Stability of the Chromosome Complement with in Vitro "Aging"

Since the original description of the finite life span of cultured human diploid cells *in vitro* by Swim and Parker (1957) and Hayflick and Moorhead (1961), these cells have been widely utilized as a model system for studying human cellular aging (Cristofalo, 1973; Hayflick, 1965; Holliday and Tarrant, 1972; Orgel, 1973; Schneider and Mitsui, 1976).

Hayflick and Moorhead (1961), in their report, examined the chromosome complement of a number of fetal lung fibroblast cultures (the WI series), and found the karyotypes to be diploid, with low levels of aneuploidy and tetraploidy. The one fetal lung fibroblast culture that was examined at different levels of *in vitro* passage ("aging") revealed no significant alterations in chromosomal number. In a later, more comprehensive study of two fetal lung fibroblast cultures (WI-26 and WI-38), significantly increased hypodiploidy as well as tetraploidy was observed when the cell cultures were in the senescent phase of their *in vitro* life span (Phase III) (Saksela and Moorhead, 1963).

As with the studies of cultured human lymphocytes, subsequent investigations of the frequency of chromosomal aneuploidy as a function of *in vitro* passage have had conflicting results. Kadanka et al. (1973) found tetraploidy without aneuploidy, while Thompson and Holliday (1975) and Benn (1976) both confirmed Saksela and Moorhead's observation of increased hypodiploidy and tetraploidy with increasing *in vitro* passage. In no case was hyperdiploidy observed as a function of *in vitro* "aging." The latter two studies involved the use of MRC-5, a fetal lung culture established by J. P. Jacobs et al. (1970). Unfortunately, no comprehensive studies were undertaken to identify the missing chromosome in the hypodiploid cells.

In addition to the finding of increased hypodiploidy as a function of *in vitro* passage, an increased frequency of chromosomal aberrations was also observed. The most frequently observed aberration was the presence of dicentric chromosomes (Benn, 1976). Examinations of these dicentric chromosomes with the new banding techniques revealed that many of these dicentric chromosomes appeared to be the result of end-to-end fusion of whole chromosomes.

In an interesting study, Thompson and Holliday (1973) examined the effect of elevated incubation temperature on the frequency of aneuploidy. They proposed that increasing temperature would accelerate *in vitro* "aging" by inducing greater error production in enzyme systems vital for macromolecular synthesis. In fact, elevation of the culture temperature to 40°C did result in significanly shortened *in vitro* life spans (Thompson and Holliday, 1973). Examination of the karyotypes of these cells cultured at 40°C revealed a marked increase in the frequency of both polyploidy and tetraploidy (Thompson and Holliday, 1973). Therefore, in both normal *in vitro* aging and accelerated *in vitro* aging, there appears to be a close association between senescence and alterations in chromosomal number.

The new chromosomal banding techniques were utilized by Chen and Ruddle (1974) to determine whether alterations in chromosomal structure or rearrangements within chromosomes occurred during *in vitro* serial passage of WI-38 fibroblasts. Although some chromosomal rearrangements were detected in these studies, no significant change in banding patterns was observed during *in vitro* fibroblast "aging."

The finite life span of human diploid fibroblasts can be extended, perhaps indefinitely, by the mechanism of virus transformation. It is of interest that this transformation of human cell cultures is accompanied by alterations in both chromosomal number and chromosomal aberrations (Koprowksi *et al.*, 1962). It therefore appears that cells at the end of their life span, as well as cells about to become immortal, manifest chromosomal alterations.

13. Chromosomal Alteration, Malignancy, and Aging

One of the most intriguing aspects of cytogenetics is the relationship between chromosomal alteration and malignancy. Since the original observation by Boveri (1914), it has been a common finding that alterations in chromosomal number accompany malignant transformation of tissues and cells (Makino *et al.*, 1964). Although there may be exceptional cases in which malignant cells appear to be diploid (Bloom *et al.*, 1974), the vast majority of malignant cells are aneuploid, and the tendency is toward hyperdiploidy. Perhaps the best example of this relationship between malignancy and aneuploidy occurs in tissue culture, in which infection of human diploid cells with SV40 virus produces both malignant transformation of cells and chromosomal abnormalities (Koprowski *et al.,* 1962; Moorhead and Saksela, 1963).

There are also several human genetic disorders that feature both chromosomal alterations and an increased frequency of malignant diseases (Miller, 1970): the Bloom syndrome (Sawitsky *et al.,* 1966), Fanconi's anemia (Swift, 1971), and ataxia–telangiectasia (Harden, 1974). Similarly, patients with the Down syndrome whose cells are aneuploid (trisomy-21) also have an increased frequency of malignant diseases (Miller, 1970).

The relationship between aging and malignancy is well documented. The studies summarized in previous sections indicate that aneuploidy and aging are closely related. These correlations suggest some intriguing possibilities. Since stability of chromosomal number is vital for maintaining normal cellular functions, perhaps age-related aneuploidy leads to two courses: cell malfunction and death or malignant transformation. Furthermore, the decline in immune function with aging (see Chapter 12) might lead to diminished selection against aneuploid malignant cells. Alternately, increased exposure with aging to agents, perhaps viruses, might lead to both aneuploidy and malignant transformation.

14. Mechanisms for the Loss of Specific Chromosomes with Aging

There are two alternative explanations for the selective loss of the specific chromosomes: (1) Loss of chromosomes is random, and only those cells that have lost chromosomes that are not essential for survival remain to be examined. (2) There is selective loss of specific chromosomes.

14.1. Survival of Cells Missing Specific Chromosomes

Diploid cells appear to have a definite selective advantage over aneuploid cells. This advantage was demonstrated by J. G. Boué and Boué (1974) and by Schneider and Epstein (1972) in their studies of the properties of human cell lines derived from patients with chromosome disorders. In these studies, aneuploid cell lines had decreased replicative abilities and shortened *in vitro* life spans in comparison with control diploid cell cultures. Further support for the concept of a selective disadvantage for aneuploid cells comes from the studies of cell cultures that were mosaic for diploid and aneuploid cells (Bloom *et al.,* 1974). In this case, the percentage of diploid cells increased as a function of culture time, indicating a selective growth advantage of these cells over aneuploid cells. There were also cases, however, of selection against the normal karyotype. This selection was most impressive in the case of an XO/XX mosaic, in which only the XO line remained. On the level of the whole organism, selection against aneuploidy was demonstrated by A. Boué *et al.* (1975), who found extremely high prenatal mortality for aneuploid fetuses.

Selection against aneuploid cell lines may be due to a variety of mechanisms. It is known that while trisomies for an extra dose of a chromosome may be relatively well tolerated, monosomies (with one important exception) are highly lethal. In man, in whom trisomies for the 13, 18, and 21 chromosomes are relatively common, the only monosomy that is commonly observed is for the X chromosome. The phenomenon of X-chromosome inactivation is probably responsible for the survival of these monosomic X infants.

The phenomenon of inactivation of one of the two X chromosomes in the female was first proposed by Lyon (1961) to explain her observations on the behavior of X-linked genes in the mouse. Subsequently, it has been demonstrated, in a wide number of species including man (Beutler *et al.*, 1962), that early in fetal development, one X chromosome is inactivated. This inactivation of the X chromosome appears to be random, and thus half the cells in any tissue contain one active X, while the remainder contain the other X as the active chromosome. By this mechanism, all females are chromosomal mosaics, and each of their cells contains only 45 active chromosomes. In effect, this process equalizes the amount of active genetic information in the male and female, since the Y chromosome in the male contains very little genetic information (McKusick, 1976*b*).

The inactivation of one X chromosome in the female and the lack of genetic information on the Y chromosome could explain the survival of cells lacking these chromosomes in the face of selection against aneuploid cells. Unfortunately, there is little evidence as yet to indicate that the inactive X (rather than the active X) is the chromosome lost in female cells. Examination of the chromosomes involved in the premature centromeric division reported by Fitzgerald (1975) revealed, however, that all three X chromosome fragments that could be identified by autoradiography were late-replicating, indicating that they were inactive X chromosomes. Further autoradiographic studies would be of great interest to determine whether the inactive X is in fact the chromosome lost with aging.

14.2. Selective Loss of Specific Chromosomes

Once again, attention should be focused on the sex chromosomes, since these are the chromosomes most frequently lost as a function of aging. In addition to the inactivation of the X chromosome and the lack of active genetic information on the Y chromosome, the sex chromosomes have other interesting properties. The X and Y chromosomes replicate later in the S phase of the cell cycle than any other chromosomes (Gilbert *et al.*, 1965; Latt, 1973; Takagi and Sandberg, 1968). Since the G2 period would be short in rapidly replicating cells, the late DNA replication of the X and Y chromosomes might interfere with normal mitotic behavior and lead to an increased frequency of missegregation of these chromosomes during mitosis.

The peripheral mitotic location of the X and Y chromosomes has also been suggested as a mechanism to explain the increased loss of the sex chromosomes. It has been proposed that increased fragility of cells from older persons coupled with this peripheral location might produce the selective loss of X and Y chromosomes that is observed as a function of aging.

Perhaps the most important finding was the observation by Fitzgerald *et al.* (1975) that the X chromosome has an increased frequency of premature centromeric division. Daughter cells of a cell that had premature centromeric division of an X chromosome would either lack an X chromosome or contain acentric X chromosome fragments. Fitzgerald and co-workers demonstrated that with increasing age, normal females had a marked increase in cells containing these acentric fragments, as well as a specific loss of the X chromosome. The identification of the acentric fragments and the absent chromosomes in these cells was achieved by the new G banding technique as well as by autoradiography. This latter technique involves pulse-labeling of cells with tritiated thymidine late in the S phase. Since the X is a late-replicating chromosome, it is heavily labeled and can easily be recognized by autoradiography.

When these same authors examined the frequency of acentric fragments in blood cultures derived from males, they found only minimal evidence for premature centromeric division. In the few cases of premature centromeric division that were observed in males, however, there appeared to be an age effect.

14.3. Effect of Aging on Selection

As for the effect of aging on the selective loss of specific chromosomes, this could occur through two mechanisms: (1) increased production of aneuploidy with age, with the selection rate against aneuploid cells being unaltered; and (2) a constant rate of the production of aneuploid cells, but with a decreased selection with aging.

It is very difficult to distinguish between these two possibilities, since most experimental data relate to the final product of both production of aneuploidy and selection. The data of Fitzgerald *et al.* (1975) would support the first mechanism, since they indicate that there is an increase in aneuploidy for specific chromosomes as a function of aging.

In regard to the second mechanism, alterations in chromosomal number were shown to have significant effects on gene expression (Tan *et al.*, 1974). Although it has not yet been demonstrated, it is also likely that aneuploidy would result in altered membrane structure, which could lead the immune system to recognize aneuploid cells as foreign. There is ample evidence to indicate that there is functional impairment of the human immune system with increasing age (see Chapter 12). Since immune surveillance is an important function of the immune system, aging could lead to dimished elimination of these "foreign" aneuploid cells. Unfortunately, experimental evidence for a decreased removal of aneuploid cells with aging is lacking. Fialkow *et al.* (1973) demonstrated, however, that mice with impaired immune systems have an increased frequency of aneuploid cells.

15. Future Research on the Cytogenetics of Aging

Unfortunately, the bulk of the studies reported in this chapter were performed without the new cytogenetic banding techniques that permit identification of all human chromosomes. Although the results of Fitzgerald's study did indicate a selective loss of the X chromosome with aging, future studies with these new techniques are necessary to identify the chromosomes involved in aneuploid cells. In addition, tritiated thymidine labeling coupled with autoradiography should be employed to determine whether the missing X chromosome is the inactive X. The recent development of the bromodeoxyuridine-differential staining techniques by Latt (1973) should permit rapid identification of the late-replicating X chromosome without autoradiography.

These new banding techniques have also added a new dimension to chromosomal analysis. Previously, only differences in chromosomal number or gross translocations or deletions could be detected. These new techniques, however, permit accurate detection of small inversions, translocations, deletions, and reduplications. Application of the techniques that produced the chromosome preparations in Fig. 5 should add even further discrimination to cytogenetic technology. It will therefore be important in future studies not only to examine aneuploidy, but also to look for alterations in banding patterns that could reflect inversions, translocations, deletions, and reduplications as a function of aging.

One of the major limitations on the study of aneuploidy with human aging is the large number of metaphase cells that must be analyzed.

Progress toward automated cytogenetic analysis has been made by several laboratories (Caspersson *et al.,* 1971; Neurath *et al.,* 1966). Perhaps the most promising new approach is the application of flow microfluorometric systems to chromosomal analysis (Gray *et al.,* 1975). Flow microfluorometry has the capability of analyzing as many as 100,000 chromosomes per minute. In the future, flow systems could be applied to examining large numbers of chromosomes from old and young donors for the detection of qualitative as well as quantitative age-related alterations.

It will also be crucial to perform large-scale cytogenetic studies on *in vivo* cell populations. The practical as well as ethical limitations of human experimentation make this task extremely difficult, since a bone marrow biopsy is not a routine procedure. It is conceivable, however, that if population studies of cancer that involve bone marrow biopsy were initiated, sufficient material might be obtained from normal subjects for chromosomal analysis. Another approach to the question of *in vivo* aneuploidy would be to use animal models.

Finally, the importance of longitudinal studies must be reemphasized. It will be crucial to determine whether aneuploidy increases gradually after puberty, or whether the increase is most dramatic in the last decades of life. It will be of particular interest to determine whether persons who have high age-related levels of aneuploidy have an increased risk of developing malignancies, immune disorders, or other disorders leading to shortened life span.

16. Summary

Cytogenetic studies of cultured human peripheral lymphocytes by a number of investigators have demonstrated an increased frequency of aneuploid cells with aging. This observed aneuploidy is due chiefly to a loss of chromosomes, and is more prominent in the female than in the male. Analysis of the missing chromosome indicates that the X chromosome is the most frequently lost chromosome in female cells and the Y chromosome in male cells.

In vivo analysis of aneuploidy by direct bone-marrow-cell preparations has also indicated an increased frequency of aneuploid cell lines with aging. Unfortunately, population studies such as those conducted on peripheral-lymphocyte cultures have not yet been performed on *in vivo* cell populations.

With *in vitro* cellular "aging," senescent fibroblast cultures have also been demonstrated to have increased frequencies of both aneuploid and polyploid cells.

Two explanations for the selective loss of specific chromosomes are proposed: (1) survival of cells with specific chromosomal loss and (2) selective loss of specific chromosomes. In addition, the potential effect of aging on selection of certain cell populations (aneuploid vs. diploid) should be considered.

Future research in cytogenetics should employ newly developed cytogenetic technology to identify the specific chromosomes that are lost as well as to examine minor chromosomal abnormalities that might occur with aging. Increased numbers of chromosomes can be processed by automating cytogenetic analysis and by utilizing flow microfluorometric systems. Finally, there is a need for longitudinal studies to define more clearly the dynamics of the age-related increase in aneuploidy.

References

Arrighi, F. E., and Hsu, T. C., 1971, Localization of heterochromatin in human chromosomes, *Cytogenetics* **10**:81.

Benn, P. A., 1976, Specific chromosome aberrations in senescent fibroblast cell lines derived from human embryos, *Am. J. Hum. Genet.* **28**:465.

Bettner, L. G., and Jarvik, L. F., 1971, Stroop color–word test, non-psychotic organic brain syndrome, and chromosome loss in aged twins, *J. Gerontol.* **26**:458.

Beutler, E., Yeh, M., and Fairbanks, V. F., 1962, The normal human female as a mosaic of X-chromosome activity: Studies using the gene for G-6PD deficiency as a marker, *Proc. Natl. Acad. Sci. U.S.A.* **48**:9.

Bloom, A. D., Archer, P. G., and Awa, A. A., 1967, Variation in the human chromosome number, *Nature (London)* **216**:487.

Bloom, A. D., McNeill, J. A., and Nakamura, F. T., 1974, Cytogenetics of lymphocyte cell lines, in: *Chromosomes and Cancer* (J. German, ed.), pp. 565–599, John Wiley & Sons, New York.

Boué, A., Boué, J., Cure, S., Deluchat, C., and Perraudin, N., 1975, *In vitro* cultivation of cells from aneuploid human embryos, initiation of cell lines and longevity of the cultures, *In Vitro* **11**:409.

Boué, J. G., and Boué, A., 1974, Anomalies chromosomiques dans les avortements spontanes, in: *Chromosomal Errors in Relation to Reproductive Failure* (A. Boué and C. Thibault, eds.), pp. 29–56, INSERM, Paris.

Boveri, T., 1914, *Zur Frage der Enstehung maligner Tumoren*, Gustav Fisher, Jena, Germany.

Cadotte, M., and Fraser, D., 1970, Étude de l'aneuploidie observée dans les cultures de sang et de moelle en fonction du nombre et de longeur des chromosomes de chaque groupe et de l'age et du sexe des sujets, *Union Med. Can.* **99**:2003.

Caspersson, T., Zech, L., Johansson, C., and Modest, E. J., 1970, Identification of human chromosomes by DNA-binding fluorescing agents, *Chromosoma* **30**:215.

Caspersson, T., Castleman, K. R., Lomakka, G., Modest, E. S., Mollar, A., Nathan, R., Wall, R. J., and Lech, L., 1971, Automated karyotyping of quinacrine mustard stained human chromosomes, *Exp. Cell Res.* **67**:233.

Chen, T. R., and Ruddle, F. H., 1974, Chromosome changes revealed by Q-band staining method during cell senescence of WI-38, *Proc. Soc. Exp. Biol. Med.* **147:**533.

Cohen, D., 1976, A behavioral–chromosome relationship in the elderly: A critical review of biobehavioral hypothesis, *Exp. Cell Res.* **2:**271.

Court Brown, W. M., Buckton, K. E., Jacobs, P. A., Tough, I. M., Kuenssberg, E. V., and Knox, J. D. E., 1966, Chromosome studies on adults, *Eugen. Lab. Mem.* **42:**1.

Cristofalo, V. J., 1973, Cellular senescence: Factors modulating cell proliferation *in vitro,* in: *Molecular and Cellular Mechanisms of Aging,* Vol. 27, pp. 65–92, INSERM, Paris.

deGalen, E. H. K., 1966, Age and chromosomes, *Nature (London)* **211:**1324.

Demoise, C. F., and Conard, R. A., 1972, Effects of age and radiation exposure on chromosomes in a Marshall Island population, *J. Gerontol.* **27:**197.

Denver Conference on the Human Karyotype, 1960, A proposed standard system of nomenclature of human mitotic chromosomes, *Lancet* **1:**1063.

Dutrillaux, B., and Lejeune, J., 1971, Sur une nouvelle technique d'analyse du caryotype humaine, *C. R. Acad. Sci.* **272:**2638.

Edwards, J. H., Harnden, D. G., Cameron, A. H., Grosse, V. M., and Wolff, O. H., 1960, A new trisomic syndrome, *Lancet* **1:**787.

Epstein, C. J., 1967, Cell size, nuclear content, and the development of polyploidy in the mammalian liver, *Proc. Natl. Acad. Sci. U.S.A.* **57:**327.

Falzone, J. A., Barrows, C. H., and Shock, N. W., 1959, Age and polyploidy of rat liver nuclei as measured by volume and DNA content, *J. Gerontol.* **14:**2.

Fang, J. S., Jagiello, G., Ducayen, M., and Graffeo, J., 1975, Aging and X chromosome loss in the human ovary, *Obstet. Gynecol.* **45:**455.

Fialkow, P. J., Paton, G. R., and East, J., 1973, Chromosomal abnormalities in spleens of NZB mice, a strain characterized by autoimmunity and malignancy, *Proc. Natl. Acad. Sci. U.S.A.* **70:**1094.

Fitzgerald, P. H., Pickering, A. F., Mercer, J. M., and Miethke, P. M., 1975, Premature centromere division: A mechanism of non-disjunction causing X chromosome aneuploidy in somatic cells of man, *Ann. Hum. Genet.* **38:**417.

Gilbert, C. W., Muldal, S., and Lathja, L. G., 1965, Rate of chromosome duplication at the end of the DNA S period in human blood cells, *Nature (London)* **208:**159.

Goodman, R. M. Fechheimer, N. S., Miller, F., Miller, R., and Zartman, D., 1969, Chromosomal alterations in three age groups of human females, *Am. J. Med. Sci.* **258:**26.

Gray, J. W., Carrano, A. V., Steinmetz, L. L., Van Dilla, M. A., Moore, D. H., Mayall, B. H., and Mendelsohn, M. L., 1975, Chromosome measurement and sorting by flow systems, *Proc. Natl. Acad. Sci. U.S.A.* **72:**1231.

Hamerton, J. L., Taylor, A. I., Angell, R., and McGuire, V. M., 1965, Chromosome investigations of a small isolated human population: Chromosome abnormalities and distribution of chromosome counts according to age and sex among the population of Tristan da Cunha, *Nature (London)* **206:**1232.

Harnden, D. G., 1974, Ataxia telangiectasia syndrome: Cytogenetic and cancer aspects, in: *Chromosomes and Cancer* (J. German, ed.), pp. 619–636, John Wiley & Sons, New York.

Hayflick, L., 1965, The limited *in vitro* lifetime of human diploid cell strains, *Exp. Cell Res.* **37:**614.

Hayflick, L., and Moorhead, P. S., 1961, The serial cultivation of human diploid cell cultures, *Exp. Cell Res.* **25:**585.

Holliday, R., and Tarrant, G. M., 1972, Altered enzymes in ageing diploid fibroblasts, *Nature (London)* **238:**26.

Honda, T., Kamada, N., and Bloom, A. D., 1969, Chromosome aberrations and culture time, *Cytogenetics* **8:**117.

Jacobs, J. P., Jones, C. M., and Baille, J. P., 1970, Characteristics of a human diploid cell designated MRC-5, *Nature (London)* **227**:168.

Jacobs, P. A., and Court Brown, W. M., 1966, Age and chromosomes, *Nature (London)* **212**:823.

Jacobs, P. A., Court Brown, W. M., and Doll, R., 1961, Distribution of human chromosome counts in relation to age, *Nature (London)* **191**:1178.

Jacobs, P. A., Brunton, M., Court Brown, W. M., Doll, R., and Goldstein, H., 1963, Change in human chromosome count distributions with age: Evidence for a sex difference, *Nature (London)* **197**:1080.

Jarvik, L. F., and Kato, T., 1969, Chromosomes and mental changes in octogenarians: Preliminary findings, *Br. J. Psychol.* **115**:1193.

Jarvik, L. F., and Kato, T., 1970, Chromosome examinations in aged twins, *Am. J. Hum. Genet.* **22**:562.

Jarvik, L. F., Yen, F. S., Fu, T. K., and Matsuyama, S. S., 1976, Chromosomes in old age: A six year longitudinal study, *Hum. Genet.* **33**:17.

Kadanka, Z. K., Sparkes, J. D., and MacMorine, H. G., 1973, A study of the cytogenetics of the human cell strain WI-38, *In Vitro* **8**:353.

Kadontani, T., Ohama, K., Nakayama, T., Takahara, H., and Makino, S., 1971, Chromosome aberrations in leukocytes of normal adults from 49 couples, *Proc. Jpn. Acad.* **47**:724.

Koprowski, H., Ponten, J. A., Jensen, F., Ravdin, R. G., Moorhead, P., and Saksela, E., 1962, Transformation of cultures of human tissue infected with simian virus SV_{40}, *J. Cell. Comp. Physiol.* **59**:281.

Latt, S., 1973, Microfluorometric detection of deoxyribonucleic acid replication in human metaphase chromosomes, *Proc. Natl. Acad. Sci. U.S.A.* **70**:3395.

Lejeune, J., Gautier, M., and Turpin, R., 1959, Étude des chromosomes somatiques de neuf enfants mongoliens, *C. R. Acad. Sci.* **248**:1721.

Lyon, M. F., 1961, Gene action in the X chromosome of the mouse, *Nature (London)* **190**:372.

Makino, S., Sasaki, M. S., and Tonomura, A., 1964, Cytological studies of tumors. XI. Chromosome studies in fifty-two human tumors, *J. Natl. Cancer Inst.* **32**:741.

Mattevi, M. S., and Salzano, F. M., 1975, Senescence and human chromosome changes, *Humangenetik* **27**:1.

McKusick, V. A., 1976a, Introduction to the Third International Workshop on Human Gene Mapping (1975), *Cytogenet. Cell Genet.* **16**:6.

McKusick, V. A., 1976b, *Mendelian Inheritance in Man,* 4th Ed., Johns Hopkins Press, Baltimore.

Miller, R. W., 1970, Neoplasia and Down's syndrome, *Ann. N. Y. Acad. Sci.* **171**:637.

Moorhead, P. S., and Saksela, E., 1963, Nonrandom chromosomal aberrations—SV40 transformed human cells, *J. Cell. Comp. Physiol.* **62**:57.

Neurath, P. W., Falek, A., Bablouzian, B. L., Warms, T. H., and Serbagi, R. C., 1966, Human chromosome analysis by computer—An optical pattern recognition problem, *Ann. N. Y. Acad. Sci.* **128**:1013.

Neurath, P., DeRemer, K., Bell, B., Jarvik, L., and Kato, T., 1970, Chromosome loss compared with chromosome size, age and sex of subjects, *Nature (London)* **225**:281.

Nielsen, J., 1970, Chromosomes in senile, presenile, and arteriosclerotic dementia, *J. Gerontol.* **25**:312.

Nielsen, J., Jensen, L., Lindhardt, H., Stottrup, L., and Sondergaard, A., 1968, Chromosomes in senile dementia, *Br. J. Psychol.* **114**:303.

Orgel, L., 1973, Aging of clones of mammalian cells, *Nature (London)* **243**:441.

Pardue, M. L., and Gall, J. G., 1970, Chromosomal localization of mouse satellite DNA, *Science* **168**:1356.

Paris Conference on the Human Karyotype, 1971, Standardization in human cytogenetics,

   Birth Defects: Orig. Artic. Ser., No. VIII, The National Foundation–March of Dimes, New York.

Patau, K., Smith, D. W., Therman, E., Inhorn, S. L., and Wagner, H. P., 1960, Multiple congenital anomaly caused by an extra autosome, *Lancet* **1**:790.

Pierre, R. V., 1974, Preleukemic states, *Semin. Hematol.* **11**:73.

Pierre, R. V., and Hoagland, H. C., 1971, 45,X cell lines in adult men: Loss of Y chromosome, a normal aging phenomenon, *Mayo Clin. Proc.* **46**:52.

Pierre, R. V., and Hoagland, H. C., 1972, Age-associated aneuploidy: Loss of Y chromosome from human bone marrow cells with aging, *Cancer* **30**:889.

Saksela, E., and Moorhead, P. S., 1963, Aneuploidy in the degenerative phase of serial cultivation of human cell strains, *Proc. Natl. Acad. Sci. U.S.A.* **50**:390.

Sandberg, A. A., Cohen, M. M., Rimm, A. A., and Levin, M. L., 1967, Aneuploidy and age in a population survey, *Am. J. Hum. Genet.* **19**:633.

Sawitsky, A., Bloom, D., and German, J., 1966, Chromosomal breakage and acute leukemia in congenital telangiectatic erythema and stunted growth, *Ann. Intern. Med.* **65**:487.

Schneider, E. L., and Epstein, C. J., 1972, Replication rate and lifespan of cultured fibroblasts in Down's syndrome, *Proc. Soc. Exp. Biol. Med.* **141**:1092.

Schneider, E. L., and Mitsui, Y., 1976, The relationship between *in vitro* cellular aging and *in vivo* human age, *Proc. Natl. Acad. Sci. U.S.A.* **73**:3584.

Sumner, A. T., Evans, H. J., and Buckland, R. A., 1971, New technique for distinguishing between human chromosomes, *Nature (London) New Biol.* **232**:31.

Swift, M., 1971, Fanconi's anemia in the genetics of neoplasia, *Nature (London)* **230**:370.

Swim, H. E., and Parker, R. F., 1957, Culture characteristics of human fibroblasts cultured serially, *Am. J. Hyg.* **66**:235.

Takagi, N., and Sandberg, A. A., 1968, Chronology and pattern of human chromosome replication. VII. Cellular and chromosomal DNA behavior, *Cytogenetics* **7**:118.

Tan, Y. H., Schneider, E. L., Tischfield, J., Epstein, C. J., and Ruddle, F. H., 1974, Human chromosome 21 dosage: Effect on the expression of the interferon induced antiviral state, *Science* **186**:61.

Thompson, K. V. A., and Holliday, R., 1973, Effect of temperature on the longevity of human fibroblasts in culture, *Exp. Cell Res.* **80**:354.

Thompson, K. V. A., and Holliday, R., 1975, Chromosome changes during the *in vitro* ageing of MRC-5 human fibroblasts, *Exp. Cell Res.* **96**:1.

Tice, R., Schneider, E. L., and Rary, J. M., 1976, The utilization of bromodeoxyuridine incorporation into DNA for the analysis of cellular kinetics, *Exp. Cell Res.* **102**:232.

Tijo, J. H., and Levan, A., 1956, The chromosome number of man, *Hereditas* **42**:1.

Yunis, J. J., 1976, High resolution of human chromosomes, *Science* **191**:1268.

Zuppinger, E., Engel, E., Forbes, A. P., Mantooth, L., and Claffey, J., 1967, Klinefelter's syndrome, a clinical and cytogenetic study in twenty-four cases, *Acta Endocrinol. Suppl.* **113**:5.

Chapter 3

Aging and DNA-Repair Capability

Raymond R. Tice

1. Introduction

The aging process is best defined as a general loss in biological competence for both the individual cell and the organism as a whole. At the cellular level, this loss is expressed as decreasing replicative ability in proliferating cells and decreasing functional activity in postmitotic cells (Little, 1976). For the organism, the aging process expresses itself as decreased viability and increased vulnerability to the normal forces of mortality (Goldstein, 1971*a*).

Current aging theories can be largely divided into two categories: those based on genetic programming and those based on error accumulation (Hayflick, 1975; Medvedev, 1976; Cutler, 1976*a*). The former theories assume that aging is actually a continuation of growth, differentiation, and morphogenesis (i.e., that aging is genetically determined). The latter theories assume that the primary aging event is stochastic (i.e., that it is not genetically determined but is governed by chance) and expresses itself by accumulation of errors in DNA, RNA, or protein or in some combination of the three.

Fundamental to most aging theories is the importance of the maintenance of DNA integrity and the possible primary role of DNA-repair processes (Samis, 1966; Alexander, 1967; Smith, 1976; Trosko and Hart, 1976). At least one aging model, in fact, is based on the possible differential repair of mutational damage in transcribed and nontranscribed DNA (Yielding, 1974). DNA-repair processes, by monitoring potential muta-

Raymond R. Tice ● Medical Department, Brookhaven National Laboratory, Upton, New York 11973

tional events, clearly represent a major homeostatic mechanism at the cellular level. Aging, then, could be the result of a declining repair capability that would permit the rapid accumulation of deleterious events at the DNA level. Alternatively, the variation in aging rates among different animal species might be due to intrinsic differences in the efficiencies of their DNA-repair systems.

Both alternatives assume that aging is a direct consequence of unrepaired mutational events. The former possibility predicts that unrepaired events will rise precipitously near the end of an organism's life span as DNA-repair capability becomes increasingly inefficient. The latter possibility predicts the presence of a direct age-related increase in unrepaired DNA lesions that should be proportional to the length of the normal life span. If one or both of these possibilities exists, then, predictably: (1) an age-related increase in unrepaired DNA lesions, whether linear or exponential, should occur; (2) genetic syndromes that express features of premature or accelerated aging should express a DNA-repair-deficiency component and vice versa; (3) the rate of the aging process itself should be subject to modification by changes in the environmental levels of DNA-damaging agents; and (4) species with different life spans could be expected to have demonstrable differences in DNA-repair capabilities, or DNA-repair capability should decline with age, or both.

This chapter will examine each of these predictions, *in vitro* as well as *in vivo,* in an attempt to assess the relationship between normal aging and DNA-repair capability.

2. DNA-Repair Processes

Investigations concerned with DNA repair in eukaryote cells are not far removed from their infancy. Slightly more than ten years have passed since the first indication of an active DNA-repair process in mammalian cells (Rasmussen and Painter, 1964). In that short time, a bewildering array of findings and conclusions have been published, and the reader is directed to some extensive reviews on this subject (Hart and Trosko, 1976; Little and Williams, 1976; Hanawalt and Setlow, 1975). What is apparent is the existence of at least four types of DNA repair—strand-break rejoining, excision repair, postreplication repair, and photoreactivation. The first two repair systems are thought to involve a large number of subcomponents, each of which may be specific for the repair of a certain type of DNA lesion. In some instances, however, the same DNA lesion can be repaired through the activity of more than one DNA-repair process. Consequently, when we speak of the DNA-repair capability of a cell, a tissue, or an organism, we are in fact speaking of the sum total of all repair processes present and the interaction among these systems to monitor and repair potential DNA lesions. The following description of these repair processes and the means by which they are assayed is meant to serve only as a basis for evaluating the possible relationship between aging and DNA repair, not as an extensive summary of the molecular mechanisms involved in DNA repair.

2.1. Strand-Breakage Rejoining

DNA strand breakage is a direct consequence of exposure of cells to ionizing radiation or to a few so-called "radiomimetic" compounds (e.g., methylmethanesulfonate). It is not known whether base and sugar damage accompanies (or precedes) strand breakage, nor is it known whether base release sometimes or always accompanies break formation (Painter, 1974). What is known is that repair of this type of lesion or these types of lesions is rapid and involves limited exonuclease activity (Dugle and Gillespie, 1975; Hart and Trosko, 1976).

2.2. Excision Repair

Excision repair is basically a process by which the cell repairs DNA base damage. It is probably the most extensively examined repair system to date, and is seemingly the most complex (Hart and Trosko, 1976). In its simplest form, excision repair involves the recognition of a base damage and the production of a nearby incision by an endonuclease, excision of the damaged base and some adjacent bases by an exonuclease, insertion of new bases to fill the excised region (repair replication), and a ligase activity to seal the loose ends (Painter, 1974). There exist at least four classes of endonucleases, each of which appears to be specific for the different types of DNA lesions induced by ionizing radiation, UV light, or chemical compounds (Hart and Trosko, 1976).

2.3. Postreplication Repair

Excision repair is not the only DNA system that acts to repair base damage. Another process, known as *postreplication* repair because of its dependence on semiconservative DNA replication, also exists (see Hanawalt and Setlow, 1975). Of the known DNA-repair systems, postreplication repair is the least understood. Presumably, it is a process by which DNA newly synthesized from a defective or damaged template is repaired (Hart and Trosko, 1976). Initially, postreplication repair was postulated as a mechanism to fill gaps in newly synthesized DNA occurring opposite base damage in the parental DNA (Lehmann, 1972; Buhl *et al.,* 1972). This model, however, has not been verified experimentally (Painter, 1974; Meneghini and Hanawalt, 1975). Postreplication repair appears to be coupled to normal semiconservative DNA replication, and the two processes might in fact share some of the same enzymes (Hart and Trosko, 1976). There is evidence to suggest that this repair process has an inducible caffeine-sensitive component in some permanent cell lines (D'Ambrosio and Setlow, 1976).

2.4. Photoreactivation

Photoreactivation is a repair process specific for UV-induced cyclobutyl pyrimidine dimers. These dimers are repaired by the photoreactivating enzyme in a two-step process. First, the enzyme binds to a dimer-containing DNA region, and then, in the presence of 300- to 600-nm light, the cyclobutane ring undergoes photolysis, producing the original two monomere pyrimidines (Sutherland *et al.*, 1974). Only recently has the presence of this enzyme been demonstrated in placental mammalian tissues such as human leukocytes and murine or human fibroblasts (Sutherland, 1974; Sutherland *et al.*, 1974).

2.5. Assay Systems for DNA Repair

The repair of strand breakage has been generally investigated by techniques based on alkaline sucrose-gradient sedimentation (McGrath and Williams, 1966). This assay system indicates not only the presence of single-strand breaks, but also the occurrence of alkali-labile bonds in DNA. The sensitivity of this assay system depends, to a large extent, on the gentleness of the preparative techniques for isolating high-molecular-weight DNA from cells.

Excision-repair capability in cells exposed to ionizing radiation, UV light, or mutagenic compounds has been examined with a number of different techniques—techniques that measure the completion of different steps in the repair process. These techniques include assaying endonuclease activity by the formation of strand breaks (Bacchetti, 1975), the excision step by the release of pyrimidine dimers from DNA (Carrier and Setlow, 1971), and the resynthesis step by repair replication (Cleaver and Painter, 1968) or unscheduled DNA synthesis (UDS) (Rasmussen and Painter, 1964). The technique most commonly used is that of UDS. This assay system involves the incorporation of tritiated thymidine into DNA of cells not actively undergoing semiconservative DNA synthesis; hence the name *unscheduled* DNA synthesis. Subsequently, this incorporation of a radioactive isotope can be measured on a cell-by-cell basis by autoradiography (Rasmussen and Painter, 1964) or for the population as a whole by scintillation counting techniques (Evans and Norman, 1968).

Techniques for the analysis of postreplication repair have largely involved measurements of DNA molecular weight by density-gradient centrifugation (Painter, 1974) or by alkaline sucrose sedimentation techniques (Lehmann, 1972). Recently, a cytogenetic technique has been developed that might permit the examination of a successful postreplication repair event—sister chromatid exchanges (SCEs) (Latt, 1973; Kato, 1977). The exact nature of SCEs and their relationship to DNA repair have not yet been fully resolved, however, and SCEs must therefore remain as a potential technique for future experimentation.

Assaying photoreactivation repair depends on the isolation of the photoreactivating enzyme from tissues and its incubation with UV-exposed DNA and the subsequent measurement of pyrimidine dimer loss (Sutherland and Chamberlin, 1973).

All these DNA-repair systems can be further assayed in proliferating cells through cytogenetic techniques. Unrepaired DNA lesions manifest themselves at the chromosomal level in metaphase cells as aberrations of one type or another, depending on the agent, the type of DNA lesion induced, and the timing in the cell cycle of the exposure to that agent (Bender *et al.*, 1973*a,b,* 1974). Consequently, a decrease in DNA-repair capability by any of the known DNA-repair systems will increase the frequency of observable chromosome aberrations in metaphase cells. This is, of course, the basis for the suggestion that human diseases characterized by increased levels of spontaneous chromosome aberrations involve a deficiency in some DNA-repair system. These diseases include such genetic syndromes as Fanconi anemia and ataxia–telangiectasia (German, 1972). What must be remembered with aberration investigations is that in most cases, the total capability of the cell to repair DNA lesions, not the efficiency of one specific repair system, is assessed.

3. Age-Related Occurrence of Unrepaired DNA Lesions

One line of evidence for a possible causal relationship between DNA-repair processes and aging is based on observations that suggest an age-related increase in the frequency of unrepaired lesions in DNA. Presumably, a dramatic increase in the frequency of unrepaired DNA lesions in aged cellular populations would indicate the absence of competent DNA-repair processes, and suggests a correlation among aging, cell death, and a decline in DNA-repair capability. Alternatively, the presence of unrepaired lesions, which increase in frequency throughout an animal's life and at a rate inversely proportional to life span, gives credence to the suggestion that aging is due to the intrinsic level of DNA repair competence, not to its decline.

3.1. DNA Strand Breakage

While many types of unrepaired lesions may be present in DNA, investigations at the DNA level have been largely concerned with assays restricted to identifying the presence of single- or double-strand breaks. In one of the earliest investigations, Price *et al.* (1971) and Modak and Price (1971) assayed the ability of isolated nuclei from brain, heart, and liver tissue of young and aged mice to provide templates for calf thymus DNA polymerase. Since this DNA polymerase requires partially denatured DNA to catalyze the incorporation of deoxyribonucleotide triphosphates and incorporation can be increased by ionizing radiation, this system presumably assays for denatured regions or strand scissions in DNA (Modak and Price, 1971). These investigators observed an age-related significant increase in mean autoradiographic grains in undenatured nuclei neurons and astrocytes, but not in Kupffer's cells or cardiac muscle. Acid denaturation of aged Kupffer's cells or cardiac muscle produced significantly increased mean grain counts in comparison with acid-denatured young cells. These results were interpreted to indicate an increase in single-stranded regions of DNA in some types of aged cells, and an increase in acid-sensitive regions in all types of aged cells examined. This increase with age was presumably the result of a decline in DNA-repair capability or an increase in the release of hydrolytic enzymes with age (Price *et al.*, 1971).

Subsequently, with more direct methods for examining single-strand lesions, Massie *et al.* (1972) hydrodynamically measured the molecular weight of both single- and double-stranded DNA isolated from rat liver cells as a function of age. Molecular weight in both types of molecules decreased approximately tenfold with increasing age, and this decrease was considered to demonstrate an increase in both single- and double-strand breaks at the molecular level. While this result might appear to be indicative of declining DNA-repair processes, it is interesting to note that the largest decrease in molecular weight took place in the first third of the animals' life span.

Supporting evidence for increased frequencies of single-strand scissions with age comes from the investigations of Karran and Ormerod (1973). DNA isolated from striated muscles of 28-day-old rats had lower molecular weights on alkaline sucrose gradients than striated muscle DNA from 1-day-old rats. As Karran and Ormerod (1973) themselves suggested, however, this apparent decrease in molecular weight might have been the result of the preparative procedure and therefore might not reflect *in vivo* conditions.

Wheeler and Lett (1974) applied zonal centrifugation alkaline sucrose gradients to DNA isolated from young and aged dog neurons. With age, the DNA was found to have decreased molecular weights, and again, this result appears to demonstrate an accumulation of unrepaired lesions. More recently, Ono *et al.* (1976) examined DNA isolated from aging mouse liver, spleen, thymus, and cerebellum by alkaline sucrose gradient centrifugation. Only hepatic DNA was observed to decrease in molecular weight with age. This decrease in molecular weight occurred, however, in mice between 1–2 and 14 months old. There was no further significant decrease in molecular weight with age.

Finally, the frequency of single-stranded DNA regions in aging mouse liver cells was measured by Chetsanga *et al.* (1975), utilizing an assay based on the single-strand-specific nuclease S_1. This assay system cannot ascertain the number of such sites present; it can ascertain only the extent to which the total genome is involved. Only after approximately half the measured life span ($\approx$30 months) did these workers note an increase in S_1 activity, which by the end of the cells' life span reached almost 25% of the total genome.

3.2. DNA Cross-Linking

The investigations discussed in preceding sections, while differing in their assay systems, have been directed exclusively at the presence in DNA of denatured regions or strand scissions or both. Other *in vivo* investigations, however, have been directed toward examining DNA cross-linking. In one study, pregnant rats were fed tritium, and the vital organs (brain and liver) of their offspring were examined at different ages for cross-linked products (Acharya, 1972). With age, not only was there an increase in the frequency of DNA–protein–RNA complexes, but also their molecular size increased. Since some of these substances retained tritium activity, it appeared as though they had remained fixed in the cells from birth and were therefore presumably immune to normal DNA-repair processes.

In a similar investigation, Cutler (1976*b*) observed an accumulation in DNA–protein cross-links with age in rodent liver tissue, and at a rate approximately inversely proportional to life span potential in two rodent species—*Mus* and *Peromycus*.

In support of the formation of DNA cross-links with age, the percentage of DNA that can readily be isolated from aging liver tissue declines (Amici *et al.*, 1974), and DNA isolated from aged organs has a higher melting temperature (von Hahn and Fritz, 1966). Also, Salser and Balis (1972) examined the extent of DNA-bound protein after extensive extraction procedures in various tissues of aging rats. They observed no change in total bound protein in rat liver, an increase in spleen and kidney, and a decrease in intestinal tissue as a function of age.

While these *in vivo* investigations have largely demonstrated an increase in cross-linking with age, one recent *in vitro* investigation proved negative. Bradley *et al.* (1976) examined levels of DNA cross-linking in WI-38 cells, an embryonic lung fibroblast cell line with a limited *in vitro* life span, and observed no increase as a function of *in vitro* passage level. Their assay system, based on filter elution rates of DNA from alkaline-lysed cells, is capable of detecting DNA cross-linked not only to complementary strands, but also to other cellular constituents (Bradley *et al.*, 1976).

3.3. Chromosome Aberrations

As another indication for an age-associated accumulation of unrepaired DNA lesions, some investigations have been directed toward examining so-called "spontaneous" levels of chromosome aberrations in metaphase cells. Chromosome aberrations can arise in cells from the presence of known unrepaired DNA lesions (Parrington *et al.*, 1971; Sasaki, 1973), and many types of DNA lesions can result in the same general classes of aberrations (Bender *et al.*, 1973a,b, 1974). Consequently, a decline in the efficiency of any DNA-repair process should give rise to an increase in spontaneous chromosome aberrations. A decrease in DNA-repair capability is not, however, the only possible mechanism by which increased spontaneous levels of aberrations could arise. Chromosome aberrations also occur as a result of interference with normal DNA synthesis (Kihlman, 1966). Secondarily, this system is, of course, limited to proliferating cellular populations and, of necessity, cannot provide information about the large variety of postmitotic tissues in the aging organism.

In vivo, two major cellular systems have been examined for spontaneous chromosome aberrations as a function of age. Both systems involve the examination of tissues that are normally quiescent—liver and peripheral lymphocytes—but that can be forced into active mitosis under the appropriate stimulus.

The liver system was initially chosen because it offered the opportunity of examining a tissue that would have the potential of accumulating DNA lesions without any loss due to normal cellular turnover (Curtis, 1963). This system involves the partial destruction of the liver either by subcutaneous injections of carbon tetrachloride (Stevenson and Curtis, 1961) or by partial hepatectomy (Brooks *et al.*, 1973). While the liver is subsequently undergoing regeneration, metaphase or anaphase cells can be examined for chromosome aberrations.

Extensive investigations have observed an age-dependent direct increase in liver chromosome aberrations in mice (Stevenson and Curtis, 1961), dogs (Curtis *et al.*, 1966), guinea pigs (Curtis and Miller, 1971), and Chinese hamsters (Brooks *et al.*, 1973). This age-dependent increase also appears to be inversely proportional to life span—increasing at a faster rate in inbred mouse strains with shorter life spans than in inbred mouse strains with longer life spans (Crowley and Curtis, 1963). While this proportionality also held true for mice, guinea pigs, and dogs, Chinese hamsters appeared to be an exception (Brooks *et al.,* 1973). This discrepancy, however, could be due to differences in ascertainment.

In another *in vivo* cellular system, peripheral lymphocytes derived from donors of different ages are stimulated to divide with a mitogen, generally phytohemagglutinin (PHA). After some specific time interval, metaphase cells are then examined for chromosome aberrations. In man, Court Brown *et al.* (1966), Tough *et al.* (1970), Jarvik and Kato (1970), Liniecki *et al.* (1971), and Ayme *et al.* (1976) observed a slight increase in aberration frequencies in the aged populations. On the other hand, Jacobs and Court Brown (1966), Sandberg *et al.* (1967), Bochkov *et al.* (1968), Goodman *et al.* (1969), and Bochkov (1972) all observed no such increase. In swine, a marginal increase in chromosome deletions was observed with increasing age, all other types of aberrations remaining constant in frequency (McFee *et al.,* (1970). This cellular system is extremely complex, however, and there are significant differences between the replicative rates of stimulated cells in young and aged lymphocyte cultures (Tice, 1976). Consequently, any difference in spontaneous aberration frequencies might be a result of metabolic alterations, not of increased frequencies in unrepaired DNA lesions.

In proliferating cellular populations *in vivo,* the data appear to be equally inconsistent. Chlebovsky *et al.* (1966) reported a dramatic increase in chromosome aberration frequencies in extremely aged rat bone marrow cells. On the other hand, Curtis and Tilley (1971) observed no such increase with age in bone marrow cells derived from either aging mice or rats.

In vitro, such investigations have been largely concerned with examining chromosome aberration frequencies in human-fetal-derived fibroblast cell lines as a function of *in vitro* passage. These cell lines have been observed to undergo increased frequencies of chromosome aberrations, aberrations largely limited to dicentric chromosome formation, during senescence (Sax and Passano, 1961; Saksela and Moorhead, 1963; Thompson, K. V. A., and Holliday, 1975; Benn, 1976). These chromosome aberrations, however, were suggested to be a consequence of defective proteins, not a major cause of death in senescent cells (Thompson K. V. A., and Holliday, 1975).

All these investigations, whether directed at single-strand scissions and cross-linking in DNA or aberrations in metaphase chromosomes, have been limited in the number of different types of tissues examined. The only *in vivo* tissue that has been clearly demonstrated to undergo an age-related increase in unrepaired DNA lesions is liver tissue. All investigations into other tissues, *in vitro* as well as *in vivo,* have been either entirely negative or not consistently positive. The frequency of cross-linked DNA and chromosome aberrations in the liver appears not to increase abruptly near the end of an animal's life span, but rather to accumulate steadily throughout. This observation would indicate that declining DNA-repair processes are not critical for aging, but rather certain proportions or types of DNA lesions escape repair and accumulate within a cell, possibly doing irreparable damage to its normal function. This increase in unrepaired lesions might be tissue-specific, however, and not reflect general *in vivo* conditions during aging.

4. DNA-Repair Capability as a Function of Age

In an attempt to correlate aging with a possible decline in DNA-repair capability, numerous investigators have examined the efficiency of various repair systems in aging cellular systems *in vitro* as well as *in vivo*. *In vitro* investigations have been primarily concerned with assessing DNA-repair levels in human- and animal-derived fibroblast cell lines as a function of the number of population doublings passed. Human cellular research has been largely directed at comparing DNA-repair capacity in cultured lymphocytes, or in a few instances cultured skin fibroblasts, derived from donors at different ages. Animal research *in vivo* has focused on a few postmitotic tissues as well as some proliferating cellular systems.

4.1. In Vitro Investigations

4.1.1. Human Cellular Systems

Goldstein (1971*b*) was the first to investigate the question of DNA-repair capability as a function of *in vitro* passage level. Using UV-induced UDS and cell survival as measurements of DNA-repair competence, he observed no decline in repair capability in human skin fibroblast cell lines until very near the end of their *in vitro* life span. This finding was soon confirmed in the human embryonic lung fibroblast cell line (WI-38) by Painter *et al.* (1973). Subsequent investigators observed some decrease in UDS-measured excision repair with increasing *in vitro* passage levels of WI-38 cell populations (Hart and Setlow, 1976; Bowman *et al.*, 1976). Both these latter two groups concluded that the observed decline correlated with the number of cells no longer capable of undergoing normal semiconservative DNA replication. While this conclusion suggests some sort of direct relationship between the two processes, it is impossible to determine which process is a consequence of the other.

Single-strand-break-rejoining has also been extensively examined in human fibroblast cultures at different *in vitro* passage levels. Clarkson and Painter (1974) examined X-ray-induced single-strand-break-rejoining in WI-

38 cells with both alkaline sucrose gradient centrifugation and UDS techniques. They observed no repair decline throughout the *in vitro* life span. In agreement with these investigators, Bradley *et al.* (1976) observed normal rates of single-strand-break-rejoining in terminally senescent WI-38 cultures as assayed by both alkaline-elution and alkaline-sedimentation techniques.

In human skin fibroblasts, J. Epstein *et al.* (1973*a*, 1974) and Little *et al.* (1975) observed a decline in the rate of strand-rejoining by alkaline sucrose gradient centrifugation as the cells approached senescence. While this decline in DNA-repair capacity was more marked in cells at the end of their *in vitro* life span, it appeared to commence prior to any indication of terminal senescence (Little, 1976).

Finally, Mattern and Cerutti (1975), in one recent study, examined aging WI-38 cell nuclei and nuclear sonicates for their ability to specifically excise osmium tetroxide- or γ-ray-induced 5,6-dihydroxydihydrothymine residues. Late-passage cells exhibited a complete loss in the ability to excise this specific type of DNA lesion, and this loss in repair occurred prior to complete cessation in growth.

4.1.2. Animal Cellular Systems

Examination of animal cellular systems for DNA-repair capability during their *in vitro* life span has been largely limited to fibroblast cell lines of fetal origin. In mouse embryo fibroblast cultures, UV-induced UDS and pyrimidine dimer release declined only in terminally senescent cultures (Ben-Ishai and Peleg, 1975). Transformed cells from these senescent cultures did not regain the loss in DNA-repair capability.

Paterson *et al.* (1974) examined UV-induced UDS in a chick fibroblast system and observed a lack of excision repair in middle- or late-passage cells in comparison with early-passage populations.

Finally, Willimas and Little (1975) investigated both UV- and γ-ray-induced UDS as well as single-strand-break-rejoining by alkaline sedimentation in primary hamster embryo cultures. Active UV- and γ-induced UDS was present throughout the *in vitro* life span of these cellular populations, ceasing only in terminally senescent cultures. Single-strand-break-rejoining rates, however, appeared to decline between early- and late-passage populations. In this cell system, transformed cells retained both the UDS activity and the single-strand-break-rejoining rates of early-passage cells.

4.1.3. Conclusions

The results of these investigations on DNA-repair capability during the *in vitro* life spans of explants derived from both human and animal tissues are somewhat conflicting. There is the possibility, however unlikely it may be, that these differences are simply a consequence of increased resolution in some of the assay systems used to examine DNA repair. The majority of investigators, however, observed no appreciable decline in either excision repair or single-strand-break-rejoining until after senescence had begun. Futhermore, through double-labeling autoradiography, the repair decline that was observed in senescent cellular populations correlated strongly with a simultaneous loss in cells of their ability to undergo normal DNA synthesis. This finding suggests that the observed *in vitro* DNA-repair decline may be a consequence of the metabolic changes in senescent cells, not the direct cause of *in vitro* senescence *per se*.

4.2. In Vivo Investigations

4.2.1. Human Cellular Systems

Research connected with examining DNA-repair capability in humans as a function of age has been limited to two cellular systems: skin fibroblast cell lines and mitogen-stimulated peripheral lymphocyte cultures. Due to their greater accessibility, cultured lymphocytes have been more often examined for alterations in DNA-repair capability. Liniecki *et al.* (1971) examined G_1 X-ray-induced chromosome aberration yields in PHA-stimulated lymphocytes from donors ranging in age from 0 to 72 years. No differences between young and aged donors in the yields of acentric fragments, rings, or intercalary deletions were observed. Only dicentric frequencies appeared to change, but negatively as a function of age.

Induction of chromosome aberrations by exposure to chemical agents has also been examined in lymphocyte cultures from young and aged persons. Bochkov and Kuleshov (1971, 1972) exposed stimulated lymphocytes to thio-tepa and degranol, and observed that the frequency of induced aberrations increased significantly in the aged population. A similar finding was that of Lambert *et al.* (1976), who measured UV-induced UDS levels and found a 25% decline in repair synthesis in lymphocytes from subjects older than 60. However, not only do stimulated lymphocytes from young and aged donors cycle at different rates (Tice, 1976) and chromosome aberration yields vary in metaphase cells depending on their replicative history (Tice and Ishii, 1977), but also levels of UV-induced excision repair in this system depend on the degree and extent of lymphocyte stimulation (Darzynkiewicz, 1971). Consequently, these results might be artifactual and not reflect the true state of DNA-repair capacity.

Only Goldstein (1971*b*) has published any data in which DNA-repair levels are compared in skin-fibroblast cultures derived from young and aged donors. He examined cell survival after UV exposure in early-passage cultures of fetal, newborn, young, and aged origin and observed no significant differences in UV sensitivity.

4.2.2. Animal Cellular Systems

Examining γ-ray-induced chromosome aberrations in swine-lymphocyte cultures from young and aged animals, McFee *et al.* (1970) observed no increase in chromosome-type aberrations (i.e., achromatic lesions, fragments, rings, or dicentrics), but did observe an increase in chromatid-type aberrations (i.e., breaks or achromatic lesions).

To assess DNA repair in an actively proliferating cellular population *in vivo,* Curtis and Tilley (1971) irradiated mice and examined chromosome-aberration frequencies in metaphase cells from the bone marrow. Not only was there no difference between young and aged mice in induced aberration yields, but also the aberration frequencies declined with time at the same rates.

Finally, two postmitotic tissues have been examined for a possible decline in DNA-repair capability. Wheeler and Lett (1974) assessed the capability of internal granular-layer neurons from beagles of different ages of repair γ-ray-induced single-strand breaks by alkaline sucrose gradient sedimentation. No age-associated decline in this type of repair ability was observed. Yet, when isolated myocardial cells isolated from newborn and adult rats were compared for UV-induced UDS levels, the adult cells exhibited a complete loss of capability (Lampidis and Schaiberger, 1975). Since, however, the newborn rat myocardial cells still evidenced some normal DNA synthesis, this finding could be attributed to the normal process of differentiation and not to aging (see Section 5).

4.2.3. Conclusions

These results derived from both human and animal models suggest that there is no appreciable age-related decline in, at least, the ability to repair damage induced by ionizing radiation in either postmitotic, proliferating, or quiescent cellular populations. There is some suggestion that there is increased sensitivity to certain chemical compounds in stimulated lymphocytes from aged humans. With these chemical agents, however, it is difficult to interpret the actual findings. The apparent differences in chromosome-aberration yields could be the result of differences in mutagen metabolism, or they could be due to differences in the replication kinetics of the cultures. Investigations examining excision repair are too few and too conflicting to be helpful. There is no doubt that more investigations are necessary in this area before any reliable conclusion can be made.

5. Tissue-Specific DNA-Repair Capability

In any discussion of a possible correlation between aging and DNA-repair capability, some consideration must be given to the possible existence of tissue-specific differences in repair levels within the organism. Several investigations have suggested that nonproliferating, terminally differentiated cells undergo a loss in DNA-repair capacity in comparison with proliferating precursor cells. Rat- or embryonic-chicken-derived skeletal muscle cells suffer a significant loss in UDS-measured repair replication as they fuse *in vitro* into multinucleated cells and myotubes (Hahn *et al.*, 1971; Stockdale, 1971; Stockdale and O'Neill, 1972). In a more extensive investigation, Chan *et al.* (1976) examined both single-strand-break-rejoining and UDS-measured repair replication in an established myoblast cell line before and after *in-vitro*-induced fusion. Both the rate and overall levels of 4-nitroquinoline (UV-like)-induced UDS were reduced by more than 50% after myotube formation. This loss was due in part to a complete cessation in the ability of myotube cells to recognize and repair alkali-sensitive lesions. On the other hand, myotubes showed no decline in their ability to repair X-ray-induced single-strand breaks. Also, developing chick retinoblasts undergo a loss in UV-induced UDS capacity (Strauss, 1976), and mouse neuroblastoma cells become increasingly sensitive to UV exposure during differentiation (McCombe *et al.*, 1976).

In at least one system, this loss in DNA-excision-repair capability with differentiation has been demonstrated to be recoverable. The mouse neuroblastoma cell system of McCombe *et al.* (1976) is capable of undergoing reversible differentiation *in vitro,* depending on serum concentration. These cells regain normal levels of resistance to UV radiation after dedifferentiation, but not until after the first mitosis has been completed.

This correlation with proliferative activity and excision-repair competence also occurs with peripheral lymphocytes. These cells exhibit dramatic increases in their ability to remove acetoxy-aminofluorene-induced damage (Strauss, 1976; Scudiero *et al.*, 1976) and undergo UV-induced UDS (Darzynkiewicz, 1971) after mitogen stimulation. Although not equal in magnitude, this increase in repair competence occurs in parallel with increasing levels of DNA polymerase activity (Scudiero *et al.*, 1976).

This loss in DNA-repair replication capacity with differentiation expresses itself in comparative tissue studies. Examinations of UV-induced UDS revealed that peripheral lymphocytes have a greater capacity than peripheral granulocytes (Darzynkiewicz, 1971) and fibroblasts have a greater capacity than pulsating cardiac cells from the same rat organ (Lampidis and Little, 1976). On the other hand, cultured bovine lens epithelial cells and lung fibroblast cells from the same animal have equal capacities for repairing X-ray-induced single-strand scissions (Treton and Courtois, 1976).

These various investigations into DNA-repair capability as a function of the proliferative state of a cellular population support the conclusion that postmitotic cells suffer a loss in excision repair, but not in DNA-strand-break-rejoining. Whether or not some positive correlation exists between DNA polymerase activity and DNA-excision-repair capability, different tissues vary qualitatively and quantitatively in their inherent abilities to repair specific DNA lesions. These differences correlate strongly with proliferative activity. This loss in excision-repair capacity concomitant with a loss in proliferation during differentiation suggests that perhaps some of the apparent decline in DNA capability observed in some proliferating cellular systems as they approach senescence (e.g., WI-38) could be due directly to a loss in proliferative activity. If DNA-repair capability is critical to the aging process, then some variation in the aging rate might be expected to occur between different tissues, since not all tissues are equally repair-competent. Because differentiated tissues exhibit the lowest repair capability, tissues such as neuronal or muscular tissue should age fastest. In fact, *in vivo* aging does appear to be more conspicuous in certain tissues, particularly those involving differentiated postmitotic cells (Franks, 1974; Aune, 1976).

6. Acceleration of the Aging Process by Exposure to DNA-Damaging Agents

The acceleration of the aging process by ionizing radiation has long been held as fundamental to the relationship among DNA repair, mutational events, and aging (Yielding, 1974). If aging is the consequence of an accumulation of unrepaired DNA lesions, then exposure of animals to agents capable of damaging DNA should accelerate the aging process. Early evidence did suggest that radiation-induced life-shortening was mechanistically related to normal aging. Exposure of animals to ionizing radiation appeared to age their physical appearance prematurely, advance the incidence of age-related biochemical changes, and increase the mortality rate by accelerating the time of onset for many diseases (Alexander, 1957; Upton, 1957; Lindop and Rotblat, 1961*a,b;* Casarett, 1964).

Extensive reassessments of all phases of radiation-induced life-shortening have suggested, however, that this phenomenon is substantially different from the normal aging process (Alexander, 1967; Walburg, 1975). While high radiation doses accelerate the appearance of nonneoplastic diseases such as nephrosclerosis, anemia, and sterility (Upton *et al.,* 1960), no evidence has been found for such effects after single, acute exposures below 300 rads when corrections for competing probabilities of death are made (Walburg, 1975). Yet, these exposure levels cause significant life-shortening in the irradiated populations (Walburg, 1975). Exposure of animals to ionizing radiation appears to increase the incidence of cancer in most organs, resulting in premature death. When survivor data are analyzed with the deaths from neoplasia removed, however, there are no differences between the life expectancy of the treated animals and of the controls (Hoel and Walburg, 1972).

In addition, there does not appear to be any proportional advancement in time of many of the morphological and physiological manifestations of the normal aging process in animals (Berech and Curtis, 1964) or in man (Conard *et al.,* 1966; Hollingworth *et al.,* 1969). Classic senescent events such as alterations in collagen, pigment accumulation, and neuromuscular function appear to be refractory to irradiation (Walburg, 1975).

Similar to radiation experiments, the possible effects of chemical mutagenic agents on life-shortening and aging have been examined. Alexander and Connell (1960) observed that chlorambucil, a nitrogen mustard compound, and Myleran, an alkylating agent, shortened the life span of mice, but did not hasten the onset of any typical aging manifestations. Conklin *et al.* (1963) concluded that midlethal doses of nitrogen mustard shortened life span, and although it was not the result of increases in specific neoplasias, the process was still not equivalent to normal aging. Curtis (1963) and Stevenson and Curtis (1961) subjected mice to either a generalized or an acute stress with nitrogen mustard or typhoid toxoid. In both instances, the life expectancy of the mice was not significantly altered. Finally, Alexander (1967) exposed mice to ethylmethanesulfonate, a known mutagen, without any evidence for life-shortening. The conclusion appears to be that while some mutagenic compounds can cause life-shortening, there exists no evidence for accelerated aging.

Radiation does, however, appear to accelerate aging at the cellular level in *in vitro* systems. Lima *et al.* (1972) examined the long-term effects of cobalt-60 on the growth potential of chick embryo fibroblastic lines, cell lines that normally have a limited potential for divisions *in vitro* and that attain lower cellular densities at confluence as a function of age. The effect of radiation exposure was both irreversible and cumulative—shortening the *in vitro* life span while also decreasing saturation densities. Macieira-Coelho *et al.* (1976) observed that exposure to ionizing radiation shortens the *in vitro* life span while concurrently accelerating the acquisition of an infinite growth potential (transformation) in those cell lines capable of such a process. It would appear that exposure to ionizing radiation has accelerated at least two normal *in vitro* aging parameters, but the possible relationship between these *in vitro* observations and *in vivo* studies has not been explored.

It would appear that the life-shortening induced by ionizing radiation or mutagenic compounds differs both quantitatively and qualitatively from the normal aging process. The life-shortening observed after exposure of

animals to agents capable of inducing DNA damage is generally a consequence of increased frequencies of neoplasia. The conclusion that many of
the normal aging parameters are not present during this life-shortening
process suggests that the accumulation of mutational events is not fundamental to the aging process. It suggests as well, however, that certain of the
age-related components, such as the observed increase in neoplasia, might
be a consequence of the presence of unrepaired DNA lesions. Perhaps this
is an indication that different tissues in an organism not only age at different
rates but also age for different reasons.

7. Human Genetic Syndromes

If DNA-repair processes are in fact basic to the aging process, then it
could be expected that genetic syndromes with known defects in specific
types of DNA repair would also express some characteristics of accelerated
aging. These characteristics could be expressed *in vivo* as premature aging
and *in vitro* as an early loss in replicative ability in fibroblast cultures.
Three genetic syndromes are known to suffer a loss in DNA repair capability: ataxia–telangiectasia, Fanconi anemia, and xeroderma pigmentosum.
These syndromes and possible related evidence for accelerated aging will
be discussed in the following sections.

In addition, two genetic syndromes that appear to predispose the
patient toward premature aging will be examined for evidence of decreased
DNA-repair capability: progeria and the Werner syndrome.

7.1. Syndromes of DNA-Repair Deficiency

7.1.1. Ataxia–Telangiectasia

Ataxia–telangiectasia (AT) (or the Louis-Bar syndrome) is an autosomal recessive trait, the general clinical manifestations of which include a
progressive cerebellar ataxia (loss of muscular control), oculocutaneous
telangiectasia (chronic dilation of small blood vessels), recurrent sinopulmonary infections, a consistent defect in cellular immunity, thymic abnormalities, and increased disposition toward neoplasia, particularly of the
reticuloendothelial system (Tadjoedin and Fraser, 1965; Kersey *et al.,*
1973; Peterson *et al.,* 1966; Bochkov *et al.,* 1974). The clinical and genetic
aspects of this syndrome are discussed in detail in Chapter 7.

This syndrome exhibits a slight but significant increase in spontaneous
chromosome-aberration frequencies in both cultured lymphocytes and
fibroblast cultures (Hecht *et al.,* 1966; Gropp and Flatz, 1967; Schroeder
and Kurth, 1971; Bochkov *et al.,* 1974; Harnden, 1974; Oxford *et al.,* 1975;

Cohen *et al.*, 1975). Some investigators, however, observed no significant increase in spontaneous aberrations in cultured lymphocytes from AT patients (Pfeiffer, 1970; Schmid and Jerusalem, 1972), suggesting possible genetic heterogeneity. Other investigators reported increased chromosome-aberration frequencies in cultured lymphocytes, but not in direct bone marrow preparations (Hecht *et al.*, 1973) or skin fibroblasts (M. A. Bender, personal communication), from the same affected person.

AT lymphocytes have been reported to display increased aberration yields after exposure to ionizing radiation in the G_0 (or G_1) part of the cell cycle (Higurashi and Conen, 1973). This increase in chromosome-aberration frequencies after ionizing radiation has its counterpart in decreased cell-survival curves *in vitro* after γ-irradiation (Taylor *et al.*, 1975) or exposure to radiomimetic chemicals (Hoar and Sargent, 1976) as well as in increased radiosensitivity *in vivo* (Oxford *et al.*, 1975).

The basic repair defect does not appear to involve rejoining of X-ray-induced single-strand breaks (Taylor *et al.*, 1975; Vincent *et al.*, 1975; Paterson *et al.*, 1976) or UV-induced excision repair (Paterson *et al.*, 1976), but rather recognition and repair of γ-ray-induced base damage (Paterson *et al.*, 1976; Taylor *et al.*, 1976).

There exists no definitive evidence for the presence of accelerated aging in persons affected with ataxia–telangiectasia. Only one report provides some indication of premature aging *in vivo* in persons affected with this syndrome. Reye and Mosman (1960) observed in one patient an advanced loss of immediate memory that was interpreted to suggest premature senility. To this author's knowledge, no published evidence suggesting accelerated aging *in vitro* exists.

7.1.2. Fanconi Anemia

Extensive investigations into the genetics of Fanconi anemia (FA) have shown that this syndrome is inherited as an autosomal recessive trait with some suggestion of genetic heterogeneity (Schroeder, 1966; Remsen and Cerutti, 1976; Schroeder *et al.*, 1976). The syndrome manifests itself as a progressive, fatal panmyelopathy associated with multiple congenital anomalies, impaired body growth, and kidney malformations (Schroeder *et al.*, 1976).

As with AT, a characteristic feature of FA is an increased frequency of spontaneous chromosome aberrations (Schroeder *et al.*, 1964). These chromosome changes have been observed in cultured lymphocytes, in skin fibroblasts, and in direct bone-marrow preparations (Swift and Hirschhorn, 1966; Schmid, 1967; Sasaki and Tonomura, 1973). Chromosome aberrations appear to consist predominantly of chromatid and chromosome breaks, with a relatively small number of exchange-type abnormalities (German, 1972).

In an attempt to correlate this increase in spontaneous chromosome aberrations with a possible defect in DNA-repair processes, Schuler *et al.* (1969) demonstrated an increased susceptibility to aberration-induction after exposure of FA cells to the alkylating agent tetramethanesulfonil-*d*-manitol. This initial observation was confirmed and extended by Sasaki and Tonomura (1973), who found that FA cells were abnormally sensitive to DNA-cross-linking agents (e.g., mitomycin C or nitrogen mustard), but not to monofunctional reacting agents (e.g., methylmethanesulfonate). Recently, Latt *et al.* (1975) demonstrated a reduced ability in cultured lymphocytes from affected subjects to complete SCEs after exposure to mitomycin C, suggesting a deficiency in replication repair.

There have also been some published reports suggesting an increased sensitivity of both G_0 (or G_1) lymphocytes and fibroblasts from affected subjects to ionizing radiation (Higurashi and Conen, 1971, 1973). This observation, however, was not confirmed by Sasaki and Tonomura (1973). Recently, FA cultured lymphocytes were demonstrated to exhibit significantly increased aberration yields over control cells after G_2 irradiation (M. A. Bender, personal communication), and two of four FA fibroblast cell lines were found to be deficient in selectively excising γ-induced products of the 5,6-dihydroxydihydrothymine type (Remsen and Cerutti, 1976). Similarly, investigations into UV sensitivity have been equally conflicting. Sasaki and Tonomura (1973) observed no increased UV sensitivity in cultured lymphocytes, yet a fibroblast cell line derived from an affected person was characterized as being inefficient in excising UV-induced pyrimidine cyclobutane dimers (Poon *et al.,* 1975).

As with AT, there are to this author's knowledge no published reports of FA that suggest any evidence for accelerated aging *in vivo* or *in vitro*. While fibroblast cell lines from affected subjects were reported to have greater population-doubling times than control cells (Elmore and Swift, 1976), Vincent and Huang (1976) observed no curtailment of *in vitro* life span.

7.1.3. Xeroderma Pigmentosum

Xeroderma pigmentosum (XP) is actually a generic term for a family of human skin diseases inherited in an autosomal recessive fashion. They are all characterized by a marked disposition to skin carcinomas and melanomas after exposure to sunlight. Associated with the skin disorders are a spectrum of neurological abnormalities ranging from mild areflexia to severe microcephaly with progressive mental deterioration (the deSanctis–

Cacchione syndrome) (Cleaver, 1974; Robbins, J. H., *et al.*, 1974; Cleaver and Bootsma, 1975; Cleaver *et al.*, 1975).

Both fibroblasts and lymphocytes from affected persons were demonstrated to display little or no UV-induced UDS (Cleaver, 1969, 1970; Burk *et al.*, 1969). Subsequent investigations have determined the basic molecular defect to be in the recognition and excision of UV-induced pyrimidine cyclobutane dimers (Setlow *et al.*, 1969; Cleaver, 1969; Cleaver and Bootsma, 1975). Recently, Sutherland *et al.* (1975) also showed XP cell lines to be deficient in photoreactivating enzyme levels. XP cells also exhibit reduced UDS repair levels after exposure to various carcinogenic *N*-oxides (Stich *et al.*, 1973). These cells are competent, however, in rejoining single-strand breaks induced by ionizing radiation (Cleaver, 1969; Kleijer *et al.*, 1973). Further extensive studies utilizing cell hybridization techniques resulted in the detection of five complementation groups, accounting for the observed heterogeneous clinical manifestations (Kraemer *et al.*, 1975; Cleaver and Bootsma, 1975). A recent report (Cleaver and Bootsma, 1975) described a class of persons who exhibit some of the clinical manifestations of XP but whose cells show normal levels of UV-induced UDS. Lehmann *et al.* (1975) determined that a DNA-repair defect existed in the postreplication repair of UV-induced damage.

In contrast to the findings in FA or AT, spontaneous chromosome-aberration frequencies do not appear to be elevated in cells from persons with XP. Reed *et al.* (1969), Cleaver and Bootsma (1975), and Parrington *et al.* (1976) observed no increase in spontaneous-aberration frequencies in fibroblast cell lines or cultured lymphocytes from affected persons. Mikhelson (1976), however, reported elevated frequencies, and Huang *et al.* (1975) found significantly increased levels of spontaneous aberrations in XP fibroblast cell lines toward the end of their *in vitro* life span.

Cleaver and Bootsma (1975), in their review of XP, concluded that neither XP patients nor XP cells *in vitro* exhibit any of the expected signs of premature aging. *In vitro,* XP cell lines show no evidence for fewer total population doublings than age-matched control cells (Goldstein, 1971*b*; Vincent and Huang, 1976). *In vivo,* however, while affected patients do not possess all the characteristics normally associated with aging, they do exhibit some clinical manifestations.

All XP patients develop pigmentation abnormalities and signs of aged skin, including cutaneous malignancies (Robbins, J. H., *et al.*, 1974; Cleaver and Bootsma, 1975). This observation would be consistent with the interpretation that the changes in the appearance of the skin associated with the aging process are largely produced by exposure to UV radiation in sunlight (Kligman, 1969). Furthermore, patients affected with the more severe neurological variants exhibit progressive abnormalities of internal organs comparable to those observed in the aged (Robbins, J. H., *et al.*,

1974). These clinical manifestations appear to correlate well with the severity in loss of excision-repair capability (Andrews *et al.,* 1976; Takebe, 1976), suggesting a causal relationship between the two processes.

7.2. Syndromes of Accelerated Aging

7.2.1. Progeria

Progeria, or the Hutchinson–Gilford syndrome, is a relatively rare autosomally recessive condition that displays a number of clinical symptoms suggestive of accelerated aging. Mean life span is dramatically shortened, and death is generally a consequence of severe atherosclerosis with cardiac and cerebral involvement (DeBusk, 1972). While thinning of the skin, atherosclerosis, and the loss of subcutaneous fat (DeBusk, 1972) are representative of accelerated aging, other features are not. These features include delayed dentition, presbyopia, articular cartilage destruction (DeBusk, 1972), and a lack of elevated tissue lipofuscin levels (Spence and Herman, 1973). The clinical features of progeria are discussed in greater detail in Chapter 7.

In vitro, progeric skin fibroblast cultures have been reported to undergo significantly fewer population doublings than control cells (Singal and Goldstein, 1973; Goldstein and Moerman, 1976). Other investigators, however, have observed relatively normal *in vitro* life spans (Martin *et al.,* 1970; Danes, 1971). Goldstein and Moerman (1976) observed significant increases in altered enzyme levels in progeric fibroblast cells, levels in excess of those normally observed in senescent fibroblasts *in vitro* (Holliday and Tarrant, 1972). There does not appear to be, however, any corresponding increase in altered morphology (Danes, 1971) such as is normally observed in aging fibroblast cultures (Robbins, E., *et al.,* 1970; Lipetz and Cristofalo, 1972).

Although these observations suggest that there are quantitative and qualitative differences between normal aging and the presumed accelerated aging observed in progeria, several investigators have used progeric cell lines to assess possible aging parameters (Epstein, J., *et al.,* 1973*b;* Goldstein and Moerman, 1976). J. Epstein *et al.* (1973*b*) proposed that the basic defect in progeria could be the result of a deficient DNA-repair capability. These investigators observed a marked decrease in the ability of progeric fibroblast cells to repair X-ray-induced single-strand breaks. This initial finding, however, was not confirmed by Regan and Setlow (1974), examining the same cell strain. Subsequently, J. Epstein *et al.* (1974) examined six progeric cell lines for single-strand-break-rejoining, and found two lines to be nearly normal and two cell lines to be markedly deficient in repair capacity. Bender and Rary (1974) observed no increase in chromosome-aberration yields of X-irradiated cultured lymphocytes from the progeric patient examined by J. Epstein *et al.* (1973b). Most recently, Bradley *et al.* (1976) observed no defective rejoining of single-strand breaks, assayed through alkaline-elution and alkaline-sedimentation techniques, in a progeric fibroblast cell line.

The evidence suggests that progeria suffers, not from an intrinsic defect in DNA repair, but rather from a loss in capability as a consequence of abnormal metabolism or some type of genetic repression or both. This interpretation would be consistent with the finding that simian-virus-40 transformation of progeric cells restores normal ability in rejoining of single-strand breaks (Little *et al.*, 1975).

7.2.2. The Werner Syndrome

This syndrome, which is inherited as an autosomal recessive trait, has its onset in persons between the ages of 15 and 20 (Epstein, C. J., *et al.*, 1966; Zucker-Franklin *et al.*, 1968). Some of the clinical features of this syndrome that resemble premature or accelerated aging include marked lymphoid depletion, glucose intolerance, cataracts, graying of the hair, increased incidence of neoplasms, and arteriosclerosis (Epstein, C. J., *et al.*, 1966; Zucker-Franklin *et al.*, 1968). As in progeria, however, there are clinical features that are qualitatively and quantitatively different from those observed in the elderly. Finally, affected persons also suffer a delayed sexual maturity (Epstein, C. J., *et al.*, 1966). The clinical manifestations of the Werner syndrome are described in Chapter 7.

In vitro, fibroblast-cell cultures routinely exhibit poor growth, decreased life span, and accelerated morphological alterations similar to those observed in senescent-normal-fibroblast cultures (Stecker and Gardner, 1970; Epstein, C. J., *et al.*, 1966; Martin *et al.*, 1970; Danes, 1971). Increased levels of altered enzymes have also been reported for these fibroblast cell lines, consistent with the notion of premature aging (Holliday *et al.*, 1974; Goldstein and Singal, 1974; Goldstein and Moerman, 1976).

There exists no published evidence of a possible defect in DNA-repair capability associated with this syndrome. While this lack cannot be considered proof that no such defect exists, it is suggestive.

7.3. Conclusions

Some tentative conclusions can be drawn from the nature of these inherited human syndromes. First, in those syndromes that appear to lack some aspect of normal DNA-repair capability, only XP exhibits any evidence of premature or accelerated aging. This accelerated aging is not of a general nature, however, but appears to be specifically limited to two tissues—skin and neural. Despite their increased frequencies of spontaneous chromosome aberrations, neither AT nor FA provides good evidence for any features resembling premature aging. These observations suggest either a lack of correlation between the two processes or possible differences in importance of specific DNA-repair systems to aging.

Secondly, while neither progeria nor the Werner syndrome can be equated in a simple fashion to premature aging *in vivo,* they do have some aspects in common with normal aging. Consequently, the lack of any definitive evidence demonstrating the presence of DNA-repair deficiencies suggests that the two processes might be intrinsically unrelated.

8. Longevity and DNA-Repair Processes

It was previously noted that different species exhibited differences in their ability to excise UV-induced thymidine dimers. Human- and bovine-derived cells were extremely competent in excision repair (Cleaver *et al.,* 1972; Regan *et al.,* 1971) in comparison with rodent-derived cells (Painter and Cleaver, 1969; Rauth, 1970). These differences led Hart and Setlow (1974) to investigate a possible correlation between extent of excision repair in an adult-derived tissue and mean life span. It was expected that differences in longevity may be a manifestation of more efficient repair processes in those species with greater life spans. Since the magnitude of excision repair depends on the state of the particular cell examined (see Section 5), these investigators examined only primary fibroblast cell lines at early *in vitro* passages. Analysis of UV-induced UDS levels in a number of different animal species resulted in a strong correlation between species' life spans and levels of excision repair (Hart and Setlow, 1974).

When, however, this correlation was further tested within primates, a closely related group of species in which total life span varies by more than 20-fold (Cutler, 1976*c*), no differences in UV-induced UDS levels were observed (H. Kato, personal communication). Consequently, the apparently strong correlation between longevity and excision repair might be nothing more than an experimental artifact. Alternatively, the data might suggest that while differences in mean life span do tend to reflect intrinsic levels of excision repair, other processes can modify the aging rate.

These studies have exclusively investigated excision-repair capability. An accurate assessment of repair capability, however, requires the examination of all DNA-repair systems present. Although rodent-derived cell lines are considered to be excision-repair-deficient, they are obviously not DNA-repair-incompetent, since they do not appear to suffer from a lack of this repair process. Also, it is difficult to firmly assess the correlation between excision repair and life span from investigations restricted to one tissue, skin fibroblasts. The possibility exists that other tissues will not express the same strong correlation between DNA repair and mean life span.

9. Summary and Conclusion

The existence of a causal relationship between DNA-repair capability and aging is based on the assumption that aging is in fact a direct consequence of the detrimental accumulation of unrepaired DNA lesions at the cellular level. Presumably, when the frequency of these lesions reaches a certain level or specific genes become inactive, or both, loss in cellular function ensues. As the proportion of such cells increases in various tissues, the organism "ages." If this assumption is valid, then the more effective a cell is in preventing or repairing DNA damage, or in doing both, the slower the aging process should be.

It is possible to envision two separate, but not mutually exclusive, mechanisms by which unrepaired DNA lesions could accumulate with time. First, a certain proportion of DNA lesions might escape detection or repair, at any one time. Assuming that both repair capabilities and environmental conditions do not vary significantly with time, unrepaired DNA lesions should then tend to accumulate in a cell at a rather constant rate. The second mechanism also assumes no significant alteration in the number of potential lesions induced, but rather that the proportion of successful repair events diminishes with time as a consequence of declining DNA-repair capability. In this event, unrepaired DNA lesions should increase at substantially faster rates as the level of repair capability becomes more inefficient with advancing age. Both mechanisms would give rise to levels of DNA lesions capable of incapacitating a particular cell. The former mechanism suggests, however, that life span is related to the intrinsic capacity of the cells in an organism to repair DNA damage and that different organisms with different repair capabilities will have different life spans. The latter mechanism, while it does not negate the former, suggests that life spans could be longer except for the decline in DNA-repair capability.

Primarily, investigations concerned with determining frequencies of unrepaired DNA lesions have compared only tissues derived from animals at the two extremes of the aging process. A further difficulty arises from the rather limited types of tissues examined. Some conclusions can be drawn, however, concerning both the occurrence and the rate of accumulation of unrepaired DNA lesions in different tissues.

First, not all tissues have been found to exhibit an age-related increase in DNA lesions. DNA strand breakage or alkaline-labile regions do not appear to increase with age in mouse spleen, thymus, or cerebellum (Ono *et al.*, 1976). Spontaneous chromosome aberrations exhibit no consistent increase in frequency in proliferating bone marrow cells with age in rats or mice (Curtis and Tilley, 1971), or in lymphocytes cultured from human donors of different ages (e.g., Sandberg *et al.*, 1967; Goodman *et al.*, 1969; Bochkov *et al.*, 1968). *In vitro* studies have proved equally negative with respect to both an increase in DNA cross-linking (Bradley *et al.*, 1976) and significant increases of spontaneous chromosome aberrations (Thompson, K. V. A., and Holliday, 1975) as a function of passage level.

Second, where unrepaired DNA lesions do exhibit increased frequencies in an aging cellular system (e.g., liver), they tend to accumulate throughout the animal's life span, not dramatically near the end of it. The increases in strand breakage observed in mouse liver cells are more significant in the early portions of the animal's life span than in the later ones (Massie *et al.*, 1972; Ono *et al.*, 1976). The increase in both DNA cross-linking and spontaneous chromosome aberrations in liver cells appears to be roughly linear with age and inversely proportional to the organism's life span (Cutler, 1976*b*; Stevenson and Curtis, 1961; Curtis *et al.*, 1966; Curtis and Miller, 1971).

These observations suggest a lack of a decline of DNA-repair capability with age, and, broadly speaking, investigations concerned with directly assessing DNA repair efficiency are in accord. *In vivo,* no significant increase in X-ray-induced chromosome aberration yields was observed in lymphocytes cultured from subjects ranging from young to aged (Liniecki *et al.*, 1971). Similarly, neurons from aged and young beagles proved equally capable of rejoining γ-ray-induced single-strand breaks (Wheeler and Lett, 1974), and skin fibroblasts from aged donors exhibited no increased sensitivity to UV light as measured by cell-killing (Goldstein, 1971*b*). Reports have appeared however, of a decline in UV-induced UDS (Lambert *et al.*, 1976) and an increase in chemically induced chromosome aberrations (Bochkov and Kuleshov, 1971, 1972) in lymphocytes from aged donors. *In vitro* investigations concerned with the efficiency of DNA-strand-break-rejoining have resulted in conflicting conclusions. Some investigations have observed no decline in this type of repair ability until *in vitro* senescence had already begun (Clarkson and Painter, 1974; Bradley *et al.*, 1976), while others have reported the presence of a decline prior to senescence (Epstein, J., *et al.*, 1973*a*, 1974; Little *et al.*, 1975; Williams and Little, 1975). Excision repair, however, appears to decline only after the onset of *in vitro* senescence, and appears to correlate with a loss in replicative ability (Hart and Setlow, 1976; Williams and Little, 1975; Bowman *et al.*, 1976).

The accumulated data, while not as extensive or as consistent as one would like, do not firmly support any age-related decline in DNA-repair capability. A large variety of cellular systems exhibit either no increase in unrepaired DNA lesions or no loss in DNA-repair capability with age.

The only cellular system to consistently exhibit an increase in DNA lesions with age is liver tissue *in vivo*. DNA strand-breakage, DNA cross-linking, and spontaneous chromosome aberrations all increase in frequency in liver tissue beginning early in the animal's life span. The importance of the conclusion that the increase of DNA lesions in liver cells is inversely proportional to the animal's life span must be examined, however, in terms of a general aging process. It is extremely difficult to demonstrate an age-related loss in liver function (Thompson, E. N., and Williams, 1965; Thung and Hollander, 1967), and liver failure is generally not a cause of death in aging animal populations (Kohn, 1966). The conclusion that life span does not depend on either the number or the percentage of altered liver cells suggests that the general accumulation of DNA lesions might rather be a consequence of liver-specific metabolic processes. It is interesting to note that a strong correlation has been found to exist between life span and the ability of cultured fibroblasts to metabolize 7,12-dimethyl-benz(a)anthracene to its mutagenic metabolites (Schwartz, 1975). Consequently, the rate of accumulation of DNA lesions in liver cells might reflect merely enzyme levels, not life-span-specific repair capabilities.

The lack of correlation between aging of the liver and age-related mortality suggests that other tissues might be of greater importance to the aging process. Aging does not appear to be a consequence of a decline in tissues that normally proliferate (e.g., bone marrow) or in tissues that retain the capacity to proliferate in response to a specific stress situation (e.g., liver) (Kohn, 1975; Franks, 1974; Cutler; 1976*b*). Aging appears to be more conspicuous in terminally differentiated postmitotic tissues such as neural or muscle tissue (Aune, 1976). In fact, a significant proportion of natural deaths can be attributed to degenerative age-associated alterations in the CNS (Burnett, 1974). Aging of these tissues does not appear to be the result of an actual loss in cell number (Kohn, 1975; Cameron and Thrasher, 1976), but rather of a continuous decline in functional capacity (Aune, 1976).

A possible significant correlation with differences in tissue-specific aging rates in an organism would be corresponding tissue differences in DNA-repair capability. The ability of any tissue to monitor and repair DNA damage depends not only on the extent, nature, and location of the induced lesion(s) (Hart and Trosko, 1976; Trosko and Hart, 1976), but also on the proliferative state of the cellular population (i.e., replicating, quiescent, or postmitotic) under examination. Postmitotic cells not only lack postreplication repair, but also exhibit a significant decrease in excision-repair capability in comparison with proliferating cells from the same organism. This difference in DNA-repair levels suggests that since postmitotic tissues should accumulate more lesions with time than proliferating tissues, they should also age at a faster rate. That they do is in fact supported by aging studies *in vivo,* suggesting that a positive correlation does exist between DNA-repair capability and life span.

   If this correlation is to be considered a strong one, then agents that induce extensive DNA damage should accelerate the aging process. Early investigators did in fact conclude that exposure to ionizing radiation accelerated the appearance of normal aging parameters. More recent extensive reassessments of the accumulated data, however, have suggested both quantitative and qualitative differences from the normal aging process (Walburg, 1975). It is apparent that exposure to ionizing radiation primarily increases the incidence of neoplasia, resulting in premature death and shortened life spans. Investigations based on exposure to chemical mutagens have been equally negative in observing an acceleration of normal aging (Alexander and Connell, 1960; Curtis, 1963; Stevenson and Curtis, 1961). These findings suggest that DNA damage is not fundamental to the aging process. It is possible, however, that aging is normally a consequence of changes in a relatively few critical tissues, and extensive exposures to DNA-damaging agents mask these important alterations.

   Of equal importance to a correlation between life span and DNA-repair capability is the expression of accelerated aging in genetic syndromes with demonstrable decreases in DNA-repair capability. Unfortunately, the findings so far have been largely inconclusive. Neither AT nor FA, both of which are syndromes of DNA-repair deficiency, expresses any significant signs of premature aging. Only XP exhibits a possible correlation between the level of repair deficiency and increased signs of accelerated aging. The more severe the loss in excision-repair capability, the greater the indications of premature aging of the skin and neural tissues (Robbins, J. H., *et al.,* 1974).

   Similarly, syndromes considered to express accelerated-aging components (e.g., progeria and the Werner syndrome) have not been demonstrated to involve DNA-repair deficiencies. Progeria was suggested to involve a defect in DNA-strand-break-rejoining capability (Epstein, J., *et al.,* 1973*b*), but subsequent investigation demonstrated that normal repair levels existed in some progeric patients (Epstein, J., *et al.,* 1974; Regan and Setlow, 1974; Bradley *et al.,* 1976). Possibly the repair loss in some progeric cell lines was a result of gene repression or altered metabolism or both, but not due to an intrinsic defect in DNA repair (Little, 1976).

   This lack of a consistent correlation between DNA-repair deficiency and premature aging suggests that the two processes are not necessarily related. One of the difficulties in making this conclusion, however, is that it assumes that all DNA-repair processes are equally important. That they are is obviously not true, since persons affected with the variant form of XP that involves a deficiency in postreplication repair exhibit milder clinical manifestations than do those with the excision-repair-deficient form (Cleaver and Bootsma, 1975). This finding might be expected, since postmitotic cells have no need for that particular repair process.

The strongest experimental finding in support of a direct correlation between life span and DNA-repair capability is the observation of Hart and Setlow (1974) that fibroblast cell lines derived from longer-lived animals show greater levels of UV-induced UDS. This correlation, however, has not been confirmed within the primates (H. Kato, personal communication). Furthermore, since aging does not appear to be a consequence of a decline in cellular systems capable of proliferation, the validity of this correlation must be questioned. It has been proposed that life span is controlled by small groups of essential postmitotic cells in critical organs and tissues such as in the brain or neuroendocrine system (Franks, 1974). If it is, then a comparison among different species of DNA-repair capability in these cells is of primary importance.

Aging does not appear to be a direct consequence of a decline in DNA-repair capability. The possibility remains that differences in life span among the various animal species are a direct result of different levels of DNA-repair capability. Current experimental support of this hypothesis, however, remains inconclusive. Also, it has yet to be proved that unrepaired DNA lesions accumulate with age in some of the tissues more critical to aging. While it is expected that DNA damage certainly contributes to the aging process, it is difficult to conclude that all of aging is a consequence of the accumulation of DNA lesions. Other factors may play an equally critical role, such as the degree of genetic redundancy for vital functions within the genome (Hart and Trosko, 1976).

This review should by no means discourage research directed at the possible relationship between DNA repair and aging; the current state of understanding concerning both these processes is still in its infancy. Rather, it should indicate the areas of interest in which research should be encouraged due to either presently conflicting results or a lack of information or both. Extensive investigations into the relationships between DNA repair and aging can only advance our understanding of the underlying molecular processes inherent in both systems.

ACKNOWLEDGMENTS

The author is supported by Grant CA 09121, awarded by the National Cancer Institute, Department of Health, Education and Welfare, and in part by the U.S. Energy Research and Development Administration.

The assistance of Ms. L. Tice and C. Hull in completing this manuscript is sincerely appreciated.

References

Acharya, P. V. N., 1972, The isolation and partial characterization of age-correlated oligo-deoxyribo-ribo-nucleotide with covalently linked aspartyl-glutamyl-polypeptides, *John Hopkins Med. J. Suppl.* **1**:254.

Alexander, P., 1957, Accelerated ageing—A long term effect of exposure to ionizing radiations, *Gerontologia* **1**:174.

Alexander, P., 1967, The role of DNA lesions in the processes leading to ageing in mice, *Symp. Soc. Exp. Biol.* **21**:29.

Alexander, P., and Connell, D. I., 1960, Shortening of the life span of mice by irradiation with x-rays and treatment with radiomimetic chemicals, *Radiat. Res.* **12**:36.

Amici, D., Gianfranceschi, G. L., Marsili, G., and Michetti, L., 1974, Young and old rats: ATP, alkaline phosphatase, cholesterol and protein levels in the blood; DNA and RNA contents of the liver—Regulation by an aqueous thymus extract, *Experientia* **30**:633.

Andrews, A. D., Barrett, S. F., and Robbins, J. H., 1976, The relationship between pathologic ageing of the nervous system and the DNA repair defects of xeroderma pigmentosum, Abstract, The Second International Workshop on DNA Repair Mechanisms in Mammalian Cells, Noordwijkerhout, The Netherlands.

Aune, J., 1976, Ultrastructure changes with age, *Interdiscip. Top. Gerontol.* **10**:44.

Ayme, S., Mattei, J. F., Mattei, M. G., Aurran, Y., and Giraud, F., 1976, Nonrandom distribution of chromosome breaks in cultured lymphocytes of normal subjects, *Hum. Genet.* **31**:161.

Bacchetti, S., 1975, Studies on DNA repair in mammalian cells; An endonuclease which recognizes lesions in DNA, in: *Molecular Mechanisms for Repair of DNA* (P. Hanawalt and R. Setlow, eds.), pp. 651–654, Plenum Press, New York.

Bender, M. A., and Rary, J. M., 1974, Spontaneous and x-ray induced chromosomal aberrations in progeria, *Radiat. Res.* **59**:181a.

Bender, M. A., Griggs, H. G., and Walker, P. L., 1973*a*, Mechanism of chromosomal aberration production. I. Aberration induction by ultraviolet light, *Mutat. Res.* **20**:387.

Bender, M. A., Bedford, J. S., and Mitchell, J. B., 1973*b*, Mechanism of chromosomal aberration production. II. Aberrations induced by 5-bromodeoxyuridine and visible light, *Mutat. Res.* **20**:403.

Bender, M. A., Griggs, H. G., and Bedford, J. S., 1974, Mechanism of chromosomal aberration production. III. Chemicals and ionizing radiation, *Mutat. Res.* **23**:197.

Ben-Ishai, R., and Peleg, L., 1975, Excision-repair in primary cultures of mouse embryo cells and its decline in progressive passages and established cell lines, in: *Molecular Mechanisms for Repair of DNA* (P. Hanawalt and R. Setlow, eds.), pp. 607–610, Plenum Press, New York.

Benn, P. A., 1976, Specific chromosome aberrations in senescent fibroblast cell lines derived from human embryos, *Am. J. Hum. Genet.* **28**:465.

Berech, J., and Curtis, H. J., 1964, The role of age and x-irradiation on kidney function in the mouse, *Radiat. Res.* **22**:95.

Bochkov, N. P., 1972, Spontaneous chromosome aberrations in human somatic cells, *Humangenetik* **16**:159.

Bochkov, N. P., and Kuleshov, N. P., 1971, Dependence of the intensity of the chemical mutagenesis in human cells on sex and age of individuals, *Genetics (USSR)* **7**:132.

Bochkov, N. P., and Kuleshov, N. P., 1972, Age sensitivity of human chromosomes to alkylating agents, *Mutat. Res.* **14**:345.

Bochkov, N. P., Kozlov, V. M., Pilosov, P. A., and Sevankaev, A. V., 1968, Spontaneous level of chromosome aberrations in cultures of human leukocytes, *Genetics (USSR)* **4**:93.

Bochkov, N. P., Lopukhin, Y. M., Kuleshov, N. P., and Kovalchuk, L. V., 1974, Cytogenetic studies of patients with ataxia telangiectasia, *Humangenetik* **24**:115.

Bowman, P. D., Meek, R. L., and Daniel, C. W., 1976, Decreased unscheduled DNA synthesis in nondividing aged WI-48 cells, *Mech. Ageing Dev.* **5**:251.

Bradley, M. O., Erickson, L. C., and Kohn, K. W., 1976, Normal DNA strand rejoining and absence of DNA crosslinking in progeroid and aging human cells, *Mutat. Res.* **37**:279.

Brooks, A. L., Mead, D. K., and Peters, R. F., 1973, Effect of ageing on the frequency of metaphase chromosome aberrations in the liver of the Chinese hamster, *J. Gerontol.* **28**:452.

Buhl, S. N., Stillman, R. M., Setlow, R. B., and Regan, J. D., 1972, DNA chain elongation in normal human and xeroderma pigmentosum cells after ultraviolet irradiation, *Biophys. J.* **12**:1183.

Burk, P. G., Lutzner, M. A., and Robbins, J. H., 1969, Decreased incorporation of thymidine into the DNA of lymphocytes from patients with xeroderma pigmentosum after UV-irradiation *in vitro, Clin. Res.* **17**:614.

Burnett, F. M., 1974, *Intrinsic Mutagenesis: A Genetic Approach to Aging,* John Wiley & Sons, New York.

Cameron, I. L., and Thrasher, J. D., 1976, Cell renewal and cell loss in the tissues of aging mammals, *Interdiscip. Top. Gerontol.* **10**:108.

Carrier, W. L., and Setlow, R. B., 1971, The excision of pyrimidine dimers (the detection of dimers in small amounts), *Methods Enzymol.* **21**:230.

Casarett, G. W., 1964, Similarities and contrasts between radiation and time pathology, *Adv. Gerontol. Res.* **1**:109.

Chan, A. C., Ng, S. K. C., and Walker, I. G., 1976, Reduced DNA repair during differentiation of a myogenic cell line, *J. Cell Biol.* **70**:685.

Chetsanga, C. J., Boyd, Y., Peterson, L., and Ruchlow, K., 1975, Single-stranded regions in the DNA of old mice, *Nature (London)* **253**:130.

Chlebovsky, O., Praslicka, M., and Horak, J., 1966, Chromosome aberrations: Increased incidence in bone marrow of continuously irradiated rats, *Science* **153**:195.

Clarkson, J. M., and Painter, R. B., 1974, Repair of x-ray damage in aging WI-38 cells, *Mutat. Res.* **23**:107.

Cleaver, J., 1969, Xeroderma pigmentosum: A human disease in which an initial stage of DNA repair is defective, *Proc. Natl. Acad. Sci. U.S.A.* **63**:428.

Cleaver, J., 1970, DNA repair and radiation sensitivity in human (xeroderma pigmentosum) cells, *Int. J. Radiat. Biol.* **18**:557.

Cleaver, J., 1974, DNA strand breaks during excision repair in human fibroblasts: Demonstration of repair defect in xeroderma pigmentosum, *Radiat. Res.* **57**:207.

Cleaver, J., and Bootsma, D., 1975, Xeroderma pigmentosum: Biochemical and genetic characteristics, *Annu. Rev. Genet.* **9**:19.

Cleaver, J., and Painter, R. B., 1968, Evidence for repair replication of HeLa cell DNA damaged by ultraviolet light, *Biochim. Biophys. Acta* **161**:552.

Cleaver, J., Thomas, G., Trosko, J., and Lett, J., 1972, Excision repair (dimer excision, strand breakage and repair replication) in primary cultures of eukaryote (bovine) cells, *Exp. Cell Res.* **74**:67.

Cleaver, J., Bootsma, D., and Friedberg, E., 1975, Human diseases with genetically altered DNA repair processes, *Genetics* **79**:215.

Cohen, M. M., Shaham, M., Dagan, J., Shmuell, E., and Kohn, G., 1975, Cytogenetic investigations in families with ataxia telangiectasia, *Cytogenet. Cell Genet.* **15**:338.

Conard, R. A., Lowrey, A., Eicher, M., Thompson, K., and Scoot, W. A., 1966, Aging studies in a Marshallese population exposed to radioactive fallout in 1954, in: *Radiation and Ageing* (P. J. Lindop and G. A. Sacher, eds.), pp. 345–360, Taylor and Frances, London.

Conklin, J. W., Upton, A. C., Christenberry, K. W., and McDonald, T. P., 1963, Comparative late somatic effects of some radiomimetic agents and x-rays, *Radiat. Res.* **19**:156.

Court Brown, W. M., Buckton, K. E., Jacobs, P. A., Tough, I. M., Kuenssberg, E. V., and Knox, J. D. E., 1966, Chromsome studies on adults, *Eugen. Lab. Mem.* **42**:1.

Crowley, C., and Curtis, H. J., 1963, The development of somatic mutation in mice with age, *Proc. Natl. Acad. Sci. U.S.A.* **49**:626.

Curtis, H. J., 1963, Biological mechanisms underlying the aging process, *Science* **141**:686.

Curtis, H. J., and Miller, K., 1971, Chromosome aberrations in liver cells of guinea pigs, *J. Gerontol.* **26**:292.

Curtis, H. J., and Tilley, J., 1971, The lifespan of dividing mammalian cells *in vivo, J. Gerontol.* **126**:1.

Curtis, H. J., Leith, J., and Tilley, J., 1966, Chromosome aberrations in liver cells of dogs of different ages, *J. Gerontol.* **21**:268.

Cutler, R. G., 1976*a,* Nature of aging and life maintenance processes, *Interdiscip. Top. Gerontol.* **9**:83.

Cutler, R. G., 1976*b,* Alteration of chromatin as a function of age in *Mus* and *Peromyscus* rodent species, Abstract, 29th Annual Meeting Gerontological Society, New York.

Cutler, R. G., 1976*c,* Evolution of longevity in primates, *J. Hum. Evol.* **2**:169.

D'Ambrosio, S. M., and Setlow, R. B., 1976, Enhancement of postreplication repair in Chinese hamster cells, *Proc. Natl. Acad. Sci. U.S.A.* **73**:2396.

Danes, S. B., 1971, Progeria: A cell culture study on aging, *J. Clin. Invest.* **50**:2000.

Darzynkiewicz, Z., 1971, Radiation induced DNA synthesis in normal and stimulated human lymphocytes, *Exp. Cell. Res.* **69**:356.

DeBusk, F. L., 1972, The Hutchinson–Gilford progeria syndrome, *J. Pediatr.* **80**:697.

Dugle, D. L., and Gillespie, C. J., 1975, Kinetics of the single-strand repair mechanism in mammalian cells, in: *Molecular Mechanisms for Repair of DNA* (P. C. Hanawalt and R. B. Setlow, eds.), pp. 685–688, Plenum Press, New York.

Elmore, E., and Swift, M., 1976, Growth of cultured cells from patients with ataxia–telangiectasia, *J. Cell. Physiol.* **89**:429.

Epstein, C. J., Martin, G. M., Schultz, A. L., and Motulsky, A., 1966, Werner's syndrome: A review of its symptomatology, natural history, pathologic features, genetics and relationship to the natural aging process, *Medicine (Baltimore)* **45**:177.

Epstein, J., Williams, J. R., and Little, J. B., 1973*a,* Deficient DNA repair in progeria and senescent human cells, *Radiat. Res.* **55**:527.

Epstein, J., Williams, J. R., and Little, J. B. 1973*b,* Deficient DNA repair in human progeroid cells, *Proc. Natl. Acad. Sci. U.S.A.* **70**:977.

Epstein, J., Williams, J. R., and Little, J. B., 1974, Rate of DNA repair in progeric and normal human fibroblasts, *Biochem. Biophys. Res. Commun.* **59**:850.

Evans, R. G., and Norman, A., 1968, Unscheduled incorporation of thymidine in ultraviolet irradiated human lymphocytes, *Radiat. Res.* **36**:287.

Franks, L., 1974, Ageing in differentiated cells, *Gerontologia* **20**:51.

German, J., 1972, Genes which increase chromosomal instability in somatic cells and predispose to cancer, *Prog. Med. Genet.* **8**:61.

Goldstein, S., 1971*a,* The biology of aging, *N. Engl. J. Med.* **285**:1120.

Goldstein, S., 1971*b,* The role of DNA repair in aging of cultured fibroblasts from xeroderma pigmentosum and normals, *Proc. Soc. Exp. Biol. Med.* **137**:730.

Goldstein, S., and Moerman, E. J., 1976, Defective proteins in normal and abnormal human fibroblasts during aging *in vitro, Interdiscip. Top. Gerontol.* **10**:24.

Goldstein, S., and Singal, D. P., 1974, Alteration of fibroblast agene products *in vitro* from a subject with Werner's syndrome, *Nature (London)* **251**:719.

Goodman, R. M., Fechheimer, N. S., Miller, F., Miller, R., and Zartman, D., 1969, Chromosome alterations in three age groups of human females, *Am. J. Med. Sci.* **258**:26.

Gropp, A., and Flatz, G., 1967, Chromosome breakage and blastic transformation of lymphocytes in ataxia–telangiectasia, *Humangenetik* **5:**77.

Hahn, G. M., King, D., and Yang, S. J., 1971, Quantitiative changes in unscheduled DNA synthesis in rat muscle cells after differentiation, *Nature (London)* **230:**242.

Hanawalt, P. C., and Setlow, R. B., 1975 (eds.), *Molecular Mechanisms for Repair of DNA,* Plenum Press, New York.

Harnden, D. G., 1974, Ataxia telangiectasia syndrome: Cytogenetic and cancer aspects, in: *Chromosomes and Cancer* (J. German, ed.), pp. 619–636, John Wiley & Sons, New York.

Hart, R. W., and Setlow, R. B. 1974, Correlation between deoxyribonucleic acid excision-repair and lifespan in a number of mammalian species, *Proc. Natl. Acad. Sci. U.S.A.* **71:**2169.

Hart, R. W., and Setlow, R. B., 1976, DNA repair in late-passage human cells, *Mech. Ageing Dev.* **5:**67.

Hart, R. W., and Trosko, J. E., 1976, DNA repair processes in mammals, *Interdiscip. Top. Gerontol.* **9:**134.

Hayflick, L., 1975, Current theories of biological aging, *Fed. Proc. Fed. Am. Soc. Exp. Biol.* **34:**9.

Hecht, F., Koler, R. D., Rigas, D. A., Dahnke, G. S., Case, M. P., Tisdale, V., and Miller, R. W., 1966, Leukemia and lymphocytes in ataxia–telangiectasia, *Lancet* **2:**1193.

Hecht, F., McCaw, B. K., and Koler, R. D., 1973, Ataxia telangiectasia—Clonal growth of translocation lymphoctyes, *N. Engl. J. Med.* **289:**286.

Higurashi, M., and Conen, P. E., 1971, Comparison of chromosomal behavior in cultured lymphocytes and fibroblasts from patients with chromosomal disorders and controls, *Cytogenetics* **10:**273.

Higurashi, M., and Conen, P. E., 1973, *In vitro* radiosensitivity in "chromosomal breakage syndrome," *Cancer* **32:**380.

Hoar, D. I., and Sargent, P., 1976, Chemical mutagen hypersensitivity in ataxia telangiectasia, *Nature (London)* **261:**590.

Hoel, D. G., and Walburg, H. E., 1972, Statistical analysis of survival experiments, *J. Natl. Cancer Inst.* **49:**361.

Holliday, R., and Tarrant, G. M., 1972, Altered enzymes in ageing human fibroblasts, *Nature (London)* **238:**26.

Holliday, R., Porterfield, J. S., and Gibbs, D. O., 1974, Werner's syndrome: Premature aging *in vivo* and *in vitro, Nature (London)* **248:**762.

Hollingworth, D. R., Hollingworth, J. W., Bogitch, S., and Keehn, R. J., 1969, Neuromuscular tests of aging Hiroshima subjects, *J. Gerontol.* **24:**276.

Huang, C. C., Banerjee, A., and Hou, Y., 1975, Chromosomal instability in cell lines derived from patients with xeroderma pigmentosum, *Proc. Soc. Exp. Biol. Med.* **148:** 1244.

Jacobs, P. A., and Court Brown, W. M., 1966, Age and chromosomes, *Nature (London)* **212:**823.

Jarvik, L. F., and Kato, T., 1970, Chromosome examinations in aged twins, *Am. J. Hum. Genet.* **22:**562.

Karran, P., and Ormerod, M. G., 1973, Is the ability to repair damage to DNA related to the proliferative capacity of a cell? The rejoining of x-ray produced strand breaks, *Biochim. Biophys. Acta.* **299:**54.

Kato, H., 1977, Spontaneous and induced sister chromatid exchanges as revealed by a BUDR-labeling method, *Int. Rev. Cytol.* **49:**55.

Kersey, J. H., Spector, B. D., and Gord, R. A., 1973, Primary immunodeficiency diseases and cancer: The immunodeficiency registry, *Int. J. Cancer* **12:**333.

Kihlman, B. A., 1966, *Actions of Chemicals on Dividing Cells,* Prentice Hall, Englewood Cliffs, New Jersey.

Kleijer, W. J., DeWeerd-Kastelein, E. A., Sluyter, M. L., Keijer, W., DeWit, J., and Bootsma, D., 1973, UV-induced DNA repair synthesis in cells of patients with different forms of xeroderma pigmentosum and of heterozygotes, *Mutat. Res.* **20**:417.

Kligman, A. M., 1969, Early destructive effects of sunlight on human skin, *J. Am. Med. Assoc.* **210**:2377.

Kohn, R. R., 1966, A possible final common pathway for natural ageing and radiation-induced life-shortening, in: *Radiation and Ageing* (P. J. Lindop and G. A. Sacher, eds.), pp. 373–392, Taylor and Frances, London.

Kohn, R. R., 1975, Intrinsic aging of postmitotic cells, in: *International Symposium on* Aging Gametes, Seattle, 1973, pp. 1–18, S. Karger, Basel.

Kraemer, K. H., DeWeerd-Kastelein, E. A., Robbins, J. H., Keijzer, W., Barrett, S. F., Petinga, R. A., and Bootsma, D., 1975, Five complementation groups in xeroderma pigmentosum, *Mutat. Res.* **33**:327.

Lambert, B., Ringborg, U., and Swanbeck, G., 1976, Repair of UV-induced DNA lesions in peripheral lymphocytes from healthy subjects of various ages, individuals with Down's syndrome and patients with actinic keratosis, Abstract, The Second International Workshop on DNA Repair Mechanisms in Mammalian Cells, Noordwijkerhout, The Netherlands.

Lampidis, T. J., and Little, J. B., 1976, Unscheduled DNA synthesis in fibroblasts and pulsating myocardial cells isolated from newborn rat heart, *Radiat. Res.* **67**:621.

Lampidis, T. J., and Schaiberger, G. E., 1975, Age-related loss of DNA repair synthesis in isolated rat myocardial cells, *Exp. Cell Res.* **96**:412.

Latt, S. A., 1973, Microfluorometric detection of deoxyribonucleic acid replication in human metaphase chromosomes, *Proc. Natl. Acad. Sci. U.S.A.* **70**:3395.

Latt, S. A., Stetten, G., Juergens, L. A., Buchanan, G. R., and Gerald, P. S., 1975, Induction by alkylating agents of sister chromatid exchanges and chromatid breaks in Fanconi's anemia, *Proc. Natl. Acad. Sci. U.S.A.* **72**:4066.

Lehmann, A. R., 1972, Postreplication repair of DNA in mammalian cells, *Life Sci.* **15**:2005.

Lehmann, A. R., Kirk-Bell, S., Arlett, C. F., Paterson, M. C., Lohman, P. H. M., De Weerd-Kastelein, E. A., and Bootsma, D., 1975, Xeroderma pigmentosum cells with normal levels of excision repair have a defect in DNA synthesis after UV-irradiation, *Proc. Natl. Acad. Sci. U.S.A.* **72**:219.

Lima, L., Malaise, E., and Macieira-Coelho, A., 1972, Aging *in vitro:* Effect of low dose-rate irradiation on the division potential of chick embryonic fibroblasts, *Exp. Cell Res.* **73**:345.

Lindop, P., and Rotblat, J., 1961*a,* Long-term effects of a single whole-body exposure of mice to ionizing radiations. I. Life-shortening, *Proc. R. Soc. London Ser. B* **154**:332.

Lindop, P., and Rotblat, J., 1961*b,* Long-term effects of a single whole-body exposure of mice to ionizing radiations. II. Causes of death, *Proc. R. Soc. London Ser. B* **154**:350.

Liniecki, J., Bajerska, A., and Andryszek, C., 1971, Chromosomal aberrations in human lymphocytes irradiated *in vitro* from donors (males–females) of varying age, *Int. J. Radiat. Biol.* **19**:349.

Lipetz, J., and Cristofalo, V. J., 1972, Ultrastructural changes accompanying the ageing of human diploid cells in culture, *J. Ultrastruct. Res.* **39**:43.

Little, J. B., 1976, Relationship between DNA repair capacity and cellular aging, *Gerontology* **22**:28.

Little, J. B., and Williams, J. R., 1976, Effects of ionizing radiation on mammalian cells, in: *Handbook of Physiology,* Vol. I, Williams and Wilkins, Baltimore.

Little, J. B., Epstein, J., and Williams, J. R., 1975, Repair of DNA strand breaks in progeric fibroblasts and aging human diploid cells, in: *Molecular Mechanisms for Repair of DNA* (P. C. Hanawalt and R. R. Setlow, eds), pp. 793–800, Plenum Press, New York.

Macieira-Coelho, A., Diatloff, C., and Malaise, E., 1976, Converse response of cells with finite and infinite life-spans to ionizing radiation, *J. Cell Biol.* **67**:253a.

Martin, G. M., Sprague, C. A., and Epstein, C. J., 1970, Replicative life-span of cultivated human cells: Effects of donor's age, tissue, and genotype, *Lab. Invest.* **23:**86.

Massie, H. R., Baird, M. B., Nicolosi, R. J., and Samis, H. V., 1972, Changes in the structure of rat liver DNA in relation to age, *Arch. Biochem. Biophys.* **153:**736.

Mattern, M. R., and Cerutti, P. A., 1975, Age-dependent excision repair of damaged thymidine from irradiated DNA by isolated nuclei from human fibroblasts, *Nature (London)* **254:**450.

McCombe, P., Lavin, M., and Kidson, C., 1976, Control of DNA repair linked to neuroblastoma differentiation, *Intr. J. Radiat. Biol.* **29:**523.

McFee, A. F., Banner, M. W., and Sherill, M. N., 1970, Influence of animal age on radiation-induced chromosome aberrations in swine leukocytes, *Radiat. Res.* **41:**425.

McGrath, R. A., and Williams, R. W., 1966, Reconstruction *in vivo* of irradiated *E. coli* deoxyribonucleic acid: The rejoining of broken pieces, *Nature (London)* **212:**534.

Medvedev, Zh. A., 1976, Error theories of aging, in: *Alterns theorien* (D. Platt, ed.), pp. 37–46, F. K. Schattauer Verlag, New York.

Meneghini, R., and Hanawalt, P. C., 1975, Postreplication repair in human cells: On the presence of gaps opposite dimers and recombination, in: *Molecular Mechanisms for Repair of DNA* (P. C. Hanawalt and R. B. Setlow, eds.), pp. 639–642, Plenum Press, New York.

Mikhelson, V. M., 1976, Deficient repair of gamma-damaged DNA in xeroderma pigmentosum cells, Abstract, The Second International Workshop on DNA Repair Mechanisms in Mammalian cells, Noordwijkerhout, The Netherlands.

Modak, S. P., and Price, G. B., 1971, Exogenous DNA polymerase-catalyzed incorporation of deoxyribonucleotide monophosphates in nuclei of fixed mouse-brain cells, *Exp. Cell Res.* **65:**289.

Ono, T., Okada, S., and Sugahara, T., 1976, Comparative studies of DNA size in various tissues of mice during the aging process, *Exp. Gerontol.* **11:**127.

Oxford, J. M. Harnden, D. G., Parrington, J. M., and Delhanty, J. D. A., 1975, Specific chromosome aberrations in ataxia telangiectasia, *J. Med. Genet.* **12:**251.

Painter, R. B., 1974, DNA damage and repair in eukaryotic cells, *Genetics* **78:**139.

Painter, R. B., and Cleaver, J. E., 1969, Repair replication, unscheduled DNA synthesis, and the repair of mammalian DNA, *Radiat. Res.* **37:**451.

Painter, R. B., Clarkson, J. M., and Young, B. R., 1973, Ultraviolet-induced repair replication on aging diploid human cells (WI-38), *Radiat. Res.* **56:**560.

Parrington, J. M., Delhanty, J. D. A., and Baden, H., 1971, Unscheduled DNA synthesis, UV-induced chromosome aberrations and SV_{40} transformation in cultured cells from xeroderma pigmentosum, *Ann. Hum. Genet.* **35:**149.

Parrington, J. M., Casey, G., West, L., and Maia, V. D. V., 1976, Frequency of chromosome aberrations and chromatid exchange in cultured fibroblasts from patients with xeroderma pigmentosum, Huntington's chorea and normal controls, Abstract, The Second International Workshop on DNA Repair Mechanisms in Mammalian Cells, Noordwijkerhout, The Netherlands.

Paterson, M. C., Lohman, P. H. M., De Weerd-Kastelein, E. A., and Westerfeld, A., 1974, Photoreactivation and excision repair of ultraviolet radiation in injured DNA in primary embryonic chick cells, *Biophys. J.* **14:**454.

Paterson, M. C., Smith, B. P., Lohman, P. H. M., Anderson, A. K., and Fishman, L., 1976, Defective excision repair of gamma-ray damaged DNA in human (ataxia telangiectasia) fibroblasts, *Nature (London)* **260:**444.

Peterson, R. D. A., Cooper, M. D., and Good, R. A., 1966, Lymphoid tissue abnormalities associated with ataxia telangiectasia, *Am. J. Med.* **41:**342.

Pfeiffer, R. A., 1970, Chromosomal abnormalities in ataxia–telangiectasia (Louis-Bar's syndrome), *Humangenetik* **8:**302.

Poon, P. K., Parker, J. W., and O'Brien, R. L., 1975, Faulty DNA repair following ultraviolet irradiation in Fanconi's anemia, in: *Molecular Mechanisms for Repair of DNA* (P. C. Hanawalt and R. B. Setlow, eds.), pp. 821–824, Plenum Press, New York.

Price, G. B., Modak, S. P., and Makinodan, I., 1971, Age-associated changes in the DNA of mouse tissue, *Science* **171:**917.

Rasmussen, R. E., and Painter, R. B., Evidence for repair of ultraviolet damaged deoxyribonucleic acid in cultured mammalian cells, *Nature (London)* **203:**1360.

Rauth, A. M., 1970, Effects of ultraviolet light on mammalian cells in culture, *Curr. Top. Radiat. Res.* **6:**193.

Reed, W. B., Landing, B., Sugarmen, G., Cleaver, J. E., and Melnyk, J., 1969, Xeroderma pigmentosum, *J. Am. Med. Assoc.* **207:**2073.

Regan, J. D., and Setlow, R. B., 1974, DNA repair in human progeroid cells, *Biochem. Biophys. Res. Commun.* **59:**858.

Regan, J. D., Setlow, R. B., and Ley, R. D., 1971, Normal and defective repair of damaged DNA in human cells: A sensitive assay utilizing the photolysis of bromodeoxyuridine, *Proc. Natl. Acad. Sci. U.S.A.* **68:**708.

Remsen, J. F., and Cerutti, P. A., 1976, Deficiency of gamma-ray excision repair in skin fibroblasts from patients with Fanconi's anemia, *Proc. Natl. Acad. Sci. U.S.A.* **73:** 2419.

Reye, C., and Mosman, N. S. W., 1960, Ataxia telangiectasia: A case report, *Am. J. Dis. Child.* **99:**238.

Robbins, E., Levine, E. M., and Eagle, H., 1970, Morphological changes accompanying senescence of cultured human diploid cells, *J. Exp. Med.* **131:**1211.

Robbins, J. H., Kraemer, K. H., Lutzner, M. D., Festoff, B. W., and Coon, H. G., 1974, Xeroderma pigmentosum: An inherited disease with sun sensitivity, multiple cutaneous neoplasms, with abnormal DNA repair, *Ann. Intern. Med.* **80:**221.

Saksela, E., and Moorhead, P. S., 1963, Aneuploidy in the degenerative phase of serial cultivation of human cell strains, *Proc. Natl. Acad. Sci. U.S.A.* **50:**390.

Salser, J. S., and Balis, M. E., 1972, Alterations in deoxyribonucleic acid-bound amino acids with age and sex, *J. Gerontol.* **27:**1.

Samis, H. V., Jr., 1966, A concept of biological aging: The role of compensatory processes, *J. Theor. Biol.* **13:**236.

Sandberg, A. A., Cohen, M. M., Rimon, A. A., and Levin, M. L., 1967, Aneuploidy and age in a population survey, *Am. J. Hum. Genet.* **19:**633.

Sasaki, M. S., 1973, DNA repair capacity and susceptibility to chromosome breakage in xeroderma pigmentosum cells, *Mutat. Res.* **20:**291.

Sasaki, M. S., and Tonomura, A., 1973, A high susceptibility of Fanconi's anemia to chromosome breakage by DNA cross-linking agents, *Cancer Res.* **33:**1829.

Sax, H. J., and Passano, K. N., 1961, Spontaneous chromosome aberrations in human tissue cells, *Am. Nat.* **95:**97.

Schmid, W., 1967, Familial constitutive panmyelocytopathy, Fanconi's anemia (F.A.). II. A discussion of the cytogenetic findings in F.A., *Semin. Hematol.* **4:**241.

Schmid, W., and Jerusalem, F., 1972, Cytogenetic findings in two brothers with ataxia–telangiectasia (Louis-Bar's syndrome), *Arch. Genet.* **45:**49.

Schroeder, T. M., 1966, Cytogenetischer Befund und Ätiologie bei Fanconi Anämie, *Humangenetik* **3:**76.

Schroder, T. M., and Kurth, R., 1971, Spontaneous chromosomal breakage and high incidence of leukemia in inherited disease, *Blood* **37:**96.

Schroeder, T. M., Anschütz, F., and Knopp, A., 1964, Spontane Chromosomenaberrationen bei familiarer Panmyelopathie, *Humangenetik* **1:**194.

Schroeder, T. M., Tilgen, D., Krüger, J., and Vogel, F., 1976, Formal genetics of Fanconi's anemia, *Hum. Genet.* **32:**257.

Schuler, D., Kiss, A., and Fabian, F., 1969, Chromosomal peculiarities and *"in vitro"* examinations in Fanconi's anemia, *Humangenetik* **7**:314.

Schwartz, A., 1975, Capacity of cultured fibroblasts from different mammalian species to metabolize 7,12-dimethylbenz(a)anthracene to mutagenic metabolities: A correlation with lifespan, *Adv. Exp. Biol. Med.* **61**:270.

Scudiero, D., Norin, A., Karran, P., and Strauss, B., 1976, DNA excision-repair deficiency of human peripheral blood lymphocytes treated with chemical carcinogens, *Cancer Res.* **36**:1397.

Setlow, R. B., Regan, J. D. German J., and Carrier, W. L., 1969, Evidence that xeroderma pigmentosum cells do not perform the first step in the repair of ultraviolet damage to their DNA, *Proc. Natl. Acad. Sci. U.S.A.* **64**:1035.

Singal, D. P., and Goldstein, S., 1973, Absence of detectable *HL-A* antigens on cultured fibroblasts in progeria, *J. Clin. Invest.* **52**:2259.

Smith, K. C., 1976, Chemical adducts to deoxyribonucleic acid: Their importance to the genetic alteration theory of aging, *Interdiscip. Top. Gerontol.* **9**:16.

Spence, A. M., and Herman, M. M., 1973, Critical re-examination of the premature aging concept in progeria: A light and electron microscopic study, *Mech. Ageing Dev.* **2**:211.

Stecker, E., and Gardner, H. A., 1970, Werner's syndrome, *Lancet* **2**:1317.

Stevenson, K. G., and Curtis, H. J., 1961, Chromosome aberrations in irradiated and nitrogen mustard treated mice, *Radiat. Res.* **15**:774.

Stich, H. F., San, R. H. C., and Kawazoe, Y., 1973, Increased sensitivity of xeroderma pigmentosum cells to some chemical carcinogens and mutagens, *Mutat. Res.* **17**:127.

Stockdale, F. E., 1971, DNA synthesis in differentiating skeletal muscle cells: Initiation by ultraviolet light, *Science* **171**:1145.

Stockdale, F. E., and O'Neill, M. D., 1972, Repair DNA synthesis in differentiated embryonic muscle cells, *J. Cell Biol.* **52**:589.

Strauss, B., 1976, Non-genetic factors affecting the quantitative repair capability of cells, Abstract, The Second International Workshop on DNA Repair Mechanisms in Mammalian Cells, Noordwijkerhout, The Netherlands.

Sutherland, B. M., 1974, Photoreactivating enzyme from human leukocytes, *Nature (London)* **248**:109.

Sutherland, B. M., and Chamberlin, M. J., 1973, A rapid and sensitive assay for pyrimidine dimers in DNA, *Anal. Biochem.* **53**:168.

Sutherland, B. M., Runge, P., and Sutherland, J. C., 1974, DNA photoreactivating enzyme from placental mammals: Origin and characteristics, *Biochemistry* **13**:4710.

Sutherland, B. M., Rice, M., and Wagner, E. K., 1975, Xeroderma pigmentosum cells contain low levels of photoreactivating enzyme, *Proc. Natl. Acad. Sci. U.S.A.* **72**:103.

Swift, M. R., and Hirschhorn, K., 1966, Fanconi's anemia: Inherited susceptibility to chromosome breakage in various tissues, *Ann. Intern. Med.* **65**:496.

Tadjoedin, M. K., and Fraser, F. C., 1965, Heredity of ataxia–telangiectasia (Louis-Bar syndrome), *Am. J. Dis. Child.* **110**:64.

Takebe, H., 1976, Decreased DNA repair activity and skin cancers in xeroderma pigmentosum, Abstract, The Second International Workshop on DNA Repair Mechanisms in Mammalian Cells, Noordwijkerhout, The Netherlands.

Taylor, A. M. R., Harnden, D. G., Arlett, C. F., Harcourt, S. A., Lehmann, A. R., Stevens, S., and Bridges, B. A., 1975, Ataxia telangiectasia: A human mutation with abnormal radiation sensitivity, *Nature (London)* **258**:427.

Taylor, A. M. R., Metcalfe, J. A., Oxford, J. M., and Harnden, D. G., 1976, Is chromatid-type damage in ataxia telangiectasia after irradiation at G_0 a consequence of defective repair?, *Nature (London)* **260**:441.

Thompson, E. N., and Williams, R., 1965, Effect of age on liver function with particular reference to bromosulphalein excretion, *Gut* **6**:266.

Thompson, K. V. A., and Holliday, R., 1975, Chromosome changes during the *in vitro* ageing of MRC-5 human fibroblasts, *Exp. Cell Res.* **96**:1.

Thung, P. J., and Hollander, C. F., 1967, Regenerative growth and accelerated aging, *Symp. Soc. Exp. Biol.* **21**:455.

Tice, R. R., 1976, Cellular kinetics of PHA-stimulated human lymphocytes from young and old human male donors, Abstract, 29th Annual Meeting Gerontology Society, New York.

Tice, R. R., and Ishii, Y., 1977, The induction of sister chromatid exchanges (SCEs) in PHA-stimulated human lymphocytes by mitomycin C (MMC), Abstract, ICN–UCLA Symposia on Molecular and Cellular Biology, Keystone, Colorado.

Tough, J. M., Smith, P. G., Brown, C., and Harden, D. G., 1970, Chromosome studies on workers exposed to atmospheric benzenes. The possible influence of age, *Eur. J. Cancer* **6**:49.

Treton, J. A., and Courtois, Y., 1976, A comparison of DNA repair in cultured bovine lens epithelial cells and lung fibroblast cells, *Exp. Cell Res.* **102**:419.

Trosko, J. E., and Hart, R. W., 1976, DNA mutation frequencies in mammals, *Interdiscip. Top. Gerontol.* **9**:168.

Upton, A. C., 2957, Ionizing radiation and the aging process—A review, *J. Gerontol.* **12**:306.

Upton, A. C., Kimball, A. W., Furth, J., Christenberry, K. W., and Benedict, W. H., 1960, Some delayed effects of atom-bomb radiations in mice, *Cancer Res.* **20**(Suppl. 8, Part 2):1.

Vincent, R. A., and Huang, P. C., 1976, The proportion of cells labeled with tritiated thymidine as a function of population doubling level in cultures of fetal, adult, mutant and tumor origin, *Exp. Cell Res.* **102**:31.

Vincent, R. A., Jr., Sheridan, R. B., III, and Huang, P. C., 1975, DNA strand breakage repair in ataxia telangiectasia fibroblast-like cells, *Mutat. Res.* **33**:357.

von Hahn, H. P., and Fritz, E., 1966, Age-related alterations in the structure of DNA. III. Thermal stability of rat liver DNA, related to age, histone content and ionic strength, *Gerontologia* **12**:237.

Walburg, H. E., Jr., 1975, Radiation-induced life-shortening and premature aging, *Adv. Radiat. Biol.* **5**:145.

Wheeler, K. T., and Lett, J. T., 1974, On the possibility that DNA repair is related to age in non-dividing cells, *Proc. Natl. Acad. Sci. U.S.A.* **71**:1862.

Williams, J. R., and Little, J. B., 1975, Correlation of DNA repair and *in vitro* growth potential in hamster embryo cells; cited in Little (1976).

Yielding, E. L., 1974, A model for aging based on differential repair of somatic mutational damage, *Perspect. Biol. Med.* **17**:210.

Zucker-Franklin, D., Rifkin, H., and Jacobson, H. G., 1968, Werner's syndrome: An analysis of ten cases, *Geriatrics* **23**:123.

Chapter 4

Somatic Mutations and Aging

G. P. Hirsch

1. Introduction

Somatic mutations have been a major focus of aging research for many years. Initial support for the view that aging in mammals was due to the accumulation of somatic mutations was the effect of radiation on life span (Prasad, 1974). This mutagenic effect of radiation has been established in several systems, including mammalian cells (Awa, 1975). A single dose of radiation in a young animal did not produce effects associated with aging such as graying until long after the administration of the radiation. That it did not led to the idea that aging had been accelerated by radiation (Finch, S. C., and Beebe, 1975).

   More recently, the thesis that aging is due to somatic mutations has received support from the relationship between mutagenesis of chemical carcinogens and the age-associated incidence of cancer in man and experimental animals. The argument is rather straightforward. Chemical compounds that produce cancer in experimental animals have been shown to be mutagenic. The spontaneous occurrence of cancer in animals and man increases logarithmically during aging. Since compounds that can cause cancer also produce mutations, the mechanism of induced cancer may be a mutagenic event. If mutations can produce cancer in experimental model systems, spontaneous mutations may be the mechanism by which cancer develops during aging. This line of reasoning led to the publication recently of two books that attempt to explain in some detail how somatic mutations can account for the decline in function associated with aging and the

G. P. Hirsch • Division of Biology, Oak Ridge National Laboratory, Oak Ridge, Tennessee 37830

increased age-associated probability of the onset of death from cancer: *Intrinsic Mutagenesis: A Genetic Approach to Aging* (Burnet, 1974) and *The Biology of Cancer: A New Approach* (Burch, 1976).

Another important reason for a focus on somatic mutations as a cause of aging is the metabolic stability of DNA in most somatic cells in mammals. Aging is generally regarded as an accumulation of deleterious changes over the period of the life span, with the accumulation occurring in proportion to the amount of elapsed metabolic time. Since DNA is a permanent component of most mammalian cells, these changes could be fixed in such a metabolically stable component. Some cell types such as neurons cannot replicate DNA after development, while other cell types such as liver cells can undergo cell division in response to stress. With the exception of cells in the GI tract, the skin, spermatogonial cells, and red and white blood cell precursors, somatic cells replicate DNA rarely or not at all. Thus, most of the DNA in a 60-year-old person is 60 years old, and has had 60 years to accumulate various kinds of damage including mutations. The metabolic stability of DNA is in sharp contrast to the majority of intracellular constituents, which are regularly replaced (Rechcigl, 1971; Menzies, 1976; Neuberger and Richards, 1964). In the mouse, for example, the ribosomes are replaced over 100 times during the life span. The only metabolically stable proteins (intracellular or membraneous) that have been identified are myelin, in the nervous system, proteins of the eye lens, and chromosomal proteins, notably histones. Since the great majority of enzymes and structural proteins are replaced regularly, the accumulation of molecular alterations and damage in these compounds can be avoided (Lewis, 1972). Thus, the potential mechanisms for age-associated loss of function are distinctly different for the metabolically stable components and those that are regularly degraded and made anew. Protein and RNA turnover emphasize the importance of DNA as the repository of information required for the normal maintenance and function of cellular processes and integrity.

The metabolic stability of DNA and the lack of cell replication in many mammalian cell types necessitates special definitions for somatic mutations. Mutations can be defined as inheritable changes that involve alterations in the quality, quantity or relationships of the DNA sequences. The main classes of mutations are base substitutions, frameshift mutations, small deletions, large deletions, exchanges, and chromosome loss. In cells that no longer go through cell division, it is not possible to demonstrate that a particular lesion is in fact heritable, since the definition of mutations involves transmission to all progeny cells. Mutations in nondividing cells can therefore only be inferred from a demonstration that the molecular changes present or induced in the nondividing cells are the same as those that occur or are induced in dividing cells and that result in the transmission of the genotype to all progeny. By restricting the definition of somatic mutations to changes in the DNA that are transmitted to all daughter cells, a distinction can be made between DNA damage that results in permanent heritable changes and DNA damage that affects only a single cell. In the nondividing cell, the end result of mutational and nonmutational damage may be the same, cell death or gene-product loss. In the somatic cell or germinal cell with a potential for cell division, the distinction between heritable and nonheritable DNA damage is important. In the dividing-cell systems, nonheritable DNA damage would not accumulate with time, whereas mutations would increase with time in the absence of selection.

Distinct criteria for somatic mutations allow definition of alternative changes that might influence gene expression. Most of the experimental data on the regulation of gene expression indicate that the regulatory mechansims do not involve a permanent alteration in the genome; thus, mutational events are not associated with differentiation (Gurdon, 1962; DiBerardino and King, 1965, 1967). The expression of gene products in differentiated cells has the characteristic of heritability, in that liver cells that are produced after partial hepatectomy have all the characteristics of other liver cells. Examples of shift in differentiation, such as repression of melanin synthesis after cell fusion, indicate that differentiation can be altered (Bernhard, 1976).

If changes in gene expression occur with aging, two alternative explanations can be considered. One would be nongenetic changes in the mechanisms controlling gene expression; another would be mutations in the gene itself or in another gene that regulates the expression of that gene (repressor or inducer). The distinction between mutational and regulatory causes of potential age-associated changes in gene expression is important in trying to elucidate the various mechanisms by which expression may fail in older animals (Wheldon and Kirk, 1973).

DNA is the major source of information fidelity in cells. Alterations in gene expression are a part of the overall scheme of information fidelity that is required for the smooth, complex transitions that occur during development and that maintain the integrity of adult organisms as environmental conditions change. A third system exists for which fidelity of information flow may be essential—the transcriptional and translational apparatus. These components consist of RNA polymerase, ribosomes, transfer RNAs (tRNAs), aminoacyl tRNA ligases, and other associated proteins and RNAs. While both protein synthesis and gene regulation are dependent on DNA for information content, either system may cause a loss in the precision of cellular function independently of DNA. Loss of information fidelity in the system of transcription and translation has been designated as *errors*. Since the protein-synthetic apparatus essentially makes copies of itself, using DNA templates as a reference, a reduction in the fidelity in this system could result in an irreversible increase in the frequency of errors. This concept is the basis for the error theory of aging (Orgel, 1963, 1970). While errors and mutations are conceptually distinct potential sources of information loss, each may interact with the other, and both result in the same kind of changes in the molecules obtained from groups of cells (Medvedev, 1976). Many experiments that were designed to estimate the fidelity of protein synthesis through determination of the quality of protein products obtained from populations of cells would also detect mutations that had occurred in a few cells. Whether age-associated changes that are detected in molecules obtained from tissues represent errors that take place in most cells or mutations that exist in only a few cells depends on the relative frequency of the two sources of aberrant molecules. Differentiating between errors and mutations can be accomplished when specific amino acid substitutions are examined on molecules obtained from cell populations or when tests of protein products are conducted on single cells.

Methods newly developed for making these distinctions and results of amino acid substitution changes after radiation and during aging constitute the central theme of this chapter. Section 2 is a brief summary of current concepts of molecular genetics for interested readers. Evidence concerning the accumulation of chromosomal aberrations with aging is discussed in Chapters 1 and 8, and is reviewed only briefly here.

2. Terminology of Mutagenesis

2.1. Concepts and Definitions

Genetics and biochemistry have converged on the study and characterization of mutations and mutagenesis to the extent that a common vocabulary has evolved. Traditionally, mutations that affected only a very small portion of the genetic material were called point mutations. With a better understanding of the nature of mutations, point mutations are now subdivided into small deletions, frameshifts, and base-substitution mutations when distinctions are possible. The base-substitution mutations can be either the missense or nonsense type, depending on whether the base change results in the coding of another amino acid (missense) or in a code word that is not normally translated by the RNA molecules (nonsense). Some real and hypothetical examples of these classes of mutations are shown for human hemoglobin variants in Table I (Weatherall and Clegg, 1976).

Table I. Examples of Mutations in Human Hemoglobins[a]

Mutations		138	139	140	141					
Base substitutions										
Missense	Hemoglobin Singapore	Ser	Lys	Tyr	Pro	(Trm)				
	Coding	UCU	AAA	UAC	CCU	UAA				
	Coding	UCU	AAA	UAC	CGU	UAA				
	Hemoglobin A—α	Ser	Lys	Tyr	Arg	(Trm)				
Nonsense	Hypothetical	Ser	Lys	(Trm)						
	Coding	UCU	AAA	UAA						
	Coding	UCU	AAA	UAC	CGU					
	Hemoglobin A—α	Ser	Lys	Tyr	Arg					
Nonsense reversion	Hemoglobin Constant Spring	Ser	Lys	Tyr	Arg	Gln	Ala	Gly	Ala	Ser
	Coding	UCU	AAA	UAC	CGU	CAA	GCU	GGA	GCC	UCG
	Coding	UCU	AAA	UAC	CGU	UAA				
	Hemoglobin A—α	Ser	Lys	Try	Arg	(Trm)				
Frameshifts										
Minus one	Hemoglobin Wayne	Ser	Asn	Thr	Val	Lys	Leu	Glu	Pro	Arg
	Coding	UCA	AAU	ACC	GUU	AAG	CUG	GAG	CCU	CGG
	Coding	UCU	AAA	UAC	CGU	UAA				
	Hemoglobin A—α	Ser	Lys	Tyr	Arg	(Trm)				

Mutations		90	91	92	93	94	95	96
Deletions								
Small	Hemoglobin Gun Hill	Leu	—	—	—	—	Lys	Leu
	Hemoglobin A—β	Leu	Leu	His	Cys	Asp	Lys	Leu
Large	Thalassemia	No product						

[a]Adapted from Weatherall and Clegg (1976).

The effect of a point mutation is either to stop the synthesis of the protein in question or to substitute one amino acid for another. For small deletions, there is a 67% probability that the sequences outside the deleted region will be joined out of register, and that soon after the point of rejoining, a "stop" code word will be generated (nonsense) and the product of the gene in question will be a shortened molecule. Statistically, for a given gene, small deletions that result in frameshifts will generate randomly distributed populations of molecules varying in size from very short to those of nearly full length. For small deletions that are joined in register (33%), nearly full-length molecules will be produced that may be distorted at some region of the molecule due to the deleted region. Frameshift mutations, which result from the insertion or deletion of bases, shift the reading frame of the DNA (except when the shift is a multiple of three bases), and will usually result in the appearance of nonsense code words after the frameshift. As in the case of deletions that are rejoined out of register, frameshifts that shift the register of translation will result in proteins of shorter than normal length. Frameshifts involving loss of one or two bases need not be distinguished from small deletions, but because insertion and deletion of a few bases probably occur by mechanisms that differ from those that produce frameshifts, they are classified separately. Frameshift mutations can often be reverted to phenotypes that are similar to normal proteins by another frameshift mutation that restores the correct translation register. Small deletions of more than five or ten bases are not reverted, since the correct genetic information is not likely to be inserted where it had been lost. Shortened gene products that are produced by frameshift mutations, and deletions rejoined out of register, could also result from base substitutions that mutate to the nonsense codons. Since only 3 to 64 codons are not translated as one or another amino acid, the frequency of production of gene fragments would be about 5% of the total base substitutions that arise.

While the mechanisms of mutagenesis may vary, the results are similar. Protein products changed in only one or a few amino acids will be produced by base substitutions of the missense type, small deletions rejoined in register, and frameshifts that occur in multiples of three bases. In contrast, base substitutions that result in nonsense coding, frameshifts, and small deletions out of register will result in the production of protein fragments. We might anticipate that for most protein fragments, there will be a critical size above which the molecule will be partially functional and below which it will be inactive. If this is true, mutations that result in protein fragments (frameshifts and nonsense) will appear as deletions if they are inactive, and as altered protein products if they are larger than the appropriate size necessary to maintain catalytic activity.

This distinction between loss of a protein product and creation of an altered product will simplify the alternative mechanism that might explain changes associated with aging and in the experimental sense distinguish the spontaneous mechanisms from one another through the use of experimental models. For example, will animal longevity be decreased by treatment with well-characterized frameshift mutagens? Deletions in the eukaryotic systems yield cells with only one copy of that particular gene (where usually two are present). Many base-substitution mutations will yield enzymes with reduced activity or substrate specificity or both. The phenotype of fidelity change deserves special consideration in aging research, since mutation in a gene involved in macromolecular synthesis could affect the functioning of many other normal genes in the same cell. For those gene products involved in the process of intracellular communications, even other nonmutant cells may be affected. Consideration of other mechanisms of information loss with aging are discussed in Section 4.3.

There are several classes of mutations that involve large chromosomal regions. These classes are discussed in detail in other chapters. We need only say here that most of the chromosomal effects observed involve the breakage or rejoining, or both, of DNA segments. There is litte evidence that the frequency of such events is sufficient to play an important role in aging, although several examples of chromosome change in tumors have been reported (Gahrton *et al.*, 1974). Chromosomal mutations, since they are easily quantitated, may serve as a sensitive and useful index for estimating molecular changes that do contribute to aging.

2.2. Mutations in Nondividing Cells

The types of molecular changes described and identified in the previous section occur in DNA and are transmitted to all progeny of a given cell. Since the majority of cells in mammalian organisms do not replicate after development, how can the mechanisms of mutagenesis be identified? In the case of base-substitution mutations, a method that could identify specifically these altered proteins could be used to quantitate the level of mutations that had accumulated in the nondividing cells in the same way that they could be used to quantitate the accumulation of mutations in dividing cells. The same argument would hold for methods that could evaluate the level of protein fragments. An increase in nonsense mutations would result in increased protein fragments in nondividing cells as well as in dividing cell types.

In nondividing cells, it is difficult to prove that the loss of a gene product was the result of mutation. If, for example an interstrand cross-link occurred in a nondividing cell, it might preclude the synthesis of messenger RNA (mRNA) and hence the protein product (Cutler, 1976). Since the event of interstrand cross-link is not heritable, however, it cannot be considered a mutation, although it could result in a mutation in a dividing cell. Although the end point of gene loss may be significant in aging, the mechanisms by which the gene loss takes place may be different for mutational events in comparison with nonheritable events. Also, the methods that might be used to identify the cause of loss of gene expression would be different for the genetic as opposed to the epigenetic and nongenetic mechanisms. In several tissues, cells of the adult organism do not normally replicate, but can be induced to do so with various forms of stimulation. For example, when two lobes of liver tissue are surgically removed, the cells in the remaining lobes will almost immediately replicate, and the mass of the liver will be regenerated rather rapidly. Normally, almost no cell division is detected in liver tissue. Liver has been used extensively to study the accumulation of mutation in "nondividing" cells. The task of demonstrating heritability has been approached by stimulating the liver tissue to regenerate and by measuring changes that remain after regeneration. Age-associated changes in liver tissue DNA that were due to mutations should be expressed after liver regeneration, while nongenetic causes would decrease in proportion to the relative mass of liver removed to stimulate regeneration.

3. Metabolic Stability of DNA: Contrast to Turnover of Intracellular Macromolecules

The extensive turnover of most intracellular components of mammalian cells poses an enigma for understanding aging at the molecular level. The question to be answered is: how can damage accumulate during aging in enzymes, structural proteins, or membranes when these molecules are being replaced regularly and often rapidly? Part of the answer seems to be that molecular turnover is the mechanism by which the accumulation of damage and limitations on longevity are avoided in these components. This is not to say that certain aspects of the process of turnover may not contribute to aging or that molecular turnover does not serve other important purposes, such as rapid physiological response capacity. The accumulaton of insoluble intracellular debris (age pigment) as a by-product of turnover may be one example of the former process. Another potential mechanism of aging that may not be overcome by macromolecular turnover is the accumulation of errors. Indeed, turnover of the protein-synthetic apparatus is a necessary ingredient of the model commonly known as *error theory,* which predicts that the fidelity of protein synthesis will decline with successive rounds of turnover of the protein-synthetic apparatus (Wiegel *et al.,* 1973). While turnover precludes the physical accumulation of damage, it does not limit the potential cumulative effects of changes in the informational integrity of cellular systems, such as fidelity of protein synthesis, and structural relationships among membranes.

The experimental data showing the extent of macromolecular turnover were often obtained for reasons other than the elucidation of aging mechanisms (Gee *et al.,* 1969; Nordgren *et al.,* 1969; Menzies *et al.,* 1969). For this reason, the majority of turnover studies have concentrated on measurements over rather short periods of the animal's life span. Only a few experiments have been designed to identify and characterize cellular components that may have characteristically long half-lives.

A summary of turnover data for several tissues is shown in Tables II–V. The turnover data summarized in these tables are designated for each tissue as to the fraction isolated or labeled, the species studied, the measured half-life of the component or fraction, the age of the animal at the initiation of the turnover study, the interval for which the measurement was made, the isotope used, the form of administration, and, in some cases, information as to the method used for calculating the half-life. In some experiments, it was possible to estimate not only the half-life but also the percentage of the total component that had a characteristic half-life, this figure being given in parentheses after the half-life value. Turnover times of many enzymes are summarized by Rechcigl (1971). Among many cellular proteins, only histones have half-lives that are long relative to the life span of the animal. These proteins and perhaps others associated with DNA in nondividing cells have a considerable metabolic stability. A few specialized tissues contain proteins of metabolic stability—the lens protein and the myelin of the brain and neural tissues (Waley, 1964; Young and Fulhorst, 1966). Extracellular matrix, consisting primarily of collagen and including elastin and proteoglycans, is relatively stable.

With the exceptions just cited, DNA and some associated proteins constitute the major intracellular entities that are metabolically stable and are therefore a primary target in nondividing cells for the accumulation of physical damage. The metabolic stability of DNA has led many researchers in aging to expect that the DNA will be the primary site for the physiological deterioration that accompanies aging. Despite considerable effort, however, no conclusive evidence has been obtained that the DNA obtained from old animals was significantly altered with aging (Zhelabovskaya and Berdyshev, 1972), although an increase in DNA cross-links was discovered by Herrmann (1975). One explanation given for the lack of DNA damage during aging is the presence of DNA-''repair'' systems. The role of DNA repair in aging is detailed in Chapter 3. It is apparent from many studies that lesions in mammalian DNA are subjected to enzymatic activity in the processes described collectively as repair. It has not been determined whether the repair events restore the DNA to its original condition or whether the repair processes produce mutations.

Table II. Brain Turnover

Fraction	Animal	Half-life (days)[a]	Age or weight	Decay interval (days)[b]	Label	Method	Ref. no.[b]	Comment
Organic hydrogen	Rat	16 (46%)	In utero: 180 days	1–300	^3H_2O	Water	26	Constant specific activity
Organic hydrogen	Rat	150 (54%)	In utero: 180 days	1–300	^3H_2O	Water	26	Constant specific activity
Protein	Rat	18.5	100–120 days	14–84	Leu-^{3}H	Ventricular	24	Intraventricular
Nonlipid carbon	Rat	9.8 (38%)	Adult	1–50	Food-^{14}C	Feeding	7	Graphic approximation, adult replacement
Nonlipid carbon	Rat	74 (30%)	Adult	1–50	Food-^{14}C	Feeding	7	Graphic approximation, adult replacement
Nonlipid carbon	Rat	100+ (32%)	Adult	1–50	Food-^{14}C	Feeding	7	Graphic approximation, adult replacement
Protein, nonproteolipid	Rat	22	11 days	1–250	Gly-^{14}C	1 i.p.	9	Brain and cord
Protein, proteolipid	Rat	NST	11 days	10–250	Gly-^{14}C	1 i.p.	9	
Protein, nonproteolipid	Rat	22	320–360	1–200	Gly-^{14}C	1 i.p.	9	Brain and cord
Protein	Mouse	10–20 (90%)	In utero: 60 days	0–60	Lys-^{14}C	Feeding	16	Constant specific activity
Lipid	Rat	77	9 and 13 days	43–125	^3H_2O	2 i.p.	8	
Lipid	Rat	66	53 days	1–82	Acetate-^{14}C	1 i.p.	8	
Phospholipid	Rat	40	10 days	10–100	Phosphate-^{32}P	1 i.p.	11	Graphic approximation
Phospholipid	Rat	NST	10 days	100–200	Phosphate-^{32}P	1 i.p.	11	
Nuclear histones	Mouse	52–56	90–105 days	1–45	Lys-^{14}C	1 i.p.	19	
Nuclear histones	Mouse	104	90–105 days	0–245	Lys-^{14}C	1 i.p.	19	
Nuclear histones	Mouse	115–117	In utero: days 5–12	110–257	Lys-^{14}C	1 i.p.	19	

	Species		Age/Weight		Label	Route	Ref.	Notes
Nuclear protein, HCl-soluble	Mouse	8–33	90–105 days	4–45	Lys-^{14}C	1 i.p.	19	
Nuclear protein, HCl-insoluble	Mouse	9–32	90–105 days	4–45	Lys-^{14}C	1 i.p.	19	
Sulfolipid	Rat	200	15 days	7–223	Sulfate-^{35}S	1 i.p.	10	Also sciatic nerve and cord
Microsomal lipid	Rat	51	9 and 13 days	43–125	^{3}H$_2$O	2 i.p.	8	
Microsomal protein	Rat	13–16	90–105 days	1–45	Lys-^{14}C	1 i.p.	19	
Ribosomal RNA	Rat	12	100–120 days	7–55	Orotate-^{14}C	1 intra-ventricular	24	
Ribosomal protein	Rat	12	100–120 days	7–58	Leu-^{14}C	1 intra-ventricular	24	
sRNA (tRNA)	Rat	12.5	180–220 g	4–24	Cytidine-^{14}C	1 intra-cysternal	6	
Supernatant protein	Rat	16	100–120 days	14–84	Leu-^{14}C	1 intra-ventricular	24	
Supernatant lipid	Rat	31	9 and 13 days	43–125	^{3}H$_2$O	2 i.p.	8	
Supernatant sulfolipid	Rat	2.7	12 days	1–31	Sulfate-^{35}S	1 i.p.	12	
Mitochondrial								
DNA	Rat	31	200–300 g	5–30	Thymidine-^{3}H	1 i.p.	13	
Protein	Rat	20	100–120 days	14–18	Leu-^{14}C	1 intra-ventricular	24	
Protein, water-soluble	Rat	18	150–180 g	1–28	Leu-^{14}C	1 i.p.	4	
Protein, water-insoluble	Rat	31	150–180 g	1–28	Leu-^{14}C	1 i.p.	4	
Myelin								
Lipid	Rat	372	53 days	1–82	Acetate-^{14}C	1 i.p.	8	
Sulfolipid	Rat	NST	4 days	12–75	Sulfate-^{35}S	1 i.p.	12	
Lipid	Rat	NST	53 days	1–51	Acetate-^{14}C	1 i.p.		
Cholesterol	Rat	210–240	15–16 days	60–360	Acetate-^{14}C	1 i.p.	25	
Protein	Rat	35	90 days	5–55	Glucose-^{14}C	1 i.p.	22	

(continued)

Table II.   (continued)

Fraction	Animal	Half-life (days)[a]	Age or weight	Decay interval (days)	Label	Method	Ref. no.[b]	Comment
Sphingomyelin	Rat	300	15–16 days	60–360	Acetate-^{14}C	1 i.p.	25	
Synaptic endings								
Vesicle protein	Rat	21	100–120 days	14–56	Leu-^{14}C	1 intra-ventricular	24	
Membrane protein	Rat	21	100–120 days	14–56	Leu-^{14}C	1 intra-ventricular	24	
Lipid	Rat	60	53 days	1–82	Acetate-^{14}C	1 i.p.	8	
Sulfolipid	Rat	19	12 days	1–31	Sulfate-^{35}S	1 i.p.	12	

[a](NST) No significant turnover.

[b]References: (1) Akeson et al. (1960); (2) Amano et al. (1965); (3) Arias et al. (1969); (4) Beattie et al. (1967); (5) Blobel and Potter (1968); (6) Bondy (1966); (7) Buchanan (1961); (8) Cuzner et al. (1966); (9) Davison (1961); (10) Davison (1962); (11) Davison and Dobbing (1960); (12) Davison and Gregson (1966); (13) Gross and Rabinowitz (1969); (14) C. A. Hirsch and Hiatt (1966); (15) Kuriyama et al. (1969); (16) Lajtha and Toth (1966); (17) Loeb et al. (1965); (18) Omura et al. (1967); (19) Piha et al. (1966); (20) Schapira et al. (1960); (21) Schimke (1964); (22) M. E. Smith (1968); (23) Swick et al. (1968); (24) von Hungen et al. (1968); (25) M. E. Smith and Eng (1965); (26) Thompson and Ballough (1956).

Table III. Kidney Turnover

Fraction	Animal	Half-life (days)	Age or weight	Decay interval (days)	Label	Method	Ref. no.[a]	Comment
Organic hydrogen	Rat	180 (8%)	In utero: 180 days	1–300	^3H_2O	Water	26	Constant specific activity
Organic hydrogen	Rat	11 (92%)	In utero: 180 days	1–300	^3H_2O	Water	26	Constant specific activity
Nonlipid carbon	Rat	8.7 (56%)	Adult	1–50	Food-^{14}C	Feeding	7	Graphic approximation, adult replacement
Nonlipid carbon	Rat	31 (35%)	Adult	1–50	Food-^{14}C	Feeding	7	Graphic approximation, adult replacement
Nonlipid carbon	Mouse	8.7 (56%)	Adult	1–50	Food-^{14}C	Feeding	7	Graphic approximation, adult replacement
Nonlipid carbon	Mouse	31 (35%)	Adult	1–50	Food-^{14}C	Feeding	7	Graphic approximation, adult replacement
Phospholipid	Rat	8–10	16 days	5–50	Phosphate-^{32}P	1 i.p.	11	Graphic approximation, no growth correction
Mitochondrial protein	Rat	8.6	150–180 g	1–28	Leu-^{14}C	1 i.v.	4	
Mitochondrial DNA	Rat	10.4	200–300 g	5–30	Thymidine-^3H	1 i.p.	13	
Mitochondrial Protein, water-soluble	Rat	6.0	150–180 g	1–28	Leu-^{14}C	1 i.v.	4	
Protein, salt-soluble	Rat	7.6	150–180 g	1–28	Leu-^{14}C	1 i.v.	4	
Protein, "structural"	Rat	9.0	150–180 g	1–28	Leu-^{14}C	1 i.v.	4	
Other cytochromes	Rat	8.4	150–180 g	1–28	Leu-^{14}C	1 i.v.	4	
Cardiolipin	Rat	11.4	200–300 g	5–30	Phosphate-^{32}P	1 i.p.	13	
Lecithin	Rat	10.0	200–300 g	5–30	Phosphate-^{32}P	1 i.p.	13	
Phosphatidyl ethanolamine	Rat	10.0	200–300 g	5–30	Phosphate-^{32}P	1 i.p.	13	

[a]See Table II, footnote b, for references.

Table IV. Liver Turnover

Fraction	Animal	Half-life (days)	Age or weight	Decay interval (days)	Label	Method	Ref. no.[a]	Comment
Protein	Rat	3.3	80–100	1–7	Arg-^{14}C(g)	1 i.p.	3	Guanido-Arg
Nonlipid carbon	Rat	4.7 (95%)	Adult	1–50	Food-^{14}C	Feeding	7	Graphic approximation, adult replacement
Nonlipid carbon	Rat	60 (5%)	Adult	1–50	Food-^{14}C	Feeding	7	Graphic approximation, adult replacement
Nonlipid carbon	Mouse	4.7 (95%)	Adult	1–50	Food-^{14}C	Feeding	7	Graphic approximation, adult replacement
Nonlipid carbon	Mouse	60 (5%)	Adult	1–50	Food-^{14}C	Feeding	7	Graphic approximation, adult replacement
Organic hydrogen	Rat	140 (3%)	In utero: 180 days	1–300	^{3}H$_2$O	Water	26	Constant specific activity
Organic hydrogen	Rat	4.5, 12 (97%)	In utero: 180 days	1–300	^{3}H$_2$O	Water	26	Constant specific activity
Nuclear protein	Rat	5.1	80–100 g	1–7	Arg-^{14}C(g)	1 i.p.	3	Guanido-Arg
Histones	Mouse	18–19	90–105 days	1–45	Lys-^{14}C	1 i.p.	19	
Histones	Mouse	56	90–105 days	50–150	Lys-^{14}C	1 i.p.	19	
Histones	Mouse	93	90–105 days	150–250	Lys-^{14}C	1 i.p.	19	
Histones	Mouse	55–58	In utero: days 5–12	69–150	Lys-^{14}C	1–5 s.q.	19	Maternal s.q.

Histones	Mouse	105	*In utero:* days 8–12	150–257	Lys-^{14}C	3 s.q.	19	Maternal s.q.
Supernatant protein	Rat	5.1	80–100 g	1–7	Lys-^{14}C	1 i.p.	3	Guanido-Arg
Arginase	Rat	4	250–275	1–16		—	21	Adult replacement
Glycogen	Rat	3–4	Adult	1–50	Food-^{14}C	Feeding	7	
Ribosomal protein	Rat	5	250–300 g	2–8	Arg-^{14}C(g)	1 i.p.	14	Guanido-Arg
Ribosomal RNA, cytoplasmic	Mouse	10.3	26–32 g	1–19	Cytidine-^{3}H	—	2	Autoradiography
Ribosomal RNA	Rat	5.1	135–150 g	3–21	Orotate-^{3}H	1 i.p.	17	
sRNA (tRNA)	Rat	3.8	155 g	2–12	Orotate-^{3}H	1 i.p.	5	
Plasma membrane	Rat	1.8	80–100 g	1–7	Arg-^{14}C(g)	1 i.p.	3	Guanido-Arg
Microsomes Protein	Rat	3.0	80–100 g	1–7	Arg-^{14}C(g)	1 i.p.	3	Guanido-Arg
Cytochrome b_5	Rat	4.3	160–180 g	2–8	Arg^{14}C	1 i.v.	15	Graphic approximation, Guanido-Arg
Smooth-membrane protein	Rat	4.7	150–200 g	1–14	Leu-^{14}C	1 i.p.	18	
Rough-membrane protein	Rat	4.6	150–200 g	1–14	Leu-^{14}C	1 i.p.	18	
Mitochondrial Protein	Rat	6.8	80–100 g	1–7	Arg-^{14}C(g)	1 i.p.	3	Guanido-Arg
Protein	Rat	8.4	150–180 g	1–28	Leu-^{14}C	1 i.v.	4	
Protein, water-soluble	Rat	4.2–5.1 (80%)	150–200 g	0–12	Ca^{14}CO$_3$	Feeding	23	Incorporation; activity of Arg relative to urea
DNA	Rat	9.4	200–300 g	5–29	Thymidine-^{3}H	1 i.p.	13	
Sphingomyelin	Rat	11.4	200–300 g	5–29	Phosphate-^{32}P	1 i.p.	13	

[a]See Table II, footnote b, for references.

Table V. Skeletal Muscle Turnover

Fraction	Animal	Half-life (days)	Age or weight	Decay interval (days)	Label	Method	Ref. no.[a]	Comment
Nonlipid carbon	Mouse	8.3 (47%)	Adult	1–50	Food-^{14}C	Feeding	7	Graphic approximation, adult replacement
Nonlipid carbon	Mouse	65 (23%)	Adult	1–50	Food-^{14}C	Feeding	7	Graphic approximation, adult replacement
Nonlipid carbon	Rat	8.3 (47%)	Adult	1–50	Food-^{14}C	Feeding	7	Graphic approximation, adult replacement
Nonlipid carbon	Rat	65 (23%)	Adult	1–50	Food-^{14}C	Feeding	7	Graphic approximation, adult replacement
Protein	Rat	b	11 days	42–250	Gly-^{14}C	1 i.p.	9	⅓ collagen
Organic hydrogen	Rat	100 (40%)	In utero: 180 days	1–300	^{3}H$_2$O	Water	26	
Organic hydrogen	Rat	16	In utero: 180 days	1–300	^{3}H$_2$O	Water	26	
Myoglobin	Rat	20	380–420 g	2–214	Gly-^{14}C	Injection	1	Moderate amount
Myoglobin	Rat	80–90	380–420 g	2–214	Gly-^{14}C	Injection	1	Majority
Aldolase	Rat	20	200–250 g	2–80	Gly-^{14}C	1 i.p.	20	Graphic approximation
Aldolase	Rat	60–100+	200–250 g	2–80	Gly-^{14}C	1 i.p.	20	Graphic approximation
Glycogen	Rat	15 (90%)	Adult	1–50	Food-^{14}C	Feeding	7	Graphic approximation, adult replacement

[a]See Table II, footnote *b*, for references.   [b] No significant turnover.

4. Accumulation of Somatic Mutations with Aging

4.1. Chromosome Aberrations

Support for the somatic mutation hypothesis of aging has come primarily from the increase in the frequency of chromosomal aberrations that occur in liver tissue (Curtis, 1966). This increase has been observed in several species, and increases linearly with aging such that the percentage of cells with aberrations reaches about 20% at the end of the life span of the species (Brooks *et al.*, 1973) (see also Table VI). The rate of chromosome-aberration accumulation is slower in long-lived species. That it is agrees with most models of aging, which predict that changes should occur more slowly in animals with greater potential life spans. Since somatic mutations are thought to arise from random processes, it has been proposed that longer-lived animals must have better repair systems that slow the rate of mutation accumulation (see Chapter 3). If somatic mutations cause aging, then processes that increase somatic mutations should accelerate aging. Indeed, radiation treatments that shorten life span do cause an increase in the number of chromosome aberrations in the treated animals, but the correspondence between the level of chromosome aberrations induced and the percentage of life-shortening is not direct. One possible explanation for the lack of correspondence between chromosome aberrations and life-shortening is that chromosome aberrations are only a partial measure of the genetic damage done by radiation. Since liver cells and other nondividing cells would not normally undergo cell division, the aberration itself might only indicate the loss of two gene products (at the site of cross-linkage) between chromosomes. The evidence that chromosome aberrations correlate with point mutations was derived from plant systems. In mammalian systems, it has been shown that chromosome aberrations in spermatogonial stem cells correlated with the radiation dose only up to a certain level of radiation, and above that point, the level of aberrations recovered is

Table VI.   Chromosome Anomalies During Aging

Anomaly	Reference
Decrease in chiasmata in CBA mice (20%) and C57BL mice (4%)	Henderson and Edwards (1968)
Increase in polyploid cells and autosomal univalents in mouse testis; no translocation difference	Leonard and Leonard (1975)
Increase in the frequency of metaphase chromosome aberrations in liver tissue of Chinese hamster	Brooks, *et al.* (1973)
Threefold increase in chromosome aberrations in mouse strains A/HEJ and C57BL/6J liver cells	Crowley and Curtis (1963)

actually reduced (Preston and Brewen, 1973). In the mouse testis for fractionated doses, a linear correlation between radiation exposure and accumulated translocations was obtained by allowing sufficient time (2 months) for repopulation of the testis (Preston and Brewen, 1976).

There are other complications involved in comparisons of chromosome aberration induction and life-shortening. One is the much greater life-shortening sensitivity of young animals to a given dose of radiation (Yuhas, 1971; Storer, 1965). Also, no life-shortening is produced by radiation, up to a certain dose, when the exposure occurs *in utero* (Upton *et al.*, 1966). Partial-body radiation is less effective than whole-body radiation in life-shortening (Sato *et al.*, 1973).

For many years, somatic mutation was discounted as a cause of aging because males and females of many species had nearly equal longevities. The argument was that since females had two copies of the X chromosome and the males had only one copy, somatic mutations on the X chromosome would increase in females only by the square root of the rate that they would increase in males. Of course, this argument applies only to recessive mutations, and only to the X chromosome. In recent years, it has been demonstrated convincingly that in the female, only one of the X chromosomes is active in a given cell and the other is inactive (Lyon, 1961; Russell, 1963: Gartler, 1976). Which chromosome remains active is determined by some random event, and it is decided at an early stage of development. Thus, the accumulation of X-linked somatic mutations would be the same for males and females.

4.2. Distinguishing Somatic Mutations from Errors

Physiological changes that have been shown to occur during mammalian aging have relied to a great extent on observations of the whole organism or tissue. In most cases, the reduced functional capacity observed with aging could not be explained by a loss in cellular elements. Reduced glucose tolerance and insulin output, for example, have not been accounted for by a concomitant loss of pancreatic beta cells. In an effort to discover molecular origin of decreased physiological function, gerontologists have concentrated on the fidelity of molecular components. The metabolic stability of DNA and the constant renewal of intracellular molecules (see Section 3) have led researchers to concentrate on examination of DNA and DNA-associated proteins. Unfortunately, only a few age-associated changes in chromatin have been reported, and the role of these changes in age-associated cellular decline has not been clarified (Hermann, 1975). Also, the sensitivity of methods that have been used to estimate DNA-associated changes has not been tested under conditions of induced life-shortening. This type of positive control is needed to demonstrate an ability to detect low levels of induced alterations. Techniques such as DNA hybridization may not be sensitive enough to detect mutation accumulated during aging.

Another way to examine DNA qualitatively is through analysis of proteins that are produced from the DNA template. If base-substitution mutations accumulate during aging, then the number of proteins containing an amino acid substitution would increase. To the extent that the mechanism of mutation is a general one (see Section 6), mutations should accumulate in most or all genes being expressed as well as those not being expressed. While amino acid substitutions should correlate with base substitutions, amino acid substitutions can arise as well from a reduced fidelity of the protein-synthetic apparatus. At the cellular level, however, mutational amino acid substitutions would be detected only in particular mutated cells, while amino acid substitutions resulting from an increase in the frequency of errors during translation or transcription would occur in essentially all cells, with the altered protein being at a much lower level than in mutant cells. This comparison can be illustrated in a model experiment designed to demonstrate the feasibility of measuring base substitutions in the hemoglobin molecules in several mammalian species (Popp *et al.*, 1978). Sheep of the *A/B* heterozygous hemoglobin genotype produce a type C hemoglobin during anemia. Only type C hemoglobin contains isoleucine, one residue in the β chain. Normal type A or B contains no genetically coded isoleucine. The reticulocyte that is synthesizing type C hemoglobin can be compared to a mutant cell in other species, including primates, cattle, and horses, in which the cell synthesizing isoleucine-containing hemoglobin represents a mutation to an isoleucine codon from another amino acid codon. Autoradiographs of isoleucine incorporated into reticulocytes in sheep *A/B* heterozygotes show a significant number of cells containing a high grain count, whereas no cells in reticulocyte preparations from sheep that do not produce the isoleucine-containing hemoglobin had high grain counts.

In estimating the frequency of amino acid substitutions by indirect methods, many experimenters have provided evidence for age-associated changes in the fidelity of protein synthesis (errors) that may have in fact resulted from accumulated somatic mutations. In those procedures that involve measurements properties of protein or enzyme obtained from whole tissue or pooled cells, the source of amino acid substitutions would be both mutations that had occurred in a few cells and errors taking place in all cells. This distinction can be further illustrated by considering the amino acid substitution of isoleucine for valine in the first position of rabbit β chain of hemoglobin. Transcriptional errors that would change the message coding from valine codons to isoleucine codons or transcriptional errors that would result from the insertion of isoleucyl tRNA in the tRNA–mRNA site at the ribosome or misacylation of valyl tRNA with isoleucine would be expected to occur at about the same frequency in most cells (illustrated as I appearing in occasional cells in Fig. 1). Mutational events that change the DNA coding of valine in the first position to isoleucine would yield a cell that contained isoleucine in half the β chain molecules (illustrated as cells containing equal numbers V's and I's). For substitutions that can take place by mutational events as well as errors, the total frequency of amino acid substitutions is the sum of errors occurring in most cells and mutations occurring in a few cells. Particular amino acid substitutions such as isoleucine for histidine cannot result from single base-substitution mutations, because the coding for these two amino acids differs by more than one base, and two base changes would be required for mutational events to cause isoleucine substitutions for histidines. By measuring the substitution of isoleucine for each amino acid at the amino terminus of highly purified hemoglobin α or β chains, one can classify isoleucine substitutions as being due to errors only—namely, those isoleucine replacements that cannot take place by single base changes in the DNA—and those substitutions that reflect the sum of both errors and mutations, which include those amino acids by triplets that can be mutated to isoleucine codons. One can expect that some lysine positions in the hemoglobin molecule will be coded by

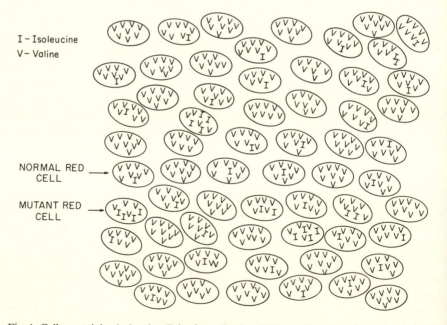

Fig. 1. Cells containing isoleucine (I) in place of valine (V) in position 1 in primate hemoglobin. Illustrated are cells produced by transcriptional errors (containing many V's and a single I) and cells produced by mutational events (containing equal numbers of V's and I's).

AAA and can thus be mutated to the isoleucine codon UAA, while other lysine positions may be coded UAG, which is not mutable to isoleucine codons by a single base change. Measurement of the substitution of isoleucine for lysine at many positions in the hemoglobin molecule after mutagenesis with base-substitution mutagens should show the frequency of isoleucine substitution for lysine to be higher for mutable lysine codons than for mutable lysine codons, and the difference in absolute frequency would be a reflection of the accumulated mutations. This particular example could be extended to other amino acid substitution pairs and to other proteins. Indications are that this procedure will eventually lead to a definitive resolution of the role of somatic base-substitution mutations in the processes of aging and the role of base-substitution mutations in the induction of cancer. The sequence-analysis method also provides information on the frequency of errors (nonmutable substitutions), and should provide conclusive evidence for or against the error theory of aging.

4.3. Base-Substitution Mutations

Base-substitution mutations have been suggested as the mechanism by which genetic variants of human hemoglobin arise. Over 90% of the substitutions of one amino acid for another can be accounted for by single base changes in the DNA (Ranney and Lehmann, 1974). During evolutionary divergence, hemoglobin sequences change more frequently by amino acid substitutions that can be explained by single base substitutions. While hemoglobin is the most-studied mammalian protein, it is assumed that mutations in other genes occur by the same mechanisms. Human hemoglobin genetic variants were most often identified by their clinical manifestations. In these cases, it is clear that the substitutions that were identified constitute a disturbance in the normal function of the organism. What is not known is whether any substitutions of one amino acid for another in a molecule such as hemoglobin will result in a product that does not distinctly decrease the function of the protein. The problem is one of definition, but also of magnitude. Are there truly neutral mutations? A neutral mutation is one in which there is no selective advantage or disadvantage of the old genotype vs. the new one. Alleles involving neutral mutations would be expected to exist in equal frequencies when sufficient time has passed after the formation of a new species for the mutant genotype to reach population equilibrium. Looking at the question from a different view, neutral mutations should accumulate in a population with time, since by definition there is no selective advantage of the progenitor genotype over the mutant one, and the excess level of progenitor genotype would undergo greater conversion to the neutral variant than the reverse. As a model of a potential neutral mutation, consider the substitution of the aliphatic amino acid isoleucine for other aliphatic amino acids—valine, leucine, or phenylalanine—in human adult hemoglobin, in which no coded isoleucine is normally found. If there were many neutral mutations of this type, one might anticipate that isoleucine would have been identified among some of more than 100 samples of human hemoglobin that have been analyzed, even though no special effort has been made to discover such variants. With the exception of a frameshift mutation, no isoleucine-containing adult human hemoglobin has been reported. This is not to say that examples of neutral mutations do not exist; some rabbit strains differ in the β chain by substitution of isoleucine for valine (Garrick *et al.,* 1974).

If many "neutral" mutations existed among mammals, the concern over some kinds of somatic base substitutions would be less than if "neutral" mutations were in fact rare. Somatic base substitutions are thought to be important because resulting amino acid substitutions alter the fidelity of enzymes and other functions that are of concern in the aging process. For the time being, we must assume that base-substitution mutations that result in amino acid changes in the protein product are not phenotypically neutral, since there exists very little sequence variation among members of a given species.

In the previous section, a theoretical method was presented to distinguish amino acid substitutions that would result from base substitutions from amino acid substitutions that would result from errors of transcription or translation. While the method has not been applied to young and old animals, it has been tested for the effect of radiation on the induction of specific amino acid changes. In particular, radiation increases the substitution of isoleucine for valine at position 1 of the rabbit β chain (valine) and position 7 (lysine, AAA coding) (Popp *et al.,* 1978) (see Table VII).

Table VII. Frequency of Substitution of Isoleucine for Coded Amino Acids

| Coded amino acid | Frequency of substitution ($\times 10^{-5}$) | | Mutable |
	Control	300 rad[a]	
1. Valine	1.6	28.0	Yes
2. Histidine	3.8	< 1.0	No
3. Leucine	0.9	1.0	Yes
4. Serine	2.0	< 1.0	Yes
5. Serine	3.7	1.5	Yes
6. Glutamic acid	0.9	6.3	No
7. Glutamic acid	3.6	5.0	No
8. Lysine	2.6	12.0	Yes

[a]150 rads exposure 14 and 11 days before assay (Popp *et al.,* 1978).

A more general method for estimating the contribution of mutations and errors was used to test the somatic mutation theory and error theory as those theories would be applied to human hemoglobin. The procedure involved chemical quantitation of trace quantities of isoleucine present in highly purified human hemoglobin. The purification scheme involved molecular sieve separation and serial rechromatography of carbonmonoxy hemoglobin, methemoglobin, and metcyanhemoglobin forms obtained from human peripheral blood. After globin preparation and hydrolysis, isoleucine was quantitated by preparative and quantitative ion-exchange chromatography methods. Verification that the isoleucine was present in hemoglobin and not in contaminating proteins was based on the recovery of isoleucine in separated α and β chains. Between the ages of 20 and 60, no significant increase in the average content of isoleucine was detected in highly purified hemoglobin (Popp *et al.,* 1976) (Fig. 2). Since isoleucine is not coded for genetically in either the α or the β chain of human hemoglobin, isoleucine incorporated would be expected to result from mutations in a few cells or a low level of errors in many cells, or both. The significance of the absence of an age-associated change in the sum of mutations and errors is demonstrated by the positive findings in radiation exposures. Persons who were exposed to radiation, especially when they were young, did have higher levels of isoleucine in their hemoglobin, even 20 years after the radiation exposure. The frequency of isoleucine substitution for the average amino acid in human hemoglobin is 30 per million. The frequency of substitution of isoleucine for particular amino acids in the rabbit hemoglobin β chain ranged from 1 to 100 per million (Loftfield and Vanderjagt, 1972). The sequence-analysis method of distinguishing errors from mutations that was applied to rabbit hemoglobin β chains should provide additional direct evidence to support the interpretation that neither somatic mutations nor errors increase with aging in human hemoglobin. By implication, other gene products in red cells and other mammalian cell lines that proliferate in the same manner as red cells should not accumulate mutations or errors during adult aging.

The low frequency of amino acid substitutions (such as that of isoleucine for leucine) indicates that the fidelity of translation and transcription is rather good in rabbit red cells. Since amino acid substitutions that result from base substitutions in the DNA yield abnormal proteins that are essentially the same as those that result from errors, experiments designed to test the error theory of aging may have at the same time provided evidence for or against the somatic mutation theory. Therefore, the observed increase in antigenically cross-reacting material present in the liver and muscle of old mice could be due to accumulation of enzymatically inactive aldolase either as a result of errors or as a result of mutations in a few cells. Changes in enzyme activity levels (Finch, C.E., 1972) or protein

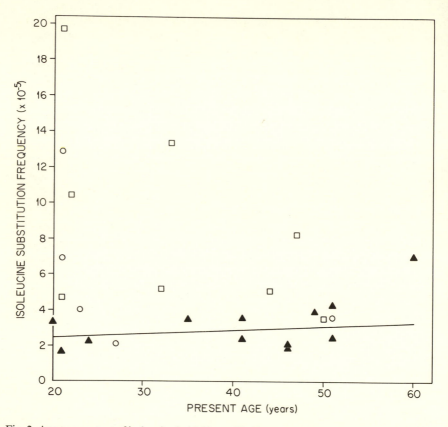

Fig. 2. Average content of isoleucine in highly purified human hemoglobin shown as a function of age at the time of assay for persons from the Marshall Islands who were unexposed (▲) or exposed to an estimated radiation dose of 69 (○) or 175 rads (□). Reproduced from Popp *et al.* (1976).

and RNA turnover could result from increased mutations as well as errors (Beauchene *et al.*, 1967; Comolli *et al.*, 1972; Menzies *et al.*, 1972). The same explanation can be applied to the alterations in the ethylation reactions and ethionine incorporation found in aging mouse tissues (Ogrodnik *et al.*, 1976). Other experimental results that may reflect mutational changes are listed in Table VIII. Special consideration should be given, however, to the suggestion that changes in the fidelity of components involved in DNA, RNA, or protein synthesis might originate from mutations. While cells may be able to tolerate a certain level of errors in these essential functions, it seems unlikely that a cell could survive if a mutation occurred in that cell such that a significant proportion of the total molecules involved in some essential step were defective. Whether a high level of errors causes cell death in mammals has not been conclusively determined (Del Monte, 1975).

To what extent is the constancy of DNA fidelity in hemoglobin from old humans representative of other gene products in other tissues? The answer to this question centers on the nature of cell proliferation in the hemotopoietic system and other replenishing tissues, and is concerned with the existence and characterization of stem cells (Cairns, 1975; Cameron, 1972a, Fliedner et al., 1970; Micklem and Ogden, 1976). Many investigators consider the hemotopoietic stem cell to be the cell that can clone in the spleen or bone marrow when transferred to an irradiated recipient (Schofield and Lajtha, 1976; Millard et al., 1973; Till and McCulloch, 1961). Thymidine killing studies indicate that some of these cells may be cell-division-arrested (G_0) cells. Experiments with busulfan, a drug that destroys nondividing cells (Millar et al., 1975; Dunn, 1974), suggest that the true stem cell is a slow- or noncycling cell that is a precusor to the cell that can produce colonies in transfer experiments. When rats were treated with busulfan and their hematopoietic systems were then repopulated with isologous bone marrow, they were able to survive more than 30 days. In

Table VIII. Aging Data Associated with Somatic Base Substitutions or Errors or Both

Supporting mutation accumulation or error increase	
Increase in enzymatically inactive mouse muscle aldolase (30%)	Gershon and Gershon (1973b)
Increase in enzymatically inactive mouse liver aldolase (50%)	Gershon and Gershon (1973a)
Increase in heat-labile glutathione reductase in aged human lens	Hardin (1973)
tRNA turnover differences in rat kidney spleen and liver	Menzies et al. (1972)
Increase in heat labile glucose-6-phosphate dehydrogenase in mouse tissues	Wulf and Cutler (1975)
Supporting fidelity in aged animals	
No difference in DNA polymerase heat lability	Barton and Yang (1975)
Only two differences in heterochronic charging reactions of aminoacyl tRNA by ligases	Frazer and Yang (1972)
No differences in leucine incorporation in place of phenylalanine in poly-U-stimulated protein synthesis	Kurtz (1975)
No age change in rat total-body methionine turnover rate	Mende and Viamonte (1965)
No age change in inactive molecules among six enzymes in human granulocytes	Rubinson et al. (1976)
No age change in RNA synthesis in nuclei from rat liver and brain	Gibas and Harman (1970)
No change in the extent of amino acid analogue incorporation in vivo in mouse liver, kidney, or brain	G. Hirsch et al. (1976)

contrast, other rats receiving as much as 50 times the amount of marrow necessary to allow 30-day survival with normal marrow could not be sustained 30 days by marrow from busulfan-treated donors. The level of cells capable of producing spleen colonies was reduced only twofold by the drug treatment. The interpretation of this experimental data is that the hemopoietic stem cell has characteristics that distinguish it from the cell that can produce spleen colonies. In mice, treatment 4 times with busulfan results in aplastic anemia, a condition that might be expected to result if these animals had only a limited number of stem cells (Morley *et al.*, 1975). The disparity between the number of colony-forming cells (CFC) and 30-day survival with busulfan treatment puts a different light on young/old comparisons of bone marrow capacity among mouse strains. While the number of CFC did not differ among many strains of young and old mice (Davis *et al.*, 1971), the longevity conferred by old donor marrow on young mice after transplantation was reduced in some genetic stocks (Harrison, 1975; Ogden and Micklem, 1976). CFC are recovered after busulfan treatment or X-rays, but only with a doubling time of about 6 days. To the extent that the hematopoietic stem cell is a long-lived, cell-division-arrested progenitor, the accumulation of mutations would compare with that in other nondividing cell types. Split neutron-dose experiments that result in selective killing of spermatogonia 16–24 hr after the first treatment suggest a similarity between hematopoietic and spermatogonial systems of cell division (de Ruiter-Bootsma *et al.*, 1976). Noncycling stem cells are also indicated in the small intestine (Withers, 1975; Withers and Elkind, 1969; Withers *et al.*, 1974). A slow rate of recovery of spermatogonial stem cells after X-ray treatment is also suggested by the lack of additivity at high split-dose exposures in translocation induction until 6 weeks or longer after the first treatment (Lyon and Cox, 1975*a,b*). Gelfant and Smith (1972) proposed that aging results from an increase in noncycling cells.

4.4. Germinal vs. Somatic Mutations

The somatic mutation theory of aging attributes the decline in physical function to loss of genes or alteration in the gene products. Because germinal cells do not contribute to the essential physiological functions, the word *somatic* is usually attached to the mutation theory of aging. Germinal cells are subjected to the same physiological changes and the same environmental effects as the somatic cells, although some transport differences exist among tissues. The proliferative nature and terminal differentiation of spermatogonia are in many ways similar to those of cells of the hemopoietic system. The absence of DNA synthesis in oogonia throughout the life span of an adult makes possible comparisons between this germ-cell type and postmitotic cells. The major difference that may be expected to exist between somatic mutations and germinal mutations is the selection that operates during development whereby a given mutation may be lethal to one organism but not lethal even to cells in another animal containing that same genetic change.

The effect of aging on mutations and chromosome alterations in these germ-cell populations is discussed in Chapter 8 (see also Vogel and Rathenberg, 1976). In the case of chromosomal interchanges, X-ray-dose–response relationships are similar for leukocytes and spermatogonia in mice and hamsters (Brewen and Preston, 1973). Base-substitution mutations in hemoglobin genes are thought to result from radiation exposure in somatic cells (see Section 4.3), but similar mutations were not recovered among 8000 progeny of mice treated with X rays (Russell *et al.*, 1976).

The fidelity of DNA polymerase and thereby the spontaneous mutation rate may be influenced by two factors: (1) the need to generate new phenotypes on which evolutionary selections can operate to allow animal species to change and survive new environmental conditions (Anderson and King, 1970) and (2) a selective advantage for individuals having a high-fidelity polymerase that causes fewer defective progeny, an energy-saving feature. The same forces may be operating at the somatic level in the form of (1) a need to generate antibody diversity by base-substitution mutations in the variable region of antibody molecules and (2) the advantage of a high-fidelity polymerase to take accurate copies of genes to progeny cells during development. If somatic mutations play an important role in aging, then long-lived species might be expected to perform more accurate replication. How selective forces govern and control the fidelity of DNA replication, including DNA polymerase and repair functions, depends on whether somatic requirements are more stringent than germinal ones or vice versa.

An approach to understanding how selective forces act on genes that influence longevity for various species (Juncker, 1971; Williams, 1957; Willson, 1971) can be gained from an analysis of survival in the wild (Charlesworth, 1973). Extensive survival data are available for the Pacific mackerel, which can serve as an example of this analysis. This survival is shown in Fig. 3 for the actual number of fish caught commercially in the age range 2–5 years (Fitch, 1951). The data shown for the age distribution of older fish, 5–9 years, are taken from a summary of all ear bones that were aged during the years 1939–1945. The sampling procedures used to estimate the total population were based on representative size classes, and since the older fish are slightly larger, there is a small bias to the older portion of the age distribution. Because the probability of survival drops exponentially for these fish, death seems to be a random event. The same interpretation can be made from survival data for several other species in the wild (Table IX) (see also Pucek and Lowe, 1973).

Genes that allow survival to greater ages gain in frequency; i.e.,

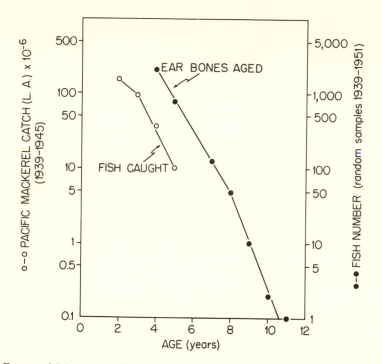

Fig. 3. Exponential decrease in life span with aging in the wild for Pacific mackerel caught by commercial fishermen in the Los Angeles–New Port area off the Southern California coast during the years 1939–1945. The actual number of fish estimated is shown for the age range 2–5 years (○). The distribution of fish of advanced age is shown from the summary of all ear bones (otoliths) aged, and the data (●) are not corrected for small differences in sampling that resulted from the fact that the average size of older fish increases 2% per year.

selection operates against those genes that cause the animal to die or otherwise fail to reproduce (see Chapter 6) (Cutler, 1976; Hamilton, 1966). Under the environmental condition of exponential survival in the wild, presumably due to random predation, an equilibrium occurring among genotypes is established only when the spontaneous mutation rate from the more favored genotype to the next less favored one just equals the selective advantage of the more favored form. In the example of the pacific mackerel, the selective advantage of genes conferring longevity to 10 years of age over that permitting 9-year longevity is 0.1%. The frequency of alleles that exist in equilibrium but limit life span to shorter times declines exponentially. Nevertheless, the majority of fish hatched will possess the genetic capacity to reach that age that is the balance point between (1) selective advantage at the extreme of survival allowed by predation and (2)

Table IX. Species That Exhibit Random Survival in the Wild

Species	Age interval examined[a]	Reference
Field mouse *(Apodemus sylvaticus)*	(12 months)	Ashby (1967)
Field mouse *(Clethrionomys glareolus)*	(12 months)	Ashby (1967)
Vole *(Microtus agrestis)*	(12 months)	Ashby (1967)
Lizard *(Amphibolurus)*	4 years	Bradshaw (1971)
Kangaroo rat *(Dipodomys)*	5 years	French *et al.* (1967)
Pocket mouse *(Perognathus)*	5 years	French *et al.* (1967)
Pocket mouse *(Perognathus formosus)*	—	French *et al.* (1974)
Pocket mouse *(Perognathus parvus)*	5 years	O'Farrell *et al.* (1975)
Coyote	9 years	Knowlton (1972)
Coyote	9 years	Nellis and Keith (1976)

[a]Exponential survival for mixed-age population shown in parentheses.

the force of spontaneous mutations. Parenthetically, the suggestion that fish age because they cease to grow should be translated to say that fish stop growing at the same time that their numbers in the wild are depleted by predation. The correlation between growth cessation and aging is that selection operates to favor growth and longevity, but only to an age related to the statistical probability of survival of a small percentage of the initial population. Of those fish that reach 2 years of age, only 600 of one million are alive 7 years later. Selection for longevity would suggest that most fish will attain this advanced age when kept in captivity. The influence that mutations might have on the balance point between mutational forces and selective forces may be judged by a knowledge of the longevity of a similar population maintained in a protected environment, where aging parameters associated with limiting longevity among other species would become apparent.

Comparisons of the fidelity of DNA polymerase among short- and long-lived mammals would provide some evidence to favor either the selective advantage of accurate DNA replication in development or the requirements of a low level of spontaneous mutations among progeny. Since large mammals accrue only 10 more cell divisions during development than smaller ones (1000 times more cells), the level of mutations accumulated during development would be only 20% greater in the larger longer-lived species. Alternative explanations for evolutionary effects are discussed in Chapter 6.

5. Mutagens, Carcinogens, Cancer, and Aging

5.1. Age-Associated Incidence of Cancer in Man and Other Mammals

One of the most startling aspects of modern biomedical science is the lack of recognition among professionals in the field of cancer research of the explicit relationship of aging and cancer. There is support for but a few research programs on the natural aging mechanisms, the understanding of which might contribute to a resolution of the etiology of cancer. That an elderly person is more likely to be diagnosed as having cancer after exploratory surgery is common knowledge. What is not appreciated is the dramatic and logarithmic increase in the probability of death from cancer in older persons (Doll, 1968; Lilienfeld et al., 1972; Smith G. S., et al., 1973). With a few exceptions, it can be said with certainty that cancer is a disease of "old age."

This logarithmic increase in cancer deaths with aging has been translated into several models of sequential molecular events. The somatic mutation hypothesis of cancer induction predicts either that a sequential series of 4–6 mutations in a single cell will result in that cell becoming cancerous or that single mutations in 4–6 individual cells that interact in a regulatory manner will allow the expression of the cancerous state. From a log/log plot of the curve, Incidence = constant X (age)^n, a nearly linear relationship between cancer incidence and age is obtained. The value of n between 4 and 6 that fits cancer-incidence data includes tumors originating in many tissues: esophagus, stomach, pancreas, bladder, rectum, colon, mouth, pharynx, and kidney. Other models involve promoters that accentuate the growth of tumors after the initial mutational event (Boutwell, 1974).

The mathematical treatment of cancer death rates has been used to predict the mechanisms that might be used to explain the cancer death data (Cook et al., 1969; Knudson et al., 1973). Some tissues show little or no increase in cancer frequencies with human aging. There are also tissues, such as the small intestine, that might be expected to yield a high level of cancer because of environmental insults, that have a cancer incidence rate a hundredfold less than comparable tissue in the stomach or colon (Lilienfeld et al., 1972).

5.2. Mutagenicity of Chemical Carcinogens

Support for the somatic mutation hypothesis of cancer has come from the demonstration that chemicals that induce cancer in experimental animals cause mutations in various test systems (Hitachi et al., 1975; Sirover and Loed, 1974). Radiation was the original mutagenic agent that was used to support the somatic mutation hypothesis (Mayneord and Clark, 1975). Much of the mutational data that show positive tests for carcinogens are derived from bacterial test systems, or tissue culture cells, in which activation of some chemicals to mutagenic metabolites is accomplished by the addition of mammalian tissue fractions (Ames *et al.,* 1973; Sugimura *et al.,* 1976).

While strong correlations have been established between carcinogens and mutagenesis in particular test systems, other mutagen assays may not be predictive to carcinogenesis. Also, not all mutagenic compounds produce cancer when administered to test animals (Philips and Sternberg, 1975). Certainly the types and levels of DNA-repair enzymes influence the carcinogenicity of particular compounds (Stich, 1974; Trosko and Chang, 1976; Frei and Venitt, 1975). The dose-administration procedure can also influence the inducibility of cancer (Beebe and Kato, 1975). To the extent that tumors arise from cell types with varying rates of cell turnover, the selectivity of particular mutagens or carcinogens may reside in the relative mutagenicity of chemicals for nondividing as opposed to dividing cells (Deschner and Bertalanffy, 1972).

Chemical- and radiation-induced carcinogenesis is influenced by aging processes almost as extensively as the spontaneously occurring cancers in man and other mammals. Cancer induction usually involves rather long periods of time between the application of the carcinogen and the appearance of tumors (Schmähl, 1975; Newberne *et al.,* 1966; Kleihues *et al.,* 1976). To further understanding of the molecular mechanisms by which chemicals produce tumors, changes that result from the treatment should occur in the same time frame as the period of latency between chemical application and the appearance of the tumor. When tumors are transplanted, their growth and spread are relatively rapid, and the time interval from transplant to death occurs is short relative to the period of latency between carcinogen treatment and the original tumor appearance. It is unlikely that latency can be explained on the basis of the time required for a mutated cell to divide enough times to produce a cell mass that can be detected as a tumor. Furthermore, in chemical and radiation carcinogenesis, higher dose results in a shorter latency between treatment and appearance of tumors.

Among species with different longevities, the latency of cancer induction for a given dose of radiation relates to a percentage of the total life span of that species, rather than to a given absolute period of time. This enigma is demonstrated dramatically by Dawe's comparison of the target size of a whale with that of a mouse for the induction of tumors based on the notion that a mutation in a given cell causes the production of a tumor (Dawe, 1969). The number of cells at risk in the blue whale is equal to the number in

3 million mice. Using the frequency of tumors present in mice after 3 years, Dawe calculated that the whale should have 100,000 tumors at 1 year of age. Species differences in the kinds and levels of DNA-repair enzymes could be used to explain the differences in latency among species in cancer induction to the extent that a given dose of chemical would produce much less permanent DNA damage in the long-lived species.

Several explanations for latency have been given. In terms of the somatic mutation theory, it is proposed that radiation or chemical treatment causes one or two of several mutations required to produce the cancerous state, and that the latent period is required for the spontaneous occurrence of the remaining somatic mutations. The higher the dose, the more mutations induced by the treatment and the shorter the latent period required for the remainder of the somatic mutations to occur.

Another favored explanation for latency involves the role of the immune system. It is suggested that mutations occur all the time during adult life, and that the immune surveillance system removes the aberrant cells as they arise. The appearance of tumors in old animals results from the failure of the immune system to recognize or remove these mutant cells. Latency of tumor induction in this model could be explained by an accelerated decline of the immune system such that failure of the immune system occurs at an earlier date. The role of the aging immune system in cancer induction is not consistent with the near-normal life span of the immunoincompetent "nude" mouse (Holland, 1977), when this mouse has been maintained in a germ-free environment. An innate genetic origin of spontaneous tumors is indicated from allophenic mouse experiments (Condamine et al., 1971). When blastocysts of a high- and a low-incidence hepatoma strain were fused and allowed to age, there arose in the old animals tumors that were predominantly of the high-tumor-incidence parent. If the immune system were responsible for the prevention of tumor induction, the immunocytes of the lower-incidence strain should have prevented the expression of tumors of the high-strain origin to the same extent as tumors of the low-strain origin, in the absence of interactive effects.

Other explanations for cancer induction involve alterations in the expression of regulatory proteins such as contact-inhibition repressors (Nery, 1976; McKinnell et al., 1969). These models cannot provide a detailed explanation for the latent period because of the lack of knowledge about mechanisms of cell-division control and gene-expression control. For these control mechanisms to be applicable, the changes in regulatory molecules should take place over the time period between carcinogen exposure and appearance of tumors. The regulatory proteins that might be altered by chemical mutagens could be expected to have a slow turnover. Turnover should be slower in long-lived species. Alternatively, the argument of multiple-step processes might be applied such that several controlling elements must be affected. A given carcinogen treatment is likely to affect only a few of the elements during a particular treatment.

Latency of cancer induction could also be explained simply by cell loss in those systems that have regulatory controls over cell division and growth. This model might include the "chalone" model, since the idea of feedback control components regulating growth control is well established. It differs from the cancer model of Bullough (1975) in the sense that the quality and quantity of chalone are adequate when considered on a cellular basis. Latency could be explained in the model through the loss of regulatory control dependent on decrease in cells that produce cell-division repressors. A dose of chemical carcinogen that results in the loss through death of a percentage of cells would shorten the period of time remaining before some critical low level of chalone production occurred. This model does not require multiple mutations or alterations in the regulatory proteins, but in fact could explain why mutagens result in cancer induction long after the chemical treatment. At high acute exposures, most mutagens kill cells, so that a cell-loss mechanism would be consistent with the carcinogen and mutagenic correlations. Since cells can be killed by other mechanisms, cancer induction might be expected to result from treatments that are clearly not mutagenic.

6. Special Genetic Mechanisms of Aging

In Sections 4.1 and 4.2, the evidence and arguments concerning the accumulation of somatic mutations during aging were discussed. Chromosome aberrations, base substitutions, and frameshift mutations are the major types of mutations that influence the availability of information or character of information fidelity. Other genetic mechanisms of aging must be considered for those genetic characteristics of cells and organisms that might contribute to the processes of aging. An example of a special genetic mechanism is that proposed by Strehler (1971), who suggested that aging results from the loss of ribosomal and other multiple-copy tandem cistrons (containing internal complementarity), due to DNA strand shifts and removal of nonpaired strands. This model proposes that where multiple copies of genes exist in a tandem arrangement, the opposite strands of the DNA can pair out of register, leaving one copy on each strand as a single-stranded sequence of DNA. Since single-stranded DNA is more susceptible to endonuclease cleavage and exonuclease degradation than the duplex DNA, these single-stranded regions have an increased probability of being removed by DNAse activity. Experimental data supporting age-associated loss of ribosomal cistrons have been obtained for human autopsy heart tissue, for tissues from dogs (Johnson and Strehler, 1972), and for very old mice. Cutler (1978), however, provided data that suggest that the decreased level of hybridization that occurs in DNA obtained from very old donors (Gaubatz *et al.,* 1976) is due, not to the loss of DNA coding for the ribosomal RNA, but rather to residual protein bound to those regions of DNA that code for the ribosomal DNA. Either mechanism, cistron loss or increased protein cross-linking, could reduce the availability of ribosomal RNA and slow the rate of protein synthesis. Age changes in the level of protein synthesis have not been demonstrated; hence, decreased ribosomal RNA production does not seem to be limiting in old animals. To the extent that the decrease in level of hybridization of ribosomal RNA to DNA is representative of loss or damage to other genes that are tandemly repeated in the genome, this mechanism of somatic genetic change may be significant. For example, tRNAs are also tandemly repeated in the mammalian genome, but there are fewer copies for each of the tRNA genes than there are for ribosomal RNA. The role of redundancy of genetic information as a protective mechanism in aging was proposed by Cutler (1974).

A special variation of the somatic mutation theory is the proposal by Yielding (1974) that the primary mechanism of somatic mutation involves damage to DNA regions not normally transcribed. He proposes that damage accumulates preferentially in these regions due to their decreased availability to repair enzymes. The effect of mutations in the inactive genes is to disrupt replication and the replenishment of cells.

Burch (1976) proposed a unique kind of somatic mutation that causes the induction of autoaggressive diseases including cancer. This mutation may be of the classic types discussed in previous sections, but causes the strand of DNA that is not normally used for transcription to serve as a template for the synthesis of RNAs that are then translated into proteins. Furthermore, the sites or genes in the DNA that contribute to the autoaggressive gene products include those involved in immune recognition (histocompatibility loci). His model presumes that the conformation of proteins that are produced from the opposite strands that normally serve as the template for transcription will bear structural similarity to the gene product that is produced from the normally transcribed DNA strands. The DNA regions involved consist of a family of repeated and inverted sequences (palindromic sequences). This model is based on observations that cell-surface mutations, especially those involved in transplantation rejection, mutate much more frequently than do other genes.

Another specialized theory of somatic mutation accumulation should be included in this discussion, although the theory has not been specifically stated. Much of the discussion of somatic mutations involves the accumulation of mutation through the errors of replication in dividing-cell types. The somatic mutation mechanism of cancer induction involves the accumulation of mutations in cell types that can or do regularly divide, since few tumors originate among "fixed" post mitotic cells such as neurons. The model of mutation induction through cell division is based on the hypothesis that the stem cells of dividing-cell types are regularly in division. Experimental results discussed in Section 4.3 suggest that stem cells are normally in a resting state, but this is not a general opinion. Thus, the mechanisms of mutation accumulation among dividing cells may have little relevance to mammalian aging. In contrast to the lack of cell division and DNA replication in adult tissues, the DNA of mitochondria undergo replication continuously during aging, even in nondividing cells (Fletcher and Sanadi, 1961). Hence, the mitochondrial genome may be only genetic material subject to the accumulation of mutations that arise independent of cell division, but by mechanisms similar to those that occur in replicating cells. The mitochondrial genome contains information for mitochondrial ribosomes, mitochondrial tRNAs, and a few other proteins. Elements involved in information fidelity are especially vulnerable to degeneration in the mitochondrial genome. Mitochondrial function has been tested during aging in rats with no significant loss in extent or control of oxidative phosphorylation. If there is any relationship between the mitochondrial protein-synthetic apparatus and that of the cytoplasm, such as mitochondrial tRNA functioning in cytoplasmic protein synthesis, then a loss in fidelity of the transfer tRNAs would influence the fidelity of nonmitochondrial constituents; otherwise, mitochondrial mutation would affect only mitochondrial function (Kurtz, 1974). An additional problem involves the magnitude of mutation accumulation that might occur during the life span of an animal. In mice, the total number of mitochondrial DNA replications would be less than 200 (7-days half-life), and the extent of additional mutations above this number that might be involved in development is about fourfold (50 cell divisions seems a good estimate for the number of divisions involved in production of particular organs containing 10^{15} cells).

The correlations that exist between the longevity of both male and female progeny and the longevity of the mother (but independently of the father's longevity) support a role for the mitochondrial genome in aging (Jalavisto, 1951). Since the mitochondrial genome is derived solely from genetic information in the egg, mitochondrial genetic characteristics that affect longevity would be expected to correspond between the mother and both sons and daughters (Dawid and Blackler, 1972).

7. Summary

New support for the somatic mutation hypothesis of aging has been obtained in recent years from the correlations that exist between the cancer-inducing nature of chemicals and their mutagenic effects. The mutagenic extrapolation to a primary mechanism of aging derives from the overwhelming occurrence of cancer among older persons, which amounts to a logarithmic increase in probability of death from cancer in human populations. Validation of this hypothesis of mutational cancer etiology can be expected to result from test systems that measure somatic mutations *in vivo,* especially in the target tissue for a given carcinogenic protocol. One such system, utilizing the hemoglobin molecule as an end point, measures base-substitution mutations and errors. The accurate synthesis of hemoglobin in older humans indicates an absence of accumulated somatic mutations, especially as contrasted with elevated amino acid substitutions in persons exposed to radiation 20 years before these measurements.

The rather accurate synthesis of proteins allows the estimation of somatic base substitutions among molecules derived from bulk tissue or populations of cells. Thus, age-associated changes that were thought to arise from an increase in the level of errors might demonstrate instead accumulated mutations. By measuring the substitution of one amino acid for others sequentially in a particular protein, a distinction can be made between those changes that might arise through errors in translation or transcription and those that would result from base substitutions as well as errors. The application of similar methods to various protein products in different species during aging and after mutation induction with chemical carcinogens should provide definitive resolution to the question of the role of somatic mutations as well as errors in the mechanisms of aging and carcinogenesis.

Measurement of the fidelity of cellular DNA replication among long- and short-lived species, i.e., species comparisons of spontaneous mutation rates, should provide some answers as to the relative selective pressures governing DNA polymerase fidelity. The mutation rate influences the balance point among alleles that determine various longevities that can be obtained in the laboratory. Equilibrium is expected for species subject to predation at an age near that of the very few long-lived survivors that occur in the wild. Genetic determinants for longevity will predominate for an age at which a fixed level of survivorship occurs in the wild if long- and short-lived species have similar spontaneous mutation rates. On the other hand, if somatic mutation accumulation by replication errors is important in aging, long-lived species would be expected to have a lower level of spontaneous mutations.

The significance of mutations in dividing cells to aging processes depends to a large degree on the nature of cellular proliferation. Selective killing of progenitor cells to the hemopoietic stem cell, a cell that can form clones in the spleens of irradiated recipients, suggests that somatic mutation accumulation by cell-division mechanisms may not be applicable in mammals. Experimental evidence indicates that noncycling stem cells may exist in the testis and in the crypts of the small intestine. If hemoglobin production in old persons is a product of clones originating from progenitors that remained in an arrested state during most of adult life, then base-substitution mutation might reflect age-associated changes in other normally nondividing cells.

In contrast to the noncycling state of some stem cells and to the preponderance of nondividing cells in the adult mammal is the continuous replication of the mitochondrial genome. Thus, the mitochondrial genome is especially susceptible to mutation accumulation through replication error mechanisms. Other specialized theories that have been proposed to explain aging include loss of ribosomal tRNA and similar tandemly repeated genes, the lack of repair lesions induced in the inactive portions of the genome, and mutation accumulation in certain genes such as histocompatibility genes, which might cause autoaggressive diseases including cancer. Nongenetic models of cancer induction can in some cases explain the latency of cancer induction and late onset of spontaneous cancer as effectively as the somatic mutation models.

References

Akeson, A., Ehrenstein, G. V., Hevesy, G., and Theorell, H., 1960, Life-span of myoglobin, *Arch. Biochem. Biophys.* **91:**310–318.

Amano, M., Lebond, C. P., and Nadler, N. J., 1965, Radioautographic analysis of nuclear RNA in mouse cells revealing three pools with different turnover times, *Exp. Cell Res.* **38:**314–340.

Ames, B. N., Durston, W. E., Yamasaki, E., and Lee, F. D., 1973, Carcinogens are mutagens: A sample test system combining liver homogenates for activation and bacteria for detection, *Proc. Natl. Acad. Sci. U.S.A.* **70:**2281–2285.

Anderson, W. W., and King, C. E., 1970, Age-specific selection, *Proc. Natl. Acad. Sci. U.S.A.* **66:**780–786.

Arias, I. M., Doyle, D., and Schimke, R. T., 1969, Studies on the synthesis and degradation of proteins of the endoplasmic reticulum of the rat, *J. Biol. Chem.* **244:**3303–3315.

Ashby, K. R., 1967, Studies on the ecology of field mice and voles (*Apodemus sylvaticus, Clethrionomys glareolus,* and *Microtus agrestis*) in Houghall Wood, Durham, *J. Zool.* **152:**389–513.

Awa, A. A., 1975, Chromosome aberrations in somatic cells, *J. Radiat. Res. Suppl.,* pp. 122–131.

Barton, R. W., and Yang, W.-K., 1975, Low molecular weight DNA polymerase: Decreased activity in spleens of old BALB/c mice, *Mech. Aging Dev.* **4:**123–136.

Beattie, D. S., Basford, R. E., and Koritz, S. B., 1967, The turnover of protein components of mitochondria from rat liver, kidney and brain, *J. Biol. Chem.* **242:**4584–4586.

Beauchene, R. E., Roeder, L. M., and Barrows, Jr., C. H., 1967, The effect of age and of ethionine feeding on the ribonucleic acid and protein synthesis of rats, *J. Gerontol.* **22:**318.

Beebe, G. W., and Kato, H., 1975, Cancers other than leukemia, *J. Radiat. Res. Suppl.,* pp. 97–107.

Bernhard, H. P., 1976, The control of gene expression in somatic cell hybrids, *Int. Rev. Cytol.* **47:**289–325.

Blobel, G., and Potter, V. R., 1968, Distribution of radioactivity between the acid-soluble pool and the pools of RNA in the nuclear, non-sedimentable and ribosomal fractions of rat liver after a single injection of labelled orotic acid, *Biochim. Biophys. Acta* **166:**48–57.

Bondy, S. C., 1966, Ribonucleic acid metabolism of the brain, *J. Neurochem.* **13:**955–959.

Boutwell, R. K., 1974, The function and mechanism of promoters of carcinogenesis, in: *CRC Critical Reviews in Toxicology,* pp. 419–443, Chemical Rubber Co., Cleveland.

Bradshaw, S. D., 1971, Growth and mortality in a field population of *Amphibolurus* lizards exposed to seasonal cold and aridity, *J. Zool.* **165:**1–25.

Brewen, J. G., and Preston, R. J., 1973, Chromosomal interchanges induced by radiation in spermatogonial cells and leukocytes of mouse and Chinese hamster, *Nature (London) New Biol.* **244:**111–113.

Brooks, A. L., Mead, D. K., and Peters, R. F., 1973, Effect of aging on the frequency of metaphase chromosome aberrations in the liver of Chinese hamsters, *J. Gerontol.* **28:**452–454.

Buchanan, D. L., 1961, Total carbon turnover measured by feeding a uniformly labelled diet, *Arch. Biochem. Biophys.* **94:**500–511.

Bullough, W. S., 1975, Chalones and cancer, in: *Host Defense Against Cancer and Its Potentiation,* (D. Mizuno *et al.,* eds.), pp. 317–335, University Park Press, Baltimore.

Burch, P. R. J., 1976, *The Biology of Cancer: A New Approach,* University Park Press, Baltimore.

Burnet, F. M., 1974, *Intrinsic Mutagenesis: A Genetic Approach to Aging,* John Wiley & Sons, New York.

Cairns, J., 1975, Mutation selection and the natural history of cancer, *Nature (London)* **255:**197–200.

Cameron, I. L., 1972a, Minimum number of cell doublings in an epithelial cell population during the life-span of the mouse, *J. Gerontol.* **27:**157–161.

Cameron, I. L., 1972b. Cell proliferation and renewal in aging mice, *J. Gerontol.* **27:**162–172.

Charlesworth, B., 1973, Selection in populations with overlapping generations. V. Natural selection and life histories, *Am. Nat.* **107:**303–311.

Comolli, R., Ferioli, M. E., and Azzola, S., 1972, Protein turnover of the lysosomal and mitochondrial fractions of rat liver during aging, *Exp. Gerontol.* **7:**369–376.

Condamine, H., Custer, R. P., and Minzt, B., 1971, Pure-strain and genetically mosaic liver tumors histochemically identified with the β-glucuronidase marker in allophenic mice, *Proc. Natl. Acad. Sci. U.S.A.* **68:**2032–2036.

Cook, P. J., Doll, R., and Fellingham, S. A., 1969, A mathematical model for the age distribution of cancer in man, *Int. J. Cancer* **4:**93–112.

Crowley, C., and Curtis, H. J., 1963, The development of somatic mutations in mice with age, *Proc. Natl. Acad. Sci. U.S.A.* **49:**626–628.

Curtis, H. J., 1966, *Biological Mechanisms of Aging,* Charles C. Thomas, Springfield, Illinois.

Cutler, R. G., 1974, Redundancy of information content in the genome of mammalian species as a protective mechanism determining aging rate, *Mech. Aging Dev.* **2:**381–408.

Cutler, R. G., 1975, On the nature of aging and life maintenance processes, in: *Interdisciplinary Topics in Gerontology,* Vol. 9 (H. P. von Hahn, ed.), pp. 88–133, S. Karger, Basel.

Cutler, R. G., 1976, Cross-linkage hypothesis of aging: DNA adducts in chromatin as a primary aging process, in: *Aging, Carcinogenesis and Radiation Biology: The Role of Nucleic Acid Addition Reactions* (K. C. Smith, ed.), pp. 443–492, Plenum Press, New York.

Cutler, R. G., 1978, Alterations with age in the informational storage and flow systems of the mammalian cell, in: *Genetics and Aging* (D. Harrison, ed.), National Foundation March of Dimes, Philadelphia (in press).

Cuzner, M. L., Davison, A. N., and Gregson, N. A., 1966, Turnover of brain mitochondrial lipids, *Biochem. J.* **101**:618–626.

Davis, M. L., Upton, A. C., and Scatterfield, L. C., 1971, Growth and senescence of the bone marrow stem cell pool in RFM/Un mice, *Proc. Soc. Exp. Biol. Med.* **137**:1452–1458.

Davison, A. N., 1961, Metabolically inert proteins of the central and peripheral nervous system muscle and tendon, *Biochem. J.* **78**:272–281.

Davison, A. N., 1962, The physiological role of cerebron sulphuric acid (sulfate) in the brain, *Biochem. J.* **85**:558–568.

Davison, A. N., and Dobbing, J., 1960, Phospholipid metabolism in nervous tissue. II. Metabolic stability, *Biochem. J.* **75**:565–570.

Davison, A. N., and Gregson, N. A., 1966, Metabolism of cellular membrane sulfolipids in rat brain, *Biochem. J.* **98**:915–922.

Dawe, C. T., 1969, Neoplasms and related disorders of invertebrate and lower vertebrate animals, National Cancer Institute Monograph No. 31, U.S. Department of Health, Education and Welfare.

Dawid, I. B., and Blacker, A. W., 1972, Maternal and cytoplasmic inheritance of mitochondrial DNA in *Xenopus, Dev. Biol.* **29**:152–161.

Del Monte, U., 1975, Altered patterns of aminoacyl-tRNA synthetases in tumors (and their possible significance), in: *Cell Biology and Tumor Immunology: Proceedings of the XIth International Cancer Congress,* Vol. 1, (P. Bucalossi, U. Veronesi, and N. Cascinelli, eds.), pp. 89–94, American Elsevier, New York.

de Ruiter-Bootsma, A. L., Kramer, M. F., de Rooij, D. G., and Davids, J. A. G., 1976, Response of stem cells in the mouse testis to fission neutrons of 1 MeV mean energy and 300 kV X-rays, Methodology, dose–response studies, relative biological effectiveness, *Radiat. Res.* **67**:56–58.

Deschner, E. E., and Bertalanffy, F. D., 1972, Mitotic indexes: Mammalian and amphibian tissues, in: *Biology Data Book,* Vol. 1 (P. L. Altman and D. S. Dittmer, eds.), pp. 119–125, Federation of American Societies for Experimental Biology, Bethesda, Maryland.

DiBerardino, M. A., and King, T. J., 1965, Transplantation of nuclei from the frog renal adenocarcinoma. II. Chromosomal and histologic analysis of tumor nuclear-transplant embryos, *Dev. Biol.* **11**:217–242.

DiBerardino, M. A., and King, T. J., 1967, Development and cellular differentiation of neural nuclear-transplants of known karyotype, *Dev. Biol.* **15**:102–128.

Doll, R., 1968, The age distribution of cancer in man, in: *Cancer and Aging* (A. Engel and T. Larsson, eds.), pp. 15–36, Nordiska Bokhandelns Forlag, Stockholm.

Dunn, C. D. R., 1974, The chemical and biological properties of busulfan (Myleran), *Exp. Hematol.* **2**:101–117.

Finch, C. E., 1972, Enzyme activities, gene function and ageing in mammals, *Exp. Gerontol.* **7**:53–67.

Finch, S. C., and Beebe, G. W., 1975, Aging, *J. Radiat. Res. Suppl.,* pp. 108–121.

Fitch, J. E., 1951, Age composition of the Southern California catch of Pacific Mackerel, 1939–40 through 1950–51, Fish Bulletin 83, State of California Department of Fish and Game.

Fletcher, M. J., and Sanadi, D. R., 1961, Turnover of rat liver mitochondria, *Biochim. Biophys. Acta* **51**:356–360.

Fliedner, T. M., Hass, R. J., and Blattmann, H., 1970, The significance of "resting" cell populations for hematopoietic regeneration after ionizing radiation or application of radiomimetic substances, *Adv. Radiat. Res.* **2**:707–739.

Frazer, J. M., and Yang, W.-K, 1972, Isoaccepting transfer ribonucleic acids in liver and brain of young and old BC3F$_1$ mice, *Arch. Biochem. Biophys.* **153**:610–618.

Frei, J. V., and Venitt, S., 1975, Chromosome damage in the bone marrow of mice treated with the methylating agents methyl methanesulphonate and *N*-methyl-*N*-nitrosourea in the presence or absence of caffeine, and its relationship with thymoma induction, *Mutat. Res.* **29**:89–96.

French, N. R., Bernardo, G. M., and Aschwanden, A. P., 1967, Life spans of *Dipodomys* and *Perognathus* in the Mojave Desert, *J. Mammal.* **48:**537–548.

French, N. R., Maza, B. G., Hill, H. O., Aschwanden, A. P., and Kaaz, H. W., 1974, A population study of irradiated desert rodents, *Ecol. Monogr.* **44:**45–72.

Gahrton, G., Lindsten, J., and Zech, L., 1974, Clonal origin of the Philadelphia chromosome from either the paternal or the maternal chromosome number 22, *Blood* **43:**837–840.

Garrick, M. D., Bricker, J., and Garrick, L. M., 1974, An electrophoretically silent polymorphism for the beta chains of rabbit hemoglobin and associated polyribosome patterns, *Genetics* **76:**99–108.

Gartler, S. M., 1976, X-chromosome inactivation and selection in somatic cells, *Fed. Proc. Fed. Am. Soc. Exp. Biol.* **35:**2191–2194.

Gaubatz, J., Prashad, N., and Cutler, R. G., 1976, Ribosomal RNA gene dosage as a function of tissue and age for mouse and human, *Biochim. Biophys. Acta* **41:**358–375.

Gee, M., Nordgren, R. A., Menzies, R. A., Hirsch, G. P., Kutsky, R., and Strehler, B. L., 1969, Evidence for long-lived lipid components in developing mouse tissues, *Exp. Gerontol.* **4:**27–32.

Gelfant, S., and Smith, Jr., J. G., 1972, Aging: Noncycling cells an explanation, *Science* **178:**357–361.

Gershon, H., and Gershon, D., 1973*a,* Inactive enzyme molecules in aging mice: Liver aldolase, *Proc. Natl. Acad. Sci. U.S.A.* **70:**909–913.

Gershon, H., and Gershon, D., 1973*b,* Altered enzyme molecules in senescent organisms: Mouse muscle aldolase, *Mech. Ageing Dev.* **2:**33–41.

Gibas, M. A., and Harman, D., 1970, Ribonucleic acid synthesis by nucleic isolated from rats of different ages, *J. Gerontol.* **25:**165–167.

Gross, N. J., and Rabinowitz, M., 1969, Synthesis of new strands of mitochondrial and nuclear deoxyribonucleic acid by semiconservative replication, *J. Biol. Chem.* **244:**1563–1566.

Gurdon, J. B., 1962, The developmental capacity of nuclei taken from intestinal epithelium cells of feeding tadpoles, *J. Embryol. Exp. Morphol.* **10:**622–640.

Hamilton, W. D., 1966, The moulding of senescence by natural selection, *J. Theor. Biol.* **12:**12–45.

Hardin, J. J., 1973, Altered heat-liability of a fraction of glutathione reductase in aging human lens, *Biochem. J.* **134:**995–1000.

Harrison, D. E., 1975, Normal function of transplanted marrow cell lines from aged mice, *J. Gerontol.* **30:**279–285.

Henderson, S. A., and Edwards, R. G., 1968, Chiasma frequency and maternal age in mammals, *Nature (London)* **218:**22–28.

Herrman, R. L., 1975, Age-related changes in nucleic acids and protein synthesis, in: *Neurobiology of Aging* (J. M. Ordy, and K. R. Brizzie, eds.), pp. 307–327, Plenum Press, New York.

Hirsch, C. A., and Hiatt, H. H., 1966, Turnover of liver ribosomes in fed and fasted rats, *J. Biol. Chem.* **241:**5936–5940.

Hirsch, G., Grunder, P., and Popp, R., 1976, Error analysis by amino acid analog incorporation in tissues of aging mice, *Interdiscip. Top. Gerontol.* **10:**1–10.

Hitachi, P. M., Yamada, K., and Takayama, S., 1975, Cytologic changes induced in rat liver cells by short-term exposure to chemical substances, *J. Natl. Cancer Inst.* **54:**1245–1247.

Holland, J. M., 1977, The thymus as a modifier of late somatic effects of X-radiation: Preliminary observations of X-irradiated and aging control germfree athymic nude mice, in: *Proceedings of the Radiation Research Society 25th Annual Meeting,* Academic Press, New York.

Jalavisto, E., 1951, Inheritance of longevity according to Finnish and Swedish genealogies, *Ann. Med. Intern. Fenn.* **40:**263.

Johnson, R., and Strehler, B. L., 1972, Loss of genes coding for ribosomal RNA in ageing brain cells, *Nature (London)* **240**:412–414.

Juncker, P., 1971, The ecological significance of death, *Biologist* **53**:66–69.

Kleihues, P., Lantos, P. L., and Magee, P. N., 1976, Chemical carcinogenesis in the nervous system, in: *International Review of Experimental Pathology*, pp. 153–232, Academic Press, New York.

Knowlton, F. F., 1972, Preliminary interpretations of coyote population mechanics with some management implications, *J. Wildl. Manage.* **36**:369–382.

Knudson, A. G., Strong, L. C., and Anderson, D. E., 1973, Heredity and cancer in man, *Prog. Med. Genet.* **9**:113–158.

Kuriyama, Y., Omura, T., Siekevitz ,P., and Palade, G. E., 1969, Effects of phenobarbital on the synthesis and degradation of the protein components of rat liver microsomal membranes, *J. Biol. Chem.* **244**:2017–2026.

Kurtz, D. I., 1974, Fidelity of protein synthesis with chicken embryo mitochondrial and cytoplasmic ribosomes, *Biochemistry* **13**:572–577.

Kurtz, D. I., 1975, The effect of ageing on *in vitro* fidelity of translation in mouse liver, *Biochim. Biophys. Acta* **407**:479–484.

Lajtha, A., and Toth, J., 1966, Instability of cerebral proteins, *Biochem. Biophys. Res. Commun.* **23**:294–298.

Leonard, A., and Leonard, E. D., 1975, Ageing and chromosome aberrations in male mammalian germ cells, *Exp. Gerontol.* **10**:309–311.

Lewis, C. M., 1972, Protein turnover in relation to Orgel's error theory of ageing, *Mech. Ageing Dev.* **1**:43–47.

Lilienfeld, A. M., Levin, M. L., and Kessler, I. I., 1972, *Cancer in the United States*, Harvard University Press, Cambridge, Massachusetts.

Loeb, J. N., Howell, R. R., and Tomkins, G. M., 1965, Turnover of ribosomal RNA in rat liver, *Science* **149**:1093–1095.

Loftfield, R. B., and Vanderjagt, D., 1972, The frequency of errors in protein biosynthesis, *Biochem. J.* **128**:1353–1356.

Lyon, M. F., 1961, Gene action in the X-chromosome of the mouse (*Mus musculus* L.), *Nature (London)* **190**:372–373.

Lyon, M. F., and Cox, B. D., 1975*a*, The induction by X-rays of chromosome aberrations in male guinea-pigs, rabbits and golden hamsters. III. Dose–response relationship after single doses of X-rays to spermatogonia, *Mutat. Res.* **29**:407–422.

Lyon, M. F., and Cox, B. D., 1975*b*, The induction by X-rays of chromosome aberrations in male guinea-pigs and golden hamsters. IV. Dose–response for spermatogonia treated with fractionated doses, *Mutat. Res.* **30**:117–128.

McKinnell, R. G., Deggins, B. A., and Labat, D. D., 1969, Transplantation of pluripotential nuclei from triploid frog tumors, *Science* **165**:394–395.

Markert, C. L., 1968, Neoplasia: A disease of cell differentiation, *Cancer Res.* **28**:1908–1914.

Mayneord, W. V., and Clark, R. H., 1975, Carcinogenesis and radiation risk: A biomathematical reconnaissance, *Br. J. Radiol., Suppl. 12.*

Medvedev, Zh. A., 1976, Error theories of aging, in: *Alternstheorien* (D. Platt, ed.), pp. 37–46, F. K. Schattauer Verlag, New York.

Mende, T. J., and Viamonte, L. M., 1965, A study of total body turnover in rats of different ages, *Gerontologia* **11**:208–213.

Menzies, R. A., 1976, Long-lived molecules and the hourglass hypothesis of aging, *Interdiscip. Top. Gerontol.* **9**:41–59.

Menzies, R. A., Press, G. D., Gold, P. H., Hendley, D. D., and Strehler, B. L., 1969, On the question of long-lived RNA in mammals, *Cell Tissue Kinet.* **2**:133–137.

Menzies, R. A., Mishra, R. K., and Gold, P. H., 1972, The turnover of ribosomes and soluble RNA in a variety of tissues of young adult and aged rats, *Mech. Ageing Dev.* **1**:117–132.

Micklem, H. S., and Ogen, D. A., 1976, Aging of haematopoietic stem cell populations in the mouse, in: *Stem Cells* (A. B. Cairnie, P. K. Lala, and D. G. Osmond, eds.), pp. 331–342, Academic Press, New York.

Millar, J. L., Hudspith, B. N., and Blackett, N. M., 1975, Reduced lethality in mice receiving a combined dose of cyclophosphamide and busulphan, *Br. J. Cancer* **32:**193–198.

Millard, R. E., Blackett, N. M., and Okell, S. F., 1973, A comparison of the effect of cytotoxic agents on agar colony forming cells, spleen colony forming cells, and the erythrocytic repopulating ability of mouse bone marrow, *J. Cell. Physiol.* **82:**309–318.

Morley, A., Trainor, D., and Blake, J., 1975, A primary stem cell lesion in experimental chronic hypoplastic marrow failure, *Blood* **45:**681–688.

Nellis, C. H., and Keith, L. B., 1976, Population dynamics of coyotes in Central Alberta, 1964–1968, *J. Wildl. Manage.* **40:**389–399.

Nery, R., 1976, Carcinogenic mechanisms: A critical review and a suggestion that oncogenesis may be adaptive ontogenesis, *Chem.-Biol. Interact.* **12:**145–169.

Neuberger, A., and Richards, F. F., 1964, Protein biosynthesis in mammalian tissues. II. Studies on turnover in the whole animal, in: *Mammalian Protein Metabolism* (H. W. Munro and T. B. Allison, eds.), pp. 243–296, Academic Press, New York.

Newberne, P. M., Harrington, D. H., and Wogan, G. N., 1966, Effects of cirrhosis and other liver insults on induction of liver tumors by aflatoxin in rats, *Lab. Invest.* **15:**962–969

Nordgren, R. A., Hirsch, G. P., Menzies, R. A., Hendley, D. D., Kutsky, R., and Strehler, B. L., 1969, Evidence for long-lived components in developing mouse tissues labelled with leucine, *Exp. Gerontol.* **4:**7–16.

O'Farrell, T. P., Olson, R. J., Gilbert, R. O., and Hedlund J. D., 1975, A population of great basin pocket mice, *Perognathus parvus,* in the shrub-steppe of South-Central Washington, *Ecol. Monogr.* **45:**1–28.

Ogden, D. A., and Micklem, H. S., 1976, The fate of serially transplanted bone marrow cell populations from young and old donors, *Transplantation* **22:**287–293.

Ogrodnik, J. P., Wulf, J. H., and Cutler, R. G., 1976, Altered protein hypothesis of mammalian ageing processes. II. Discrimination ratio of methionine versus ethionine in the synthesis of ribosomal protein and RNA of C57BL/6J mouse liver, *Exp. Gerontol.* **10:**119–136.

Omura, T., Siekevitz, P., and Palade, G. E., 1967, Turnover of constituents of the endoplasmic reticulum membranes of rat hepatocytes, *J. Biol. Chem.* **242:**2389–2396.

Orgel, L. E., 1963, The maintenance of the accuracy on protein synthesis and its relevance to ageing, *Proc. Natl. Acad. Sci. U.S.A.* **49:**517–521.

Orgel, L. E., 1970, The maintenance of the accuracy of protein synthesis and its relevance to ageing: A correction, *Proc. Natl. Acad. Sci. U.S.A.* **67:**1476.

Philips, R. S., and Sternberg, S. S., 1975, Tests for tumor induction by antitumor agents, in: *The Ambivalence of Cytostatic Therapy* (E. Grundmann and R. Gross, eds.), pp. 29–35, Springer-Verlag, New York.

Piha, R. S., Cuenod, M., and Waelsch, H., 1966, Metabolism of histones of brain and liver, *J. Biol. Chem.* **241:**2397–2404.

Popp, R. A., Bailiff, E. G., Hirsch, G. P. and Conrad, R. A., 1976, Errors in human hemoglobin as a function of age, *Interdiscip. Top. Gerontol.* **9:**209–218.

Popp, R. A., Hirsch, G. P., and Bradshaw, B. S., 1978, Amino acid substitution: Its use in detection and analysis of genetic variants, *Genetics* (in press).

Prasad, K. N., 1974, *Human Radiation Biology,* Harper & Row, Hagerstown, Maryland.

Preston, R. J., and Brewen, J. G., 1973, X-ray-induced translocation in spermatogonia. I. Dose and fractionation response in mice, *Mutat. Res.* **19:**215–223.

Preston, R. J., and Brewen, J. G., 1976, X-ray-induced translocations in spermatogonia. II. Fractionation responses in mice, *Mutat. Res.* **36:**333–344.

Pucek, Z., and Lowe, V. P. W., 1973, Age criteria in small mammals, in: *Small Mammals:*

Their Productivity and Population Dynamics, (F. B. Golley, K. Petrusewicz, and L. Ryszkowski, eds.), Chapter 3, Cambridge University Press, London.

Ranney, H. M., and Lehmann, H., 1974, The hemoglobinopathies, in: *The Red Blood Cell,* Vol 1, 2nd Ed. (D. MacN. Surgenor, ed.), Chapter 21, pp. 873–908, Academic Press, New York.

Rechcigl, M., Jr., 1971, Intracellular protein turnover and the roles of synthesis and degradation in regulation of enzyme levels, in: *Enzyme Synthesis and Degradation in Mammalian Systems* (M. Rechcigl, Jr., ed.), pp. 236–310, S. Karger, Basel.

Rubinson, H., Kahn, A., Boivin, P., Schapira, F., Gregori, C., and Dreyfus, J.-C., 1976, Aging and accuracy of protein synthesis in man: Search for inactive enzymatic crossreacting material in granulocytes of aged people, *Gerontology* 22:438–448.

Russell, L. B., 1963, Mammalian X-chromosome action: Inactivation limited in spread and in region of origin, *Science* **140**:976–978.

Russell, L. B., Russell, W. L., Popp, R. A., Vaughn, C., and Jacobson, K. B., 1976, Radiation-induced mutations at mouse hemoglobin loci, *Proc. Natl. Acad. Sci. U.S.A.* **73**:2843–2846.

Sato, F., Tsuchihashi, S., and Kawashima, N., 1973, Life-shortening of mice by whole or partial body X-irradiation, *J. Radiat. Res.* **14**:115–119.

Schapira, G., Kruh, J., Dreyfus, J. C., and Schapira, F., 1960, The molecular turnover of muscle aldolase, *J. Biol. Chem.* **235**:1738–1741.

Schimke, R. T., 1964, The importance of both synthesis and degradation in the control of arginase levels in rat liver, *J. Biol. Chem.* **239**:3803–3817.

Schmähl, D., 1975, Experimental investigations with anti-cancer drugs for carcinogenicity with special reference to immunodepression, *Recent Results Cancer Res.* **52**:18–28.

Schofield, R., and Lajtha, L. G., 1976, Cellular kinetics of erythropoiesis, in: *Congenital Disorders of Erythropoiesis, Ciba Found. Symp.* **37**:3–24.

Sirover, M. A., and Loeb, L. A., 1974, Erroneous basepairing induced by a chemical carcinogen during DNA synthesis, *Nature (London)* **252**:414–416.

Smith, G. S., Walford, R. L., and Mickey, M. R., 1973, Lifespan and incidence of cancer and other diseases in selected long-lived inbred mice and their F_1 hybrids, *J. Natl. Cancer Inst.* **50**:1195–1213.

Smith, M. E., 1968, The turnover of myelin in the adult rat, *Biochim. Biophys. Acta* **164**:285–293.

Smith, M. E., and Eng., L. F., 1965, Turnover of the lipid components of myelin, *J. Am. Oil Chem. Soc.* **42**:1013.

Stich, H. F., 1974, DNA repair as a possible link between carcinogenesis and mutagenesis, in: *XIth International Cancer Congress of Chemical and Viral Oncogenesis,* Vol. 2 (P. Bucalossi, U. Veronesi, and N. Cascinelli, eds.), pp. 58–61, Excerpta Medica, Amsterdam.

Storer, J. B., 1965, Radiation resistance with age in normal and irradiated populations of mice, *Radiat. Res.* **25**:435–459.

Strehler, B. L., 1971, Aging at the cellular level, in: *Clinical Geriatrics* (I. Rossman, ed.) pp. 49–81, Lipponcott, Philadelphia.

Sugimura, T., Sato, S., Nagao, M., Yahagi, T., Matsushima, T., Seino, Y., Takeuchi, M., and Kawachi, T., 1976, Overlapping of carcinogens and mutagens, in: *Fundamentals in Cancer Prevention* (P. N. Magee, S. Takayama, T. Sugimura, and T. Matsushima, eds.), pp. 191–215, University Park Press, Baltimore.

Swick, R. W., Rexroth, A. K., and Stange, 1968, The metabolism of mitochondrial proteins. III. The dynamic state of rat liver mitochondria, *J. Biol. Chem.* **243**:3581–3587.

Thompson, R. C., and Ballou, J. E., 1956, Studies of metabolic turnover with tritium as a tracer. V. The predominantly nondynamic state of body constituents in the rat, *J. Biol. Chem.* **233**:795–809.

Till, J. E., and McCulloch, E. A., 1961, A direct measurement of the radiation sensitivity of normal mouse bone marrow cells, *Radiat. Res.* **14**:312–322.

Trosko, J. E., and Chang, C.-C., 1976, Role of DNA repair in mutation and cancer production, in: *Aging, Carcinogenesis, and Radiation Biology* (K. C. Smith, ed.), pp. 399–442, Plenum Press, New York.

Upton, A. C., Conklin, J. W., and Popp, R. A., 1966, Influence of age at irradiation on susceptibility to radiation-induced life-shortening in RF mice, in: *Radiation & Ageing* (P. J. Lindop and G. A. Sacher, eds.), pp. 337–344, Taylor & Francis, London.

Vogel, F., and Rathenberg, R., 1976, Spontaneous mutation in man, in: *Advances in Human Genetics* (H. Harris and K. Hirschhorn, eds.), pp. 223–318, Plenum Press, New York.

von Hungen, K., Mahler, H. R., and Moore, W. J., 1968, Turnover of protein and ribonucleic acid in synaptic subcellular fractions from rat brain, *J. Biol. Chem.* **243**:1415–1423.

Waley, S. G., 1964, Metabolism of amino acids in the lens, *Biochem. J.* **91**:576–583.

Weatherall, D. J., and Clegg, J. B., 1976, Molecular genetics of human hemoglobin, *Annu. Rev. Genet.* **10**:157–178.

Wheldon, T. E., and Kirk, J., 1973, An error cascade mechanism for tumor progression, *J. Theor. Biol.* **42**:107–111.

Wiegel, D., Beier, W., and K.-H. Brehme, 1973, Vitality and error rate in biological systems: Some theoretical considerations, *Mech. Ageing Dev.* **2**:117–124.

Williams, G. C., 1957, Pleiotropy, natural selection, and the evolution of senescence, *Evolution* **11**:398–411.

Willson, M. F., 1971, Life history consequences of death rates, *Biologist* **53**:49–56.

Withers, H. R., 1975, Cell cycle redistribution as a factor in multifraction irradiation, *Radiology* **114**:199–202.

Withers, H. R., and Elkind, M. M., 1969, Radiosensitivity and fractionation response of crypt cells of mouse jejunum, *Radiat. Res.* **38**:598–613.

Withers, H. R., Mason, K., Reid, B. O., Dubravsky, N., Barkley, H. T., Brown, B. W., and Smathers, J. B., 1974, Response of mouse intestine to neutrons and gamma rays in relation to dose fractionation and division cycle, *Cancer* **34**:39–47.

Wulf, J. H., and Cutler, R. G., 1975, Altered protein hypothesis of mammalian ageing processes. I. Thermal stability of glucose-6-phosphate dehydrogenase in C57BL/6J mouse tissue, *Exp. Gerontol.* **10**:101–118.

Yielding, K. L., 1974, A model for aging based on differential repair of somatic mutational damage, *Perspect. Biol. Med.* **17**:201–208.

Young, R. W., and Fulhorst, H. W., 1966, Regional differences in protein synthesis within the lens of the rat, *Invest. Ophthalmol.* **5**:288–297.

Yuhas, J. M., 1971, Age and susceptibility to reduction in life expectancy: An analysis of proposed mechanisms, *Exp. Gerontol.* **6**:335–343.

Zhelabovskaya, S. M., and Berdyshev, G. D., 1972, Composition, template activity and thermostability of the liver chromatin in rats of various age, *Exp. Gerontol.* **7**:313–320.

Part II

Organism Level

Chapter 5

Genetics of Aging in Lower Organisms

James R. Smith

1. Introduction

One of the major problems confronting investigators in the field of aging is identifying the proper experimental organisms for study. The organism should have a short enough life span to facilitate experiments on duration of life span and progressive changes occurring during aging, and ideally, the results should be applicable to problems of human aging.

We certainly do not know whether lower organisms age by the same mechanisms as do humans. In fact, one could argue that they most likely would not (Danielli, 1978), since they are evolutionarily very distant. We anticipate, however, that the more we learn about the mechanisms of aging in any organism, the better equipped we will be to understand aging in humans.

One advantage of using lower organisms for studying the mechanisms of aging is their short life spans. An example is the life span of insects, which range from a few days to almost 3 years.

The variety of aging patterns found in lower organisms also presents some potential advantages. Of the filamentous fungi, only two species are known to undergo vegetative "senescence." The situation is similar in the protozoa, of which only a few species undergo clonal senescence. In the latter organisms, senescence occurs only when they are prevented from reorganizing their genetic material. Other potentially interesting traits are the induction of "spanning" in otherwise immortal clones of *Amoebae* by food restriction and the induction of "senescence" phenomena in *Neurospora* by certain mutations.

James R. Smith • W. Alton Jones Cell Science Center, Lake Placid, New York 12946

An important consideration in the study of aging is the effect of environment and diet on longevity. Great differences in life span have been noted when organisms are kept at different temperatures or reared on different diets (Loeb and Northrop, 1917; Maynard-Smith, 1958; Gardner, 1948*a,b;* Rockstein, 1959). The sensitivity of such organisms, especially the insects, to diet and temperature makes it difficult to interpret the results obtained by varying the genotype. Although environmental factors may not be directly related to genetic effects on longevity, they should be closely examined to ensure proper interpretation of the work of various investigators on lower organisms.

Although it is very clear that the longevity of an organism is determined by its genotype, the genetics of longevity appears to be very complex, and the mechanisms of this relationship remain to be elucidated. At present, the basic question rests: is the life span of an organism predetermined by a set of "aging genes" that function properly, or, alternatively, does an organism age because its genetic program is damaged?

To cover all aspects of aging in lower organisms would require an entire volume. In this chapter, therefore, we will discuss the genetic control of aging in a few representative organisms.

2. Inheritance of Life Span

2.1. Effect of Chromosome Number on Longevity

The females of most insect species have a greater longevity than the males. A possible explanation is that males are heterogametic (XY and XO) and females homogametic (XX). A deleterious gene would therefore be more likely to be expressed in the haploid state than when the organism is diploid for a specific chromosome.

In *Drosophila,* the diploid chromosome number is eight, with two sex chromosomes and six autosomes. The normal diploid female has two X chromosomes and the normal male one X and one Y chromosome. Triploid females have been produced (Gowen, 1931) with three X chromosomes and three sets of autosomes. In the same experiment, Gowen produced "sex intergrades" with two X chromosomes, one Y, and three sets of autosomes. These experiments were performed with a stock (cx.) that had been laboratory bred for at least 300 generations. The balanced triploid females had the same life span as normal diploid females (33 days). Normal males were somewhat shorter-lived (29 days). In contrast to the normal life span of triploid females, the sex intergrades had a markedly reduced life span (15 days). These experiments suggest that chromosome quantity *per se* is not important in determining longevity, but chromosome balance must be maintained to obtain optimum life span.

Experiments involving haploid and diploid male wasps (*Habrobracon* sp.) also yielded some interesting insight into the effect of chromosome number (Clark and Rubin, 1961; Clark *et al.*, 1963). Haploid males can be produced in this species by parthenogenesis from unfertilized eggs. Two strains of haploid males, wild type and the veinless (*vl*) mutant, were examined along with wild type (+/*vl*) diploid males. Both haploid strains had the same life span as the diploid. Furthermore, the survival curves for all three populations were essentially identical. After X-ray irradiation, however, the haploid strains had a much shorter life span than the diploid. X-irradiation apparently causes life-shortening by producing deleterious mutations and chromosome damage. These findings therefore confirm the expectation that recessive mutations have much greater effects on the haploid genome. If life span were determined by a simple accumulation of deleterious recessive mutations, as has been suggested by some investigators (Failla, 1957; Szilard, 1959; Curtis, 1963), the life span of unirradiated haploids should also be shorter than that of unirradiated diploids. That this difference was not observed in haploid male *Habrobracon* would indicate that life span is not simply determined by recessive mutations. The increased life span of hybrid *Drosophila* suggests, however, that recessive mutations may be a contributing factor in life span determination (Clarke and Maynard-Smith, 1955).

2.2. Effect of Genotype on Longevity

It is difficult if not impossible to approach the genetics of longevity directly. To do so, one would have to be able to select for the desired phenotype, i.e., short or long life span. The phenotype of interest is not expressed, however, until long after reproduction ceases. Most of the work on this subject has therefore been indirect, and has not yet led to an elucidation of the genetic control of life span.

Several species of insects have been well studied with respect to aging (Clark and Rockstein, 1964). *Drosophila* has proved to be most useful because of its detailed genetic characterization.

One of the most elaborate studies of the effect of genotype on the longevity of *Drosophila* was conducted by Gonzalez (1923) (Table I). Gonzales determined not only the effect of each of five mutations on life span, but also the life span for various combinations of the mutations. The data obtained are quite complex and are not subject to any simple interpretation. Nevertheless, these data form a good starting point for investigations on the genetics of longevity. The wild-type male and female have

Table I.   Effect of Five Specific Recessive Mutations on Life Span of
Drosophila melanogaster[a]

Phenotype	Mean life span (days)		
	Female and male	Male	Female
Wild	39	38	40
Quintuple	10	9	12
Black (*b*)	40	41	40
Purple (*pr*)	24	27	21
Vestigial (*vg*)	18	14	20
Arc (*a*)	26	25	28
Speck (*sp*)	42	46	38
b–pr	27	30	24
b–vg	20	16	24
b–a	21	20	23
b–sp	31	32	29
pr–vg	15	11	19
pr–a	33	36	31
pr–sp	23	23	22
a–sp	36	38	34
b–pr–a	32	35	30
b–pr–sp	27	31	24
b–a–sp	30	33	26
pr–a–sp	39	38	40
vg–a–sp	18	12	25
pr–vg–sp	10	9	12
b–pr–vg–a	18	14	22
b–vg–a–sp	16	13	19
b–pr–a–sp	22	22	23

[a]From Gonzalez, (1923).

almost the same mean life span—38 and 40 days, respectively. There was no consistency, however, in the way the different mutations affected the different sexes.

It is interesting that the male black mutant had a mean life span about 10% longer than the wild type, while the life span of the speck mutant in the male was about 20% longer. All other mutants in the male and all the mutants in the female had a decreased or unchanged life span.

This work raises many interesting but as yet unanswered questions concerning combinations of genes on life span. For example, as noted, both black and speck males were longer-lived than wild type, but in combination they resulted in about a 15% decrease in life span, while purple and arc both decreased the life span in the male, but in combination resulted in a life span much longer than that of either alone and only slightly less than that of the wild type.

In a similar series of experiments using the Oregon R strain of *Droso-phila* as wild type, Gedda and Brenci (1969) found that three phenotypic mutants all had shorter life spans than wild types (Table II). These investi-gators also reported that combinations of mutants had a slightly shorter life span than the individual single mutants. For example, the combination of brown (*bw*) and cinnabar (*cn*) decreased the life span by 10.5 days, while *bw* and *cn* separately decreased the life span by 5.3 and 7.8 days, respec-tively. In this case, both mutations contributed significantly to life-shorten-ing. Vestigial (*vg*), however, caused a decrease in life span of 19.2 days, and the addition of *bw* or *cn* caused an additional 0.7- or 1.0-day decrease, respectively, while a strain with all three mutations had a life span 21.8 days shorter than wild type. These mutant strains were selected on the basis of phenotypic departures from wild type, and all the mutants were recessive to the wild-type allele. The total physiological state of the organism also appears to be involved in life-span determination, since black and speck females (Table I) had a life span essentially the same as that of a wild type, while the males were longer-lived than the wild type.

In a study on the effect of heterozygous mutant genes on longevity, Pearl *et al.* (1923) crossed the wild-type strain of *Drosophila* "Old Fal-mouth" with a strain homozygous for five genes, "quintuple." Although the quintuple had a much shorter life span than that of the wild type, the F_1 hybrids had a life span even longer than that of the wild type (Table III). In this case, a series of mutations that shorten life span when homozygous actually appear to increase the life span in the heterozygous state.

Another interesting approach along these lines involved the crossing of different strains of *Drosophila*. Using two inbred strains of *D. subobscura*,

Table II.   Life Span of the Homozygous F_8
Strains of Drosophila melanogaster (Obtained
by Back-Crossing F_1 Individuals)[a]

Strain	Number of flies	Mean life span (days)
Oregon R	634	43.4
bw	561	38.1
cn	504	35.6
vg	255	24.2
bw–cn	166	32.9
bw–vg	294	23.5
cn–vg	168	23.2
bw–cn–vg	185	21.6

[a]From Gedda and Brenci, (1969).

Table III.   Life Span of Parent Stocks and Hybrids of
Drosophila melanogaster[a]

Stock	Mean age at death (days)
Old Falmouth	46.26 ± 0.44
Quintuple	14.08 ± 0.23
Old Falmouth (male) × quintuple (female)	51.12 ± 0.84
Quintuple (male) × Old Falmouth (female)	51.73 ± 0.57
All F_1's	51.55 ± 0.47

[a]From Pearl *et al.* (1923).

Clarke and Maynard-Smith (1955) and Maynard-Smith (1959) found that the hybrid F_1 populations had a greater life span than did the parent strains (Table IV). These results are essentially the same as those obtained earlier by Pearle and Parker (1922*a,b*), and suggest that in particular strains of *Drosophila,* life span is limited by homozygous recessive mutations. That haploid and diploid wasps have the same life span (Clark and Rubin, 1961) suggests, however, that this phenomenon may not be a general one. Clarke and Maynard-Smith (1955) also found that females from the B♀ × K♂ hybrids had a longer life span than that of the K♀ × B♂ hybrids. This result suggests some component of extrachromosomal inheritance in life-span determination (see Section 3).

2.3. Cytoplasmic Inheritance of Aging in Fungi

Most of the filamentous fungi are capable of unlimited vegetative growth. Two species are known that are capable of only limited vegetative growth, *Aspergillus glaucus* (Jinks, 1959) and *Podospora anserina* (Mar-

Table IV.   Effect of Hybridization on Life
Span of Drosophila subobscura[a]

Strain	Life span (days)	
	Female	Male
B	35.1	27.7
K	25.0	39.2
B♀ × K♂	70.6	63.4
K♀ × B♂	62.0	67.3

[a]From Clarke and Maynard-Smith, (1955).

cou, 1961). "Senescence" has been studied in more detail in *P. anserina,* and will be discussed here.

In *P. anserina,* the fungal organism (mycelium) is made up of septate filaments (hyphae) that are connected by cytoplasmic bridges. The nuclei are contained in the small region between septa, but the cytoplasm can move through the septa and cytoplasmic bridges and is common to the whole mycelium. The mycelium grows by elongation of the hyphal tips at a rate of about 0.7 cm/day. The organism is haploid, and in the simpler case, all the nuclei are identical. In some cases, the mycelium is composed of a mixture of two nuclear types, differing only at the "mating-type" allele. The equivalent of the male sexual organs in this organism is the spermatia. The spermatia are loosely attached to the mycelium and can be easily detached. They contain one haploid nucleus and essentially no cytoplasm. The equivalent of the female sexual organs is the ascogonia. These are much larger than the spermatia, and contain one haploid nucleus and a large amount of cytoplasm. Sexual crossing occurs when a spermatium of one mating type fuses with an ascogonium of the other mating type. The spermatial nucleus migrates to the ascogonial nucleus, they fuse, and the diploid nucleus is replicated several times. The diploid nuclei then undergo meiotic reduction, and spores are formed in the ascogonium. Both mononucleate and binucleate spores are formed. The cytoplasm of these spores is derived from the ascogonial cytoplasm. In most cases, the binucleate spores contain nuclei that differ at the mating-type allele. These spores give rise to "self-fertile" mycelia. In the other cases, mycelia grow from a mononuclear spore or one that contains two nuclei of the same mating type. These mycelia are "self-sterile," and can be fertilized only by spermatia collected from another mycelium of the other mating type. By fertilizing ascogonia of one mycelium with spermatia of the other, crosses can be made that produce a mixed nuclear genetic complement from both parents and a cytoplasmic genetic complement of only one (the ascogonial) parent.

Mycelia of *P. anserina* have a limited ability to grow in vegetative culture (Rizet, 1953). A mycelium that has exhausted or nearly exhausted its growth potential is referred to as *senescent.* Several strains of *Podospora* have been isolated. The mean life span of these different strains ranges from 15 to 150 days, depending on the strain. The work of Smith and Rubenstein (1973*a,b*), Rizet (1957), and Marcou (1961) resulted in the following model of "senescence" in these organisms: From growth and cytoplasmic fusion experiments, Rizet and Marcou suggested that "senescence" in this organism was due to some cytoplasmic factor. Some permanent heritable change occurs in a cytoplasmic component of the mycelium at a rate of 10^{-6}–10^{-7} per cell division. The abnormal or mutant component replicates at a slightly higher rate than the normal cellular components, and spreads throughout the cytoplasm via the septa and hyphal anastomoses. Several days after its initial appearance in the cytoplasm, the abnormal component is present at a high enough level to cause the mycelium to stop growing and eventually die.

In a series of back crosses between strains with different life spans, Smith and Rubenstein (1973*a,b*) found that the median life span of the progeny was determined by cytoplasmic determinants, and was affected only slightly, if at all, by the nuclear genetic composition. This fungus represents the only case known in which life span is determined almost exclusively by the cytoplasm. This phenomenon may be due to the much larger differences in life span among different wild-type strains of *Podospora* than are found in other organisms. In most cases, the nuclear sex differences in life span outweigh possible differences in cytoplasmic determinants.

2.4. Effect of Parental Age on Longevity

If life span were determined by the accumulation of deleterious mutations, then one might expect the offspring from older parents to be shorter-lived than those from young parents. Some of the work on the effect of parental age is reviewed in this section. As in the case of other hypotheses of aging, the results are both supportive and contradictory.

Lansing (1947, 1954) was the first to observe the effect of parental age on life span. In rotifers, the life span of successive generations from old mothers progressively decreased, while that of successive generations from young mothers progressively increased. The effect was reversible, however, indicating no increase in deleterious mutations, but rather a nongenetic aging factor transmitted through the maternal cytoplasm.

O'Brian (1961) found that both male and female *D. melanogaster* offspring from older parents had a shorter life span than those from younger parents. He selected through nine generations, but found progressive changes only during the first three generations. On the other hand, Comfort (1953) found no difference in life span among the progeny from young and old *D. subobscura* selected over eight generations. The relationship between parental age and life span is further complicated by the observations of Glass (1960). He established two lines from the Oregon R strain of *D. melanogaster*. One was obtained by mating very young ("early-line") flies and the other by mating 21-day-old ("late-line") flies. The progeny life span for each subline was then determined under two mating conditions, "early" and "late." For the "early-line," the progeny from the early mating had a longer life span than those from the later mating. The opposite result was obtained for the "late-line"—the progeny from the later mating had the longer life span. Thus, each subline gave rise to longer-lived progeny under the conditions of mating by which it was selected.

3. Induction of Aging in Immortal Organisms

As a general rule unicellular organisms, given a proper environment, can live and proliferate indefinitely. When *Paramecia* are prevented from reorganizing their genetic material by autogamy or conjugation, however, or when the food supply of *Amoeba* is restricted, a finite life span is exhibited. Most species of filamentous fungi can also grow indefinitely, though certain mutants of *Neurospora* have a limited life span.

These cases are especially interesting to the study of aging, since they represent alternative physiological states of organisms, one of which results in limited life span and the other in unlimited life span.

3.1. "Spanning" of Amoeba

Clones of *A. proteus* and *A. discoides* grown under normal culture conditions are apparently immortal. When their food intake is sufficiently restricted for 3–5 weeks, however, they enter a state in which they have a definite life span (Muggleton and Danielli, 1958; Danielli and Muggleton, 1959). Individual clones exhibit one of two types of behavior. "Type A," or stem-cell-like, behavior occurs when at each division one of the two daughter cells dies within a few days of division, while the other divides again into daughters, one of which soon dies. This process is repeated until both daughter cells of a division fail to divide. The alternate mode, "Type B," occurs when clones grow exponentially until all the cells of a clone die at approximately the same time.

The role of *Amoeba* nuclear and cytoplasmic determinants of life span was studied in an elegant series of experiments by Muggleton and Danielli (1968) involving nuclear transplantation and cytoplasmic transfer. When normal nuclei were transplanted into enucleated "spanned" cells of either Type A or Type B, all the resultant cells were "spanned" and exhibited Type B behavior. It appears, therefore, that the cytoplasm contains the determinants for Type B spanning. Furthermore, the determinants are most likely self-replicating, since several divisions occurred between transfer of the normal nucleus and death of the clone. On the other hand, when nuclei from "spanned" *Amoeba* were transplanted into enucleated normal cells, the cells all exhibited Type A "spanning" behavior. From these observations, it seems that both the nuclei and the cytoplasm of "spanned"

Amoeba participate in determining the life span, but in different ways: "spanned" nuclei cause a stem-cell-like behavior, while "spanned" cytoplasm results in the death of an exponentially growing clone.

3.2. Mutants of Neurospora

Wild-type *Neurospora* can be grown by mycelial transfer for an indefinite period of time. Only two mutants of *Neurospora* have a limited life span in vegetative culture. One mutant, *leu-5* (Printz and Gross, 1967), which is auxotrophic for leucine, can grow indefinitely at 20–25°C. When it is transferred to 37°C, however, growth continues normally for 3–4 days and suddenly ceases. Lewis and Holliday (1970) reported evidence that the limited life span of this mutant is due to errors in protein synthesis leading to an error catastrophe (Orgel, 1963).

The other mutant (Sheng, 1951), natural death (*nd*), is in some ways more interesting for aging research, since it causes growth stoppage of *Neurospora* at all temperatures and does not seem to be due to a single enzyme deficiency. The *nd* mutation is at a single locus on the mating-type chromosome about 15 map units from the centromere. As yet, the function of the wild-type allele is not known. Although life span is limited at all temperatures, it decreases as the temperature is increased.

In heterocaryons between *nd* and non-*nd* nuclei, an indefinite life span was obtained when the ratio of *nd* to non-*nd* nuclei was 3.5 or less. From experiments on rejuvenation of *nd* by heterocaryon formation or by sexual crossing with non-*nd*, Sheng suggested that a cytoplasmic determinant might be involved in life-span determination. Further work is needed, however, to confirm this hypothesis.

3.3. Autogamy-Deprived Paramecia

One other example of organisms that can exist in both aging and nonaging modes is worth mentioning. Until 1954 (Sonneborn, 1954), clones of *Paramecium aurelia* were considered to be immortal. It was then found that if *Paramecia* were prevented from undergoing genetic reorganization, they eventually stopped dividing and the whole clone died. The organism could be rejuvenated by either conjugation or autogamy. The process of conjugation involves exchange of genetic material between different organisms. During autogamy, a single organism undergoes internal reorganization of its genetic material. The metabolically active macronucleus fragments, the micronuclei replicate, and all but one of these micronuclei disintegrate. This micronucleus regenerates new micronuclei and the macronucleus.

This process of genetic reorganization resets the clock to zero, and the clone can go through an additional 200–300 divisions before senescence sets in. The mechanisms by which rejuvenation occurs is not known. There is some evidence, however (Sonneborn and Schneller, 1960), that there is an accumulation of dominant lethal mutations in old clones.

Fukushima (1975) recently published evidence for increased mutations in the micronuclei as a function of clonal age. These mutations caused a decrease in fission rate in the progeny after autogamy. It was also reported (Smith-Sonneborn, 1974) that older clones are more sensitive to UV irradiation than young clones, and that the dark repair system for DNA damage was more sensitive to caffeine in old clones. These results suggest that increased mutations and damage to DNA occur as clones of *Paramecia* age. It is not known, however, whether these are the primary mechanisms by which life span is limited. More work is needed on the effect of specific biochemical mutations on the life span of this organism.

4. Summary and Conclusions

Because there has been little recent work in this area, much of the work on genetic aspects of aging reviewed in this chapter was done in the early part of this century. The results that have been obtained are not easy to interpret and have not provided much insight into the mechanisms of aging. It is clear, however, that life span is an inherited trait, and that it can be modified by single gene mutations. The amount of background information available on the genetics of *Drosophila* would appear to make this organism a prime candidate for further studies on aging. Since the biochemical basis for many phenotypic mutants is known, detailed studies correlating various biochemical lesions with life span might add considerably to our understanding of the mechanisms of aging.

References

Clark, A. M., and Rockstein, M., 1964, Aging in insects, in: *Physiology of Insecta I* (M. Rockstein, ed.), pp. 227–281, Academic Press, New York.

Clark, A. M., and Rubin, M. A., 1961, The modification by X-irradiation of the life span of haploids and diploids of the wasp, *Habrobracon, Radiat. Res.* **15**:244.

Clark, A. M., Bertrand, H. A., and Smith, R. E., 1963, Life span differences between haploid and diploid males of *Habrobracon serinopae* after exposure as adults to X-rays, *Am. Nat.* **97**:208.

Clarke, J. M., and Maynard-Smith, J., 1955, The genetics and cytology of *Drosophila subobscura*. XI. Hybrid vigor and longevity, *J. Genet.* **53**:172.

Comfort, A., 1953, Absence of a Lansing effect in *Drosophila subobscura, Nature (London)*
   172:83.
Curtis, H. J., 1963, Biological mechanisms underlying the aging process, *Science* **141**:686.
Danielli, J. F., 1978, Cell state transitions and aging and senescence of cells, *J. Theor. Biol.* (in
   press).
Danielli, J. F., and Muggleton, A., 1959, Some alternative states of amoeba with special
   reference to life-span, *Gerontologia* **3**:76.
Failla, G., 1957, Considerations bearing on permissible accumulated radiation doses for
   occupational exposure: The aging process and carcinogenesis, *Radiology* **69**:23.
Fukushima, S., 1975, Clonal age and the proportion of defective progeny after autogamy in
   Paramecium aurelia, Genetics **79**(3):377.
Gardner, T. S., 1948*a*, Use of *Drosophila melanogaster* as screening agent for longevity
   factors: Pantothenic acid as longevity factor in royal jelly, *J. Gerontol.* **3**:1.
Gardner, T. S., 1948*b*, Use of *Drosophila melanogaster* as screening agent for longevity
   factors: Effects of biotin, pyridoxine, sodium yeast nucleate, and pantothenic acid on life
   span of fruit fly, *J. Gerontol.* **3**:9.
Gedda, L., and G. Brenci, 1969, Biology of the gene: The ergon/chronon system, *Acta Genet.
   Med. Gemellol.* **18**(4):329
Glass, B., 1960, The influence of immediate versus delayed mating on the life span of
   Drosophila, in: *Biology of Aging* (B. L. Strehler, ed), pp. 185–187, Publication No. 6,
   American Institutes of Biological Sciences, Washington, D.C.
Gonzalez, B. M., 1923, Experimental studies on the duration of life. VIII. The influence upon
   duration of life of certain mutant genes of *Drosophila melanogaster, Am. Nat.* **57**:289.
Gowen, J. W., 1931, Metabolism as related to chromosome structure and the duration of life,
   J. Gen. Physiol. **14**:463.
Jinks, J. L., 1959, Lethal, suppressive cytoplasms in aged clones of *Aspergillus glaucus, J.
   Gen. Microbiol.* **21**:397.
Lansing, A. I., 1947, A transmissible, cumulative, and reversible factor in aging, *J. Gerontol.*
   2:228–239.
Lansing, A. I., 1954, A nongenic factor in the longevity of rotifers, *Ann. N.Y. Acad. Sci.*
   57:455.
Lewis, C. M., and Holliday, R., 1970, Mistranslation and ageing in *Neurospora, Nature
   (London)* **228**:877.
Loeb, J., and Northrop, J. H., 1917, On the influence of food and temperature upon the
   duration of life, *J. Biol. Chem.* **32**(1):103.
Marcou, D., 1961, Notion de longévité et nature cytoplasmique du déterminant de la sénes-
   cence chez quelques champignons, *Ann. Sci. Nat. Bot. Ser. 12e* **2**:653.
Maynard-Smith, J., 1958, Prolongation of the life of *D. subobscura* by a brief exposure of
   adults to a high temperature, *Nature (London)* **181**:496.
Maynard-Smith, J., 1959, The rate of ageing in *Drosophila subobscura,* in: *Ciba Found.
   Colloq. Ageing* (G. E. W. Wolstenholme and M. O'Connor, eds.), Vol. 5, *The Lifespan
   of Animals,* pp. 269–280, Churchill, London.
Muggleton, A., and Danielli, J. F., 1958, Aging of *Amoeba proteus* and *A. discoides* cells,
   Nature (London) **181**:1738.
Muggleton, A., and Danielli, J. F., 1968, Inheritance of the "life-spanning" phenomenon in
   Amoeba proteus, Exp. Cell Res. **49**:116.
O'Brian, D. M., 1961, Effects of parental age on the life cycle of *Drosophila melanogaster,
   Ann. Entomol. Soc. Am.* **54**:412.
Orgel, L. E., 1963, The maintenance of the accuracy of protein synthesis and its relevance to
   ageing, *Proc. Natl. Acad. Sci. U.S.A.* **49**:517.
Pearl, R., and Parker, S. L., 1922*a*, Experimental studies on the duration of life. II. Hereditary
   differences in duration of life in line-bred strains of *Drosophila, Am. Nat.* **56**:174.

Pearl, R., and Parker, S. L., 1922*b,* Experimental studies on the duration of life. V. On the influence of certain environmental factors on duration of life in *Drosophila, Am. Nat.* **56:**385.

Pearl, R., Parker, S. L., and Gonzalez, B. M., 1923, Experimental studies on the duration of life. VII. The Mendelian inheritance of duration of life in crosses of wild type and quintuple stocks of *Drosophila melanogaster, Am. Nat.* **57:**153.

Printz, D. B. and Gross, S. R., 1967, An apparent relationship between mistranslation and an altered leucyl-tRNA synthetase in a conditional lethal mutant of *Neurospora crassa, Genetics* **55:**451.

Rizet, G., 1953, Sur la longévité des souches de *Podospora anserina, C. R. Acad. Sci.* **237:**838.

Rizet, G., 1957, Les modifications qui conduisent a la senescence chez *Podospora* sont-elles de nature cytoplasmique, *C. R. Acad. Sci.* **244:**663.

Rockstein, M., 1959, The biology of aging in insects, in: *Ciba Found. Colloq. Ageing* (G. E. W. Wolstenholme and M. O'Connor, eds.), Vol. 5, pp. 247–264, Churchill, London.

Sheng, T. C., 1951, A gene that causes natural death in *Neurospora crassa, Genetics* **36:**199.

Smith, J. R., and Rubenstein, I., 1973*a,* The development of "senescence" in *Podospora anserina, J. Gen. Microbiol.* **76:**283.

Smith, J. R., and Rubenstein, I., 1973*b,* Cytoplasmic inheritance of the timing of "senescence" in *Podospora anserina, J. Gen. Microbiol.* **76:**297.

Smith-Sonneborn, J., 1974, Age-correlated effects of caffeine on nonirradiated and UV-irradiated *Paramecium aurelia, J. Gerontol.* **29**(3):256.

Sonneborn, T. M., 1954, The relation of autogamy to senescence and rejuvenescence in *Paramecium aurelia, J. Protozool.* **1:**38.

Sonneborn, T. M., and Schneller, M., 1960, Age-induced mutations in *Paramecium,* in: *The Biology of Aging* (B. L. Strehler, ed.), pp. 286–287, Publication No. 6, American Institute of Biological Sciences, Washington, D.C.

Szilard, L., 1959, A theory of ageing, *Nature (London)* **184:**956.

Chapter 6

Evolution of Longevity and Survival Characteristics in Mammals

George A. Sacher

1. Introduction

The comparative analysis of aging patterns in mammals is at present in a highly fragmented state, because the data now available were gathered by investigators from various disciplines for various purposes, and are not all equally suitable for the purposes of this survey. Nevertheless, it is possible to discern evidence of a consistent pattern of longevity and aging in the class Mammalia. This brief review will examine this pattern, although the paucity of data in some areas limits the discussion to a semiquantitative examination of the possibilities.

An important outcome of the evolutionary-comparative approach is the realization that "aging" should not be the sole focus of biogerontological thinking and research. There is increasing evidence that longevity—in fact, every aspect of the survival characteristic of a species—has significance for evolutionary fitness, and evidence also that there is natural selection for longer life, mediated by positive, genetically controlled mechanisms. That evidence is a sufficient basis for the development of an alternative paradigm for biogerontology, centered on the identification and control of constitutive enzymatic and physiological mechanisms for longevity assurance. The main outlines of that new paradigm are sketched in the following sections.

George A. Sacher • Division of Biological and Medical Research, Argonne National Laboratory, Argonne, Illinois 60439

2. Evolutionary Gerontology: What Evolved, Aging or Longevity?

2.1. Allometry of Vertebrate Life Span

The wide range of mammalian life spans is by now well documented (Sacher, G. A., and Jones, 1972), and it has been shown that the use of maximum life span as a measure of the longevity potential of a species is justified from both the biological and the statistical point of view (Sacher, G. A., 1975). Only in recent years, however, have biogerontologists begun to face the scientific challenge presented by the wide variation of longevity in mammals, and in other tetrapod classes. The first step was to determine whether species longevity has anatomical or biochemical correlates (Sacher, G. A., 1959, 1975, 1976; Mallouk, 1975). The allometric relationships of species longevity to a set of anatomical and physiological variables were estimated by means of multiple regression analysis of large samples of homeothermic mammalian species representing all the major orders. Maximum life span (Sacher, G. A., and Jones, 1972) is allometrically related to adult brain weight and body weight; i.e., there is a linear relationship of logarithm of life span (log L) to the logarithm of brain weight (log E) and of body weight (log S) (Sacher, G. A., 1959):

$$\log L = 0.64 \,(\log E) - 0.23 \,(\log S) + 1.035 \tag{1}$$

This regression relationship accounts for 85% of the total life-span variance in the sample of 63 species. Similar relationships hold within single taxonomic groups of mammals; in particular, the suborder Anthropoidea, which includes the monkeys, apes, and man, has a relationship of L to E and S that does not differ significantly from these relationships for all mammals or for rodents (Sacher, G. A., 1975). The accuracy of prediction is further improved if the resting metabolic rate and body temperature are also taken into account (Sacher, G. A., 1976).

These results support the conclusion that *the longevity of mammals is a constitutional characteristic,* i.e., a parameter that has close functional relationships to other anatomical and physiological species dimensions; not different in kind from the allometric relationships among body dimensions (Gould, 1966), or of metabolic rate to body weight (Brody, 1945). The next stage of investigation must focus on discovering why these relationships subsist, a considerably more difficult problem.

2.2. "Senescence Gene" Hypothesis of the Evolution of Aging

The analysis of the factors governing the evolution of longevity and aging has until recently been almost entirely speculative, and characterized by a fixation on theories that postulate the accumulation in the genome of late-acting genes for deleterious senescent change. The adherents to this position are split into two main camps. One camp, following Weismann (1882, 1891), postulates that senescence is an adaptive characteristic, and concludes, therefore, that the senescence genes become fixed in the genome by natural selection. The opposing view, espoused by Medawar (1957) and Williams (1957), is that senescence is not adaptive, but that senescence traits nevertheless accumulate in the genome by random genetic drift, because traits that are expressed after the end of the reproductive span are not accessible to natural selection.

There are serious theoretical objections to both the selectionist and the nonselectionist position, which arise from their mutual acceptance of the postulate that aging evolved by the accumulation of genes with late-acting deleterious expression. One paradox this postulate engenders is that if these genes accumulate during the course of evolution, then tracing the evolutionary process backward would lead to an original genome that lacks all senescence genes, and therefore is presumably somatically immortal. The implication that the living state is intrinsically perfect, and that organisms are mortal only because of the accumulation of adventitious senescence genes, is more easily reconciled with a cosmology of special creation than with current scientific conceptions about the origin of terrestrial life from organic precursors through a sequence of long-extinct primitive life-forms.

The theory of late-acting senescence genes, as developed by Williams (1957) and Medawar (1957), contains as one of its major structural elements the assumption that the senescence genes have the property of *serial pleiotropy,* in that they have a benign or innocuous expression during early life, and then acquire another injurious expression at a later life stage (Sacher, G. A., 1968). A critical problem for the theory that is not explicitly faced by Medawar or Williams is the mechanism that determines when the pleiotropic genes "switch" from a benign to a detrimental expression. The alternative possibilities are that the switch occurs as a function of time or that it occurs as a result of a change of the internal environment. Medawar seems to entertain the former view when he speaks of "precession" and "recession" in the time of onset of the senescent expression from generation to generation. It is difficult, however, to find a physically plausible mechanism whereby genes can measure the passage of time.

The other alternative—that the switch occurs as a result of a change in the environment of the gene—is much more easily reconciled with the accepted principles of molecular genetics, but it raises a fatal logical difficulty for the senescence gene theory, because the prior environmental change would then be the proximate cause of the pleiotropic switch, which thereby becomes an effect of a prior age change, rather than a cause. If that prior age change is in turn postulated to be due to a pleiotropic gene switch, then the same argument applies to it and so on, back to conception. Although this process is theoretically feasible, it is a developmental hypothesis that bears little relationship to the original senescence gene hypothesis.

One of the salient findings of modern molecular genetics is that many, or even most, of the genes in a cell nucleus are repressed at any given time, and are derepressed, or activated, by specific molecules that are produced under specific environmental influences (Watson, 1976). The assumption of serial pleiotropy in the Medawar–Williams theory can be replaced by the assumption that senescence genes switch from a repressed to a derepressed state. This replacement would give the theory a much more contemporary sound, but would not alter the objections raised above in the slightest degree.

The rejection of the senescence gene hypothesis for the evolution of aging does not imply a denial of the existence of genes that lead to specific metabolic disorders, and to increased vulnerability to neoplastic and degenerative diseases. It does reject, however, the view that the aging process is shaped by such genes to more than a minor degree. Detrimental genes are rare in natural populations (McKusick, 1975), but have been given artificial prominence by the use of inbred animal strains in which they have been fixed by selection. The importance of mutant forms for the analysis of the etiology of the diseases of senescence is beyond question (Martin, 1977), but it does not necessarily follow that senescence exists only because of the presence in the genome of fixed deleterious genes with similar expression.

In most groups of mammals, there has been an overall evolutionary trend toward increase in body size and brain size, and decrease of reproductive rate. In view of the relationships discussed above, it follows that there was necessarily an increase of life span over the course of evolution of many mammalian taxa. This increase was a dramatic feature in the rapid evolution of *Homo sapiens* (Sacher, G. A., 1975; Cutler, 1975). According to the senescence gene hypothesis, this longevity increase was accomplished by the selective elimination of life-shortening genes. Although such elimination is not a logical impossibility, it is neither plausible nor aesthetically appealing, and it provides the worst possible basis for the development of a research strategy for gerobiology. Fortunately, there is support for the alternative hypothesis that longevity evolved by selection of positive longevity-assurance systems. The evidence for this hypothesis is given in the next section.

2.3. Evolution of Longevity by Means of Longevity-Assurance Genes

The evidence presented above that longevity is a constitutional characteristic supports the neo-Weismannian hypothesis of Hamilton (1966) that the survival characteristic of a species is an aspect of its extended fitness. It also gives justification for the hypothesis developed here, that the control of longevity by natural selection is mediated by genetic systems that govern positive enzymatic mechanisms for the protection, regulation, and repair of the longevity-assurance systems at all levels of organization (Sacher, G. A., 1966*a*, 1968; Sacher, G. A., and Hart, 1977).

This hypothesis is the dialectical antithesis to the view that aging evolved as the result of the accumulation of deleterious genes. These two classes of theories have profoundly different implications for the strategy of biogerontological research, and for the definitions and disciplinary structure of biogerontology. In particular, the hypothesis that longevity evolved as a positive characteristic leads naturally to an interest in the comparative approach to biogerontology, and to the search for the set of enzymatic systems that constitute the mechanisms of genetically controlled longevity assurance.

If longevity is an aspect of fitness, then the selective forces acting on the life table are strongly influenced by the reproductive pattern. Reproductive histories are of many types, but the fundamental distinction is between the *semelparous* species that have a single reproductive act per lifetime and the *iteroparous* species that reproduce repeatedly (Cole, 1954). Semelparous forms, such as annual plants, which do not complete their reproduction until the very end of life (and, in many cases, not until after somatic death), can be expected to have fundamentally different somatic aging processes, and different genetic mechanisms for their control, than iteroparous organisms, such as the mammals, the reproductive success of which is contingent on producing and rearing several small litters over an extended span of adult reproductive life.

Extensive research on the senescence processes of plants has established that plant senescence is subject to highly specific control by humoral substances—e.g., auxin, kinetin, and abscisic acid—and that these substances are in turn regulated by internal maturational sequences and by environmental factors (Leopold, 1961; Sacher, J. A., 1973; Woolhouse, 1974). The specific senescence processes, such as ripening or abscision, are mediated by hydrolytic enzymes that are in part synthesized *de novo* in response to the humoral signals (Sacher, J. A., 1967; De Leo and Sacher, 1970). In the interest of better semantics, it should be noted that the term *senescence,* with all its implications of deterioration, is inappropriate when applied to an event that is vitally important to reproductive success, that is temporally and physiologically integrated with the reproductive process, and that is carried out by specific enzymatic mechanisms under systemic humoral control. It is preferable to denote processes that satisfy these criteria as *programmed life termination* (Sacher, G. A., 1966*a*).

In the case of the annual plants, programmed life termination contributes directly to reproductive success by facilitating seed dispersal, rather than indirectly, by decreasing competition with succeeding generations, as postulated by Weismann. Nevertheless, this evidence supports the general view that the survival characteristic is a constituent of fitness. In iteroparous organisms, there is no evidence that life termination (death) of the individual contributes to increased fitness of the population, and in the absence of such evidence, the hypothesis of genetically programmed aging—particularly in application to mammalian aging—lacks necessity, and hence should not be entertained without some justification.

3. Evolution of Longevity in Man and the Other Mammals

The existence of programmed life termination cannot be ruled out in the iteroparous mammals, but no specific mechanism for its achievement has yet been demonstrated. The postreproductive death of salmon after the completion of their semelparous reproduction may be an instance, but the specificity of mechanism is still an open question. The termination of fertility by menopause in the human female is not a senescent change—its selective advantage may indeed be to increase life expectation—but the comparatively recent evolution of such a programmed change in late life is an indication that the genetic potentiality for programmed life termination exists in mammals. It becomes pertinent to ask why that potentiality is not utilized. An examination of the population biology of species that employ the iteroparous reproductive strategy—and of mammals in particular—does not indicate a useful role for programmed life termination. On the contrary, the need for an extended reproductive span to assure a sufficiently high rate of increase per generation places a premium on maximizing longevity.

The specific causal factors of reproductive and population biology that generate the close functional relationships between longevity and body dimensions expressed in equation (1) have not yet been investigated in detail. G. A. Sacher and Staffeldt (1974) showed that increase in species brain size necessarily leads to decrease of reproductive rate. Given this finding, selection for increased brain size, which has occurred independently as an anagenetic trend in several groups of mammals (Rensch, 1959; Jerison, 1973), must be accompanied by selection for increased reproductive span, and hence for increased life span, to maintain an adequate intrinsic rate of increase. The cases in which brain size evolved rapidly—such as the threefold increase of brain weight during the few million years of hominid evolution (Sacher, G. A., 1975; Cutler, 1975)—are therefore important because they may eventually enable us to set an upper limit to the number of gene substitutions required to bring about the approximate doubling of life span in the same few million years.

In regard to the molecular-genetic basis for the increase of longevity in mammals by natural selection (Sacher, G. A., and Hart, 1977), the first demonstrative evidence came from the work of Hart and Setlow (1974), who measured the activity of the enzymatic system for excision repair of UV-ray injury to the DNA of cultured cells from seven species ranging in life span from about 2 years (shrew and mouse) to 70 or more years (elephant and man). They found a close relationship of the rate of repair to the logarithm of life span, and this finding has since been reinforced by data on rate of excision repair in several additional species (Hart, personal communication), and by evidence that several other variables affecting the stability of fibroblasts in culture show differences between two rodent species, *Mus musculus* and *Peromyscus leucopus,* that are consistent with the twofold species difference in longevity (Sacher, G. A., and Hart, 1977).

In recapitulation, longevity in mammals has a close multivariate allometric relationship to brain and body size, metabolic rate, and body temperature. In the case of brain size, the increase of life span has been shown to be a necessary compensation for the depressive influence of brain size on reproductive rate. Moreover, the correlation of mammalian life span with certain specific genetically controlled mechanisms for maintenance of cell survival, such as the mechanism for DNA repair, has been demonstrated, so that all the requirements are satisfied for the hypothesis that longevity (1) is a positive performance of mammals (and other vertebrates); (2) is a significant factor in fitness; and (3) is maintained or increased by the action of natural selection on genetically modifiable enzymatic mechanisms that regulate, protect, and repair the genetic information, and the cell and tissue structure, of the organism.

The discussion in the following sections carries this analysis one step further by showing that there is a correlated variation across species of two actuarial parameters, leading to an association between the life expectation for a species and the shape of its survivorship curve. Consistent with the hypothesis of longevity as a fitness character, the correlation of these two actuarial parameters contributes to increased fitness.

4. Life Tables for Natural Populations

Life tables have been determined for a diverse group of species in the wild. General reviews and critiques of life tables for wild populations are given by Bourliére (1964), Caughley (1966), and Deevey (1947). Three general methods are employed: (1) age determinations by measurement of wear of teeth or other structures that experience statistically uniform wear; (2) age determination by counting anatomical features that accumulate discretely and regularly with age, such as the layered deposition of dentine and cementum in teeth, or the accumulation of corpora albicantia, which are the permanent fibrotic remnants of corpora lutea in the ovaries of certain species; and (3) censusing of survival by the method of marking and recapture. The two methods based on anatomical age determination require an external calibration based on measurements of animals of known age. The method of marking and recapture presents the serious methodological problem of determining whether failure of an animal to return to the record is due to emigration or to death. The statistical procedures required to infer life tables from recapture data have been extensively investigated (Haldane, 1954; Jolly, 1965).

In addition to the reviews cited above, useful information is contained in the following publications. Life tables for several African ungulate species are given by Spinage (1972), based on counts of annual layers in the dentine and cementum of the teeth. The African elephant has been thoroughly studied (Laws, 1967*a*,*b*; Laws and Parker, 1968), as has the hippopotamus (Laws, 1968). Life tables for several species of whales have been determined because analysis of population structure is an important aspect of the management of the whale fisheries (Laws, 1961; Sergeant, 1962). Excellent life tables for seals are available for the same reason (Hewer, 1963). Recapture records for banded bats are extensively reported, but population analysis is rarely undertaken. Perry (1965) provides a study of the age structure of populations of the guano bat. Many studies of the population dynamics of rodent species have provided life tables based on marking and recapture (Blair, 1948; Stickel and Warbach, 1960; Manville, 1949; Snyder, 1956; Bendell, 1959; Tryon and Snyder, 1973; Barkalow *et al.*, 1970).

One conclusion from these studies is that aging can no longer be considered to be an artifact of civilization or captivity. Wild populations of many of the long-lived species have convex curves of logarithm of survival vs. age in adult life, indicating that the rate of mortality in the wild increases with age (Fig. 1). Most small rodents, on the other hand, have approximately linear decrease of log survival with age, indicating that their death rates are independent of age over their short ecological life spans.

5. Evolutionary Change of the Parameters of the Gompertzian Survival Characteristic

The *survival characteristic* of a population is defined as a mathematical model that provides an adequate representation of the survival data for the population (Sacher, G. A., 1977). Evidence has been offered that the survival of well-nourished and protected populations of several mammalian species, including *Homo sapiens,* can be described quite well by the *Gompertz equation* (Gompertz, 1825; Sacher, G. A., 1966*b*), which has the

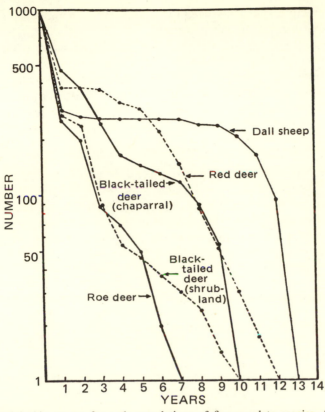

Fig. 1. Survivorship curves for male populations of five ungulate species. Survivorship normalized to 1000 at birth and plotted on a semilogarithmic grid. A convex upward curve on this grid indicates that mortality rate increases with age. Note that three of the five populations have convex curves. Reproduced by permission from Bourlière (1959).

property that the logarithmic derivative of the survival N increases exponentially with age x:

$$M_x \equiv \frac{d \ln N}{dx} = M_0 e^{\alpha x} \qquad (2)$$

This is equivalent to the statement for a real population that its age-specific death rate q_x increases exponentially:

$$q_x \equiv \frac{d_x}{h L_x} = q_0 e^{\alpha x} \qquad (3)$$

where d_x is the number of deaths in a brief interval h at age x, and L_x is the number living at age x. Equation (2) integrates to yield a negatively skewed survivorship curve, as is observed for well-nurtured homogeneous populations of experimental animals and man.

The parameter q_0, the death rate extrapolated back to birth, is an estimate of *initial vulnerability* of the population to the causes of senescent death in adults; i.e., it measures the vulnerability of the population *before* the onset of aging. The parameter α, the rate of increase of the death rate, is a measure of the *actuarial aging rate*. An alternative form, more convenient for some uses, is the doubling time of mortality rate T_d:

$$T_d = 0.693\alpha^{-1} \tag{4}$$

Figure 2 gives the survivorship curves for two rodent species of the superfamily Muroidea. *Mus musculus* is a member of the Old World family Muridae, and *Peromyscus leucopus* belongs to the cosmopolitan family Cricetidae (Simpson, 1945; Wood, 1955). These two species have been extensively investigated in relation to the comparative biology of aging and cancer susceptibility (Sacher, G. A., and Hart, 1977). *Mus* is short-lived,

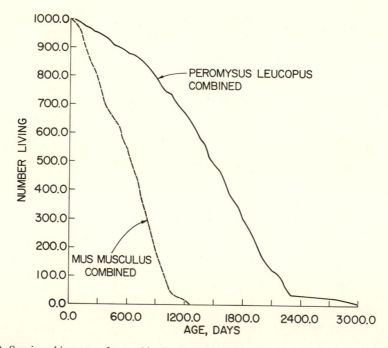

Fig. 2. Survivorship curves for combined sexes of two muroid rodent species, *Mus musculus* and *Peromyscus leucopus*, bred and maintained in captivity (Sacher, G. A., and Staffeldt, 1972; Sacher, G. A., and Hart, 1977). *Peromyscus*, though similar in size and ecological adaptation to *Mus*, lives about 2.5 times as long. Reproduced by permission from G. A. Sacher and Hart (1977).

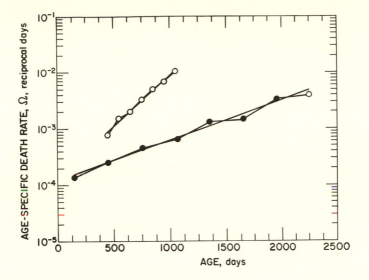

Fig. 3. Plots of logarithm of age-specific mortality rate (Gompertz function), on a logarithmic scale, vs. age for combined sexes for *Mus musculus* (○) and *Peromyscus leucopus* (●). Both species have approximately linear Gompertz function plots, signifying that their actuarial aging processes obey the Gompertz equation (Eq. 3). They have comparable q_0 values, but *Peromyscus* has a slope (actuarial aging rate) about half that for *Mus* (see Table I).

with a life expectancy of about 600 days, while *Peromyscus leucopus* lives 1400 days on the average. Figure 3 gives the Gompertz function plots for these two species. It can be seen that in both species, the Gompertz function is a straight line, and that the slope is lower for *Peromyscus* than for *Mus*.

Table I gives the life expectation E_0, the initial vulnerability parameter q_0, and the doubling time of mortality rate T_d for captive populations of nine species of mammals drawn from five orders (Andersen, 1970; Andersen and Rosenblatt, 1974; Blus, 1971; Comfort, 1956, 1957, 1958*a,b*, 1959*a,b*, 1960, 1961; Sacher, G. A., and Staffeldt, 1972). The relationship of q_0 to T_d is graphed in Fig. 3, which shows that while the aging rate α decreases by about a factor of 30 from the small insectivores and rodents to man, the initial vulnerability q_0 decreases by a factor on the order of 1000. As noted above, these data were obtained from homogeneous noninbred populations maintained under good conditions, so that mortality of environmental origin is relatively unimportant and the Gompertz equation parameters can be well estimated. Nevertheless, it would not be proper to assume that the nine populations were exposed to equivalent environmental pressures. In particular, individual caging of the rodent populations, together with improved sanitation and increased opportunity for environment selec-

Table I. Life Expectation E_0, Initial Vulnerability q_0, and Doubling Time of Mortality Rate T_d for Nine Mammalian Species.[a]

Species	E_0 (days)	q_0 (day)$^{-1}$	T_d (days)
Blarina brevicauda (short-tailed shrew)	240[b]	4.4×10^{-4}	87
Mus musculus (house mouse)	602	3.0×10^{-4}	220
Sigmodon hispidus (cotton rat)	514	2.2×10^{-4}	125
Oryzomys palustris (rice rat)	789	1.1×10^{-4}	197
Peromyscus leucopus (white-footed mouse)	1,475	1.2×10^{-4}	447
Peromyscus californicus (California mouse)	1,100	2.4×10^{-4}	441
Canis familiaris (beagle dog)	3,617	2.7×10^{-5}	812
Equus caballus (thoroughbred mare)	6,329	6.0×10^{-6}	1332
Homo sapiens (U.S. white female, 1969)	27,700	1.5×10^{-7}	3100

[a]Life expectations are from birth; in the cases of the rodents and the shrew, they do not include the deaths from birth to weaning. Data for all rodent species from Sacher and Staffeldt (unpublished); for short-tailed shrew, from Blus (1971); for beagle dog, from Andersen (1970), Andersen and Rosenblatt (1974), and Norris *et al.* (1976); for thoroughbred mare, from Comfort (1958*a,b*). Reproduced, with modifications, from G. A. Sacher (1977).
[b]Median survival time.

tion and for choice of diet, could perhaps decrease vulnerability, and hence q_0, by a substantial factor. Moreover, all nonhuman populations are in some degree at a disadvantage in comparison with well-nurtured human populations. These differences in environmental morbidity pressures give rise to a bias in the slope of the relationship of q_0 to T_d in Fig. 3, but at worst the distortion of the overall relationship is minor, because these inequalities of environmental morbidity pressure may be responsible for bias in q_0 by no more than a factor of 10, whereas the overall variation of q_0 from shrew and mouse to man is on the order of 1000. As the product $q_0 T_d$ decreases, the effect is to lengthen the shoulder phase of the survivorship curve relative to the duration of the declining phase. This means that the individual population member can expect to have a longer period of assured survival before the onset of failure, both in absolute time and as a fraction of his maximum life span.

Increased determinateness of the survival curve* is a necessary concomitant of the evolution of large body size and brain size, for these changes in body dimensions lead to a reduced reproductive rate because of reduction of litter size and increase of gestation time and maturation time (Sacher, G. A., and Staffeldt, 1974). All these trends contribute to an increase of the *replacement time,* i.e., the minimum age at which a female

---

*G. A. Sacher (1966*a*) defines determinateness as $D = \mu_1^2/\mu_2$, where μ_1 and μ_2 are the first and second moments of survival from birth. It has a range from unity for a rectangular curve to zero for all distributions with infinite variance and finite mean.

can replace herself in the population, both in absolute terms and as a fraction of the maximum life span (Table II).

The ratio of replacement time to life span is about 3 times greater for man than for the mouse, with horse and dog occupying intermediate positions. The approximately 1000-fold decrease of q_0 from mouse to man in Table I is quantitatively consistent with the approximate threefold increase in the relative replacement time, as the following argument shows. The life expectation from age zero, E_0, for a population with a Gompertz survival characteristic is (Sacher, G. A., 1960)

$$E_0 = \tau \exp(q_0\tau)[- Ei(-q_0\tau)] \tag{5}$$

where $\tau = \alpha^{-1}$ and $Ei(-z)$ is the exponential integral of argument z (WPA, 1940). To a satisfactory approximation, this can be replaced by

$$E_0 = -\tau \ln(\gamma q_0\tau) \tag{6}$$

where γ is a pure number, $\gamma = 1.781. . . .$

Equation (6) indicates that if the product $q_0\tau$ is a constant, life expectation is directly proportional to τ. This is the case in which the life tables of different species are similar in form, and differ only in a single scaling factor.

Table II. Estimation of Replacement Time for Mus musculus and Homo sapiens[a]

| | Mus musculus | | | Homo sapiens | | | |
Parameter	N	Days	%	N	Days	%	Formula
Gestation time		20	1.7		267	0.8	
Time to weaning		28	2.3		730	2.1	
Time to self-sufficiency		28	2.3		~ 4,700	13.8	
Time to sexual maturity		36	3.0		5,100	15.0	
Interval between births		~ 60	5.0		~ 365	1.1	
Litter size	5			1.01			
Number of litters for replacement[b]	1			4			
Parous period for replacement		~ 60	5.0		~ 1,460	4.3	5 × 7
Life expectation							
Wild		~120			~11,000		
Nurtured		600			25,500		
Maximum life span		1,200			34,000		
Replacement time		124	10.3		11,300	33.1	4 + 8 + 3

[a]Reproductive data from Asdell (1964); longevity data from Table I and G. A. Sacher and Hart (1977). Data preceded by an approximate sign (~) are estimates made by the author, either because published data are very scattered or because no data were known. The ratio of relative replacement times for man/mouse is 3.2 : 1. This ratio has a large uncertainty, but it surely lies in the interval 2.0–4.5.
[b]Assuming 50% survival to maturity.

The quantity $q_0\tau$, using the values of q_0 and τ in Table I, is lower in man than in the house mouse by a factor of 100. The increase in life expectation due to this decrease is given [equation (6)] by the ratio of $\ln(\gamma q_0\tau)$ for man and mouse. This quantity is 3.2, which says that according to the Gompertz model, omitting neonatal and age-independent mortality, the human life expectation is 3.2 times longer than if $q_0\tau$ had remained constant at the mouse level. This is in good agreement with the observed increase of relative replacement time by a factor of 3 from mouse to man (Table II).

Under the conditions in the wild in which the species evolved, there is no such thing as an assured period of survival, because of the high age-independent mortality rate from predation, accident, starvation, and other environmental contingencies. This raises a question about the evolutionary significance of an assured period of survival if the environmental conditions for it never exist in nature. This is an important question, and the lack of a satisfactory answer in the past has been a deterrent to the development of a consensus about the evolutionary origin of the sigmoid survival curves observed for well-nourished and protected populations of experimental animals and *Homo sapiens*.

There is an answer to this question, and it can account for the evolution of the survival characteristic of captive animals, and for its quantitative change from mouse to man. The explanation draws on the independently established fact that the disease *morbidity* rate as a function of age in well-nurtured populations has the same general exponentially increasing trend, and about the same slope coefficient, as the mortality rate (Dublin *et al.*, 1949). Even a brief period of illness or disability in a parous female would, with high probability, lead to the loss of all her dependent progeny, either through predation or starvation. Because of the accelerating trend of the morbidity rate curve, the probability of loss of litters would also increase exponentially with age.

Insofar as the probability of loss of litters as a result of limitations on intrinsic vigor and stress resistance is independent of the probability of death of the dam from age-independent environmental contingencies, natural selection can operate independently on the gene systems governing vulnerability to the intrinsic age-related degenerative diseases and disabilities. The reproductive success of iteroparous organisms is dependent on the maintenance of successful reproduction for a time period sufficient for replacement and an adequate rate of increase. As the litter size decreases, the length of this interval increases. The evolutionary trend in the mammals toward increase of brain size is just such as would lead to an increase of the replacement time. This increase is accomplished in part by selection toward decreased random death from environmental contingencies, but the additional requirement for the maintenance of a very high degree of physiological performance over the full duration of the replacement time gives rise to independent selection for increased physiological stability and resistance to failure, and this selection is reflected in a change of survival parameters. That the survival characteristic so selected can be observed only under good captive conditions is not important, for that survival characteristic is a consequence of selection for an extended period of physiological and reproductive vigor, and these characteristics *are* important in the wild state.

6. Conclusion

This discussion of life-table evolution in terms of factors of change from mouse to man is simple and approximate, but it is appropriate to the quality of the available data, and it suffices to prove the point that the evolution of the mammalian life table is more than a matter of increase of longevity. The shape of the survival characteristic also changed in the direction of increased determinateness of survival, as required by the evolutionary changes in reproductive pattern brought about by increase of brain and body size. It is important to realize that only about half the increase of longevity from mouse to man is due to decrease in the aging rate. The other half is due to the great decrease of initial vulnerability. Longevity is a two-dimensional function.

The comparative analysis of mammalian life tables, and of their relationship to reproductive patterns, supports the hypothesis that the mammalian life-table parameters, as observed in captive populations, evolved in nature as a consequence of natural selection for a longer reproductive replacement time.

ACKNOWLEDGMENT

The author's work is supported by the U.S. Department of Energy.

References

Andersen, A. C. (ed.), 1970, General pathology, in: *The Beagle as an Experimental Dog,* pp. 520–546, Iowa State University Press, Ames.

Andersen, A. C., and Rosenblatt, L. S., 1974, Survival of beagles under natural and laboratory conditions, in: *Dogs and Other Large Mammals in Aging Research: I* (A. C. Andersen, E. A. Boyden, and J. H. Dougherty, eds.), pp. 18–23, MSS Information Corp., New York.

Asdell, S. A., 1964, *Patterns of Mammalian Reproduction,* 2nd Ed., Cornell University Press, New York.

Barkalow, F. S., Jr., Hamilton, R. B., and Soots, R. F., Jr., 1970, The vital statistics of an unexploited gray squirrel population, *J. Wildl. Manage.* **34**:489.

Bendell, J. F., 1959, Food as a control of a population of white-footed mice, *Peromyscus leucopus noveboracensis* (Fischer), *Can. J. Zool.* **37**:173.

Blair, W. F., 1948, Population density, life span and mortality rates of small mammals in the blue-grass meadow and blue-grass field association of Southern Michigan, *Am. Midl. Nat.* **49**:395.

Blus, L. J., 1971, Reproduction and survival of short-tailed shrews *(Blarina brevicauda)* in captivity, *Lab. Anim. Sci.* **21**:884.

Bourlière, F., 1959, Lifespans of mammalian and bird populations in nature, in: *Ciba Found. Colloq. Ageing* (G. E. W. Wolstenholme and M. O'Connor, eds.), Vol. 5, *The Lifespan of Animals,* pp. 99–103, Churchill, London.

Bourlière, F., 1964, *The Natural History of Mammals,* 3rd Ed., Knopf, New York.

Brody, S., 1945, *Bioenergetics and Growth,* Reinhold, New York.

Caughley, G., 1966, Mortality patterns in mammals, *Ecology* **47**:906.

Cole, L. C., 1954, The population consequences of life history phenomena, *Q. Rev. Biol.* **29**:103.

Comfort, A., 1956, Longevity and mortality of Irish wolfhounds, *Proc. Zool. Soc. London* **127**:27.

Comfort, A., 1957, Survival curves of mammals in captivity, *Proc. Zool. Soc. London* **128**:349.

Comfort, A., 1958*a,* The longevity and mortality of thoroughbred mares, *J. Gerontol.* **13**:342.

Comfort, A., 1958*b,* Coat color and longevity in thoroughbred mares, *Nature (London)* **182**:1531.

Comfort, A., 1959*a,* The longevity and mortality of thoroughbred stallions, *J. Gerontol.* **14**:9.

Comfort, A., 1959*b,* Studies on the longevity and mortality of English thoroughbred horses, in: *Ciba Found. Colloq. Ageing* (G. E. W. Wolstenholme and M. O'Connor, eds.), Vol. 5, *The Lifespan of Animals,* pp. 35–54, Churchill, London.

Comfort, A., 1960, Longevity and mortality in dogs of four breeds, *J. Gerontol.* **15**:126.

Comfort, A., 1961, A life table for Arabian mares, *J. Gerontol.* **17**:14.

Cutler, R. G., 1975, Evolution of human longevity and the genetic complexity governing aging rate, *Proc. Natl. Acad. Sci. U.S.A.* **72**:4664.

Deevey, E. S., Jr., 1947, Life tables for natural populations of animals, *Q. Rev. Biol.* **22**:283.

De Leo, P., and Sacher, J. A., 1970, Control of ribonuclease and acid phosphatase by auxin and abscisic acid during senescence of *Rhoeo* leaf sections, *Plant Physiol.* **46**:806.

Dublin, L. I., Lotka, A. J., and Spiegelman, M., 1949, *Length of Life,* Rev. Ed., Ronald Press, New York.

Gompertz, B., 1825, On the nature of the function expressive of the law of human mortality and on a new mode of determining life contingencies, *Philos. Trans. R. Soc. London* **1825**:513.

Gould, S. J., 1966, Allometry and size in ontogeny and phylogeny, *Biol. Rev. Cambridge Philos. Soc.* **41**:587.

Haldane, J. B. S., 1954, The calculation of mortality rates from ringing data, *Acta XI Congr. Ornithol.,* Basel **1954**:454.

Hamilton, W. D., 1966, The moulding of senescence by natural selection, *J. Theor. Biol.* **12**:12.

Hart, R. W., and Setlow, R. B., 1974, Correlation between deoxyribonucleic acid excision–repair and life-span in a number of mammalian species, *Proc. Natl. Acad. Sci. U.S.A.* **71**:2169.

Hewer, H. R., 1963, The determination of age, sexual maturity, longevity and a life-table in the grey seal *(Halichoerus grypus), Proc. Zool. Soc. London* **142**:593.

Jerison, H. J., 1973, *Evolution of the Brain and Intelligence,* Academic Press, New York.

Jolly, G. M., 1965, Explicit estimates from capture–recapture data with both death and immigration: Stochastic model, *Biometrika* **52**:225.

Laws, R. M., 1961, Reproduction, growth and age of southern fin whales, *Discovery Rep.* **31**:327.

Laws, R. M., 1967*a*, Eye lens weight and age in African elephants, *East Afr. Wildl. J.* **5**:46.

Laws, R. M., 1967*b*, Occurrence of placental scars in the uterus of African elephant *(Loxodonta africana), J. Reprod. Fertil.* **14**:445.

Laws, R. M., 1968, Dentition and ageing of the hippopotamus, *East Afr. Wildl. J.* **6**:19.

Laws, R. M., and Parker, I. S. C., 1968, Recent studies on elephant populations in East Africa, *Symp. Zool. Soc. London* **21**:319.

Leopold, A. C., 1961, Senescence in plant development, *Science* **134**:1727.

Mallouk, R. S., 1975, Longevity in vertebrates is proportional to relative brain weight, *Fed. Proc. Fed. Am. Soc. Exp. Biol.* **34**:2102.

Manville, R. H., 1949, *A Study of Small Mammal Populations in Northern Michigan,* Miscellaneous Publication No. 73, 83 pp., Museum of Zoology, University of Michigan, Ann Arbor.

Martin, G. M., 1977, Genetic disorders in man with relevance to aging, in: *Genetic Effects on Aging* (D. Bergsma and D. E. Harrison, eds.), pp. 7–42, A. R. Liss, New York.

McKusick, V. A., 1975, *Mendelian Inheritance in Man,* 4th Ed., Johns Hopkins University Press, Baltimore.

Medawar, P. B., 1957, Old age and natural death, and An unsolved problem of biology, in: *The Uniqueness of the Individual,* Methuen and Co., London.

Norris, W. P., Tyler, S. A., and Sacher, G. A., 1976, An interspecies comparison of responses of mice and dogs to continuous ^{60}Co gamma irradiation, in: *Biological and Environmental Effects of Low-Level Radiation,* Vol. 1, pp. 147–155, International Atomic Energy Agency, Vienna.

Perry, A., 1965, Population analysis of the guano bat *Tadarida brasiliensis mexicana* (Saussure) using the lens-weight method of age determination, Ph.D. dissertation, Oklahoma State University of Agriculture and Applied Science, Stillwater.

Rensch, B., 1959, *Evolution Above the Species Level,* Methuen and Co., London.

Sacher, G. A., 1959, Relation of lifespan to brain weight and body weight in mammals, in: *Ciba Foundation Colloquia on Ageing* (G. E. W. Wolstenholme and M. O'Connor, eds.), Vol. 5, *The Lifespan of Animals* pp. 115–133, Churchill, London.

Sacher, G. A., 1960, Problems in the extrapolation of long term effects from animals to man, in: *The Delayed Effects of Whole-Body Radiation* (B. B. Watson, ed.), pp. 3–10, Johns Hopkins University Press, Baltimore.

Sacher, G. A., 1966*a*, Abnutzungstheorie, in: *Perspectives in Experimental Gerontology* (N. W. Shock, ed.), pp. 326–335, Charles C. Thomas, Springfield, Illinois.

Sacher, G. A., 1966*b*, The Gompertz transformation in the study of injury–mortality relationship: Application to late radiation effects and ageing, in: *Radiation and Ageing: Proceedings of a Colloquium Held in Semmering, Austria, June 1966* (P. J. Lindop and G. A. Sacher, eds.), pp. 411–441, Taylor and Francis, London.

Sacher, G. A., 1968, Molecular versus systemic theories on the genesis of ageing, *Exp. Gerontol.* **3**:265.

Sacher, G. A., 1975, Maturation and longevity in relation to cranial capacity in hominid evolution, in: *Antecedents of Man and After,* Vol. I, *Primates: Functional Morphology and Evolution* (R. Tuttle, ed.), pp. 417–441, Mouton and Co., The Hague.

Sacher, G. A., 1976, Evaluation of the entropy and information terms governing mammalian longevity, *Interdiscip. Top. Gerontol.* **9**:69.

Sacher, G. A., 1977, Life table modification and life prolongation, in: *Handbook of the Biology of Aging* (C. E. Finch and L. Hayflick, eds.), pp. 582–638, Van Nostrand-Reinhold, New York.

Sacher, G. A., and Hart, R. W., 1977, Longevity, aging and comparative cellular and molecular biology of the house mouse, *Mus musculus,* and the white-footed mouse, *Peromyscus leucopus,* in: *Genetic Effects on Aging* (D. H. Harrison, ed.), pp. 73–98, A. R. Liss, New York.

Sacher, G. A., and Jones, M. L., 1972, Life span: Mammalia, in: *Biology Data Book* (P. L. Altman and D. S. Dittmer, eds.), 2nd Ed., Vol. 1, pp. 229–230, Federation of American Societies for Experimental Biology, Bethesda, Maryland.

Sacher, G. A., and Staffeldt, E., 1972, Life tables of seven species of laboratory-reared rodents, *Gerontologist* **12**(3)(Part III):39.

Sacher, G. A., and Staffeldt, E. F., 1974, Relation of gestation time to brain weight for placental mammals: Implications for the theory of vertebrate growth, *Am. Nat.* **108**:593.

Sacher, J. A., 1967, Control of synthesis of RNA and protein in subcellular fractions of *Rhoeo discolor* leaf sections by auxin and kinetin during senescence, *Exp. Gerontol.* **2**:261.

Sacher, J. A., 1973, Senescence and postharvest physiology, *Annu. Rev. Plant Physiol.* **24**:197.

Sergeant, D. E., 1962, The biology of the pilot or pothead whale *Globicephala melaena* (Traill) in Newfoundland waters, Bulletin No. 132, pp. vii + 84, Fisheries Research Board, Ottawa, Canada.

Simpson, G. G., 1945, The principles of classification and a classification of mammals, *Bull. Am. Mus. Nat. Hist.* **85**:xvi + 350.

Snyder, D. P., 1956, *Survival Rates, Longevity and Population Fluctuations in the White-Footed Mouse, Peromyscus leucopus, in Southeastern Michigan,* Miscellaneous Publication No. 95, pp. 1–33, Museum of Zoology, University of Michigan, Ann Arbor.

Spinage, C. A., 1972, African ungulate life tables, *Ecology* **53**:645.

Stickel, L. F., and Warbach, O., 1960, Small-mammal populations of a Maryland woodlot, *Ecology* **41**:269.

Tryon, C. A., and Snyder, D. P., 1973, Biology of the eastern chipmunk, *Tamias striatus:* Life tables, age distribution, and trends in population numbers, *J. Mammal.* **54**:145.

Watson, J. D., 1976, *Molecular Biology of the Gene,* 3rd Ed., W. A. Benjamin, New York.

Weismann, A., 1882, *Über die Dauer des Lebens,* G. Fischer, Jena.

Weismann, A., 1891, *Essays upon Heredity and Kindred Biological Problems,* Oxford University Press, London.

Williams, G. C., 1957, Pleiotropy, natural selection, and the evolution of senescence, *Evolution* **11**:398.

Wood, A. E., 1955, A revised classification of rodents, *J. Mammal.* **36**:165.

Woolhouse, H. W., 1974, Longevity and senescence in plants, *Sci. Prog. (Oxford)* **61**:123.

WPA, 1940, *Tables of Sine, Cosine and Exponential Integrals,* Vols. 1 and 2, Works Projects Administration, New York.

Part III

Human Genetics

Human Genetic Disorders That Feature Premature Onset and Accelerated Progression of Biological Aging

Samuel Goldstein

1. Introduction

Despite a burgeoning number of recent investigations and increasingly rigorous scrutiny, a universally acceptable definition of normal biological aging is still not available. The origins of senescence remain enigmatic, and little agreement exists regarding its true nature. While most would accept as genuine aging phenomena the diverse processes of hair graying, wrinkling of skin, and arteriosclerosis, they would, on the other hand, reserve embryogenesis, somatic growth, and pubescence for development. Both kinds of phenomena are clearly time-dependent, but the interface between them is often blurred (Goldstein, S., 1971*a*). The conceptual difficulty is exemplified by the frequent juxtaposition of involution and new development, even at early and middle stages of the life span (Saunders and Fallon, 1966). Cogent examples are the placenta vs. the fetus during gestation and the replacement of deciduous teeth by permanent dentition during infancy. During childhood, atrophy of the thymus occurs when virtually all other organs are growing and maturing, while the menopausal ovary involutes relatively abruptly in comparison with other organs in the middle-aged female. One could invoke examples of involution at the molecular level such as the loss during fetal life of various proteins including γ-hemoglobin,

Samuel Goldstein • Departments of Medicine and Biochemistry, McMaster University, Hamilton, Ontario, Canada L8S 4J9

carcinoembryonic antigen, α-fetoprotein, and others (Gold, 1971). In short, attempts to delineate the point at which development is succeeded by aging may be futile, since both processes probably operate along the same continuum.

Perhaps the major distinction that can be identified is that during aging, in contrast to development, no proteins, matrices, or organs with essentially new structures or functions arise. It must be accepted, however, that this area remains fraught with pitfalls and semantic difficulties. A useful definition for purposes of orientation is that aging is a progressive unfavorable loss of adaptation and a decreasing expectation of life with the passage of time; it is expressed in measurement as decreased viability and increased vulnerability to the normal forces of mortality (Comfort, 1964).

2. Specific Criteria of Aging

2.1. Physiological Markers

2.1.1. General Test Battery

Comfort (1969) elaborated a test battery of several diverse physiological, cellular, and biochemical parameters that collectively define the aging rate of the subject. This battery would provide three major benefits, since it (1) allows the establishment of normal ranges; (2) enables objective evaluation of suspected cases of premature aging; and (3) expedites the evaluation of the effects of various regimens on normal and abnormal human aging, especially as they affect variables other than mortality. Such tests are generally noninvasive and readily available, but would require, in total, a substantial expenditure of time and money, even in relatively small surveys. Additionally, repetition of screening tests would be necessary at intervals to determine trends.

What would be desirable is a single, relatively simple test that encompasses aging of the whole organism. Although such a test is proving unattainable, it is instructive to present two examples of physiological tests that illustrate the problem.

2.1.2. Specific Tests

a. Creatinine Clearance. Creatinine clearance is a standard measure of the renal glomerular filtration rate. This parameter declines with age after maturity in both cross-sectional and longitudinal studies (Lindeman, 1975; Rowe *et al.*, 1976), even after subjects with specific diseases or those taking medications that might alter the test are excluded. The value of this kind of marker is that it summates the age-dependent decline of a number of individual physiological systems, including cardiac output, renal plasma flow, and the effective renal vascular bed. Two major limitations, however, are its inability to measure functional reserve and its lack of sensitivity in predicting trends and outcomes in specific persons.

b. Glucose Intolerance and Insulin Resistance. Although the correlation is also imperfect, one index that frequently declines with age is glucose tolerance. There is a progressive inability to maintain glucose homeostasis in aging persons either in the fasting state or following the challenge of an administered glucose load. Indeed, hyperglycemia is so common in the elderly that Andres *et al.* (1975) formulated a percentile system to rank a subject with age-matched cohorts. This system avoids labeling a disquietingly high proportion of people as diabetics. It seems clear that glucose disposition involves every cell in the body; hence, one would expect glucose tolerance to provide an excellent summation of whole-organism aging. This parameter is complex, however, and is determined by the relative balance among several metabolic and hormonal components, particularly insulin. There is also the likelihood that some cells actually increase their glucose consumption with age (Goldstein, S., and Trieman, 1975).

Several disorders, most of them inherited in a classic Mendelian sense, are associated with glucose intolerance or insulin resistance or both (Table I). Many also feature stunted growth and precocious and accelerated aging. The high correlation between abnormal glucose metabolism and aging in a widely assorted group of genetic disorders substantiates the idea of a common denominator at the cellular level.

3. Premature Aging

3.1. General Criteria

An objective set of prerequisites has been formulated to qualify extrinsic or intrinsic agents as inducers of premature aging (Rubin and Casarett, 1968; Walburg, 1975). Each agent should:

1. Bring about an earlier increase in mortality in comparison with a nontreated control group without altering the shape of the entire mortality curve.
2. Bring forward proportionately in time the age of onset and the time of development of all diseases or causes of death that affect the control group without altering degree, sequence, or absolute incidence of diseases and causes of death, and without induction of new diseases.

3. Cause all the morphological and physiological manifestations of aging to appear and develop at proportionately earlier chronological ages to degrees and rates in the various organs proportional to those degrees and rates in organs of control organisms.

There is a further refinement in the definition: if the agent causes these manifestations to occur early in life without altering their rate of development, this occurrence is regarded as "precocious or premature aging." If the rate of development is increased, the effect is one of "accelerated aging."

These definitions are conceptually useful, but impose severe constraints if rigidly applied. In fact, most cases of abnormal aging have not

Table I.   Genetic Disorders Associated with Glucose Intolerance or Insulin Resistance or Both and Many Also with a Decreased Life Span[a]

Familial	
Alstrom syndrome	Laurence–Moon–Biedl syndrome
Ataxia–telangiectasia	Lipoatrophic diabetes (Seip
Cockayne syndrome	syndrome)
Cervical lipodisplasia	Muscular dystrophy
(Launois–Bensaude	Myotonic dystrophy
adenolipomatosis)[b]	Ocular hypertension induced by
Cystic fibrosis	dexamethasone
Fanconi anemia	Optic atrophy and diabetes
Friedreich ataxia	Optic atrophy, diabetes insipidus, and
Glucose-6-phosphate dehydrogenase	diabetes mellitus
deficiency	Hereditary relapsing pancreatitis
Type 1 glycogen storage disease	Photomyoclonus, diabetes, deafness,
Gout	nephropathy, and cerebral
Hemochromatosis	dysfunction
Huntington disease	Pineal hyperplasia and diabetes
Hutchinson–Gilford syndrome	Acute intermittent porphyria
(progeria)	Pheochromocytoma
Hyperlipidemia, diabetes,	Prader–Willi syndrome
hypogonadism, and short stature	Retinitis pigmentosa, neuropathy,
syndrome	ataxia, and diabetes
Hyperlipoproteinemia III, IV, and V	Schmidt syndrome
Isolated growth hormone deficiency	Werner syndrome

Nonfamilial (chromosomal)		
Down syndrome[c]	Klinefelter syndrome	Turner syndrome

[a]From S. Goldstein et al. (1975) and S. Goldstein (1978a,b).
[b]Greene et al. (1970).
[c]A small percentage of cases, e.g., balanced translocation, are familial. Further details on the familial disorders can be found in McKusick (1975).

Table II.   Selected Pathophysiological and Cellular Criteria of Aging[a]

1. Intrinsic mutagenesis hypothesis of aging[b]
2. Increased frequency of nonconstitutional chromosomal aberrations
3. Increased susceptibility to one or more types of neoplasms relevant to aging
4. Defects in stem-cell populations or in the kinetics of stem-cell proliferation
5. Premature graying or loss of hair or both
6. Dementia or certain types of related degenerative neuropathology or both
7. Increased susceptibility to "slow virus"
8. Increased amyloid deposition
9. Increased deposition of lipofuscin pigments
10. Diabetes mellitus
11. Disordered lipid metabolism
12. Hypogonadism
13. Autoimmunity
14. Hypertension
15. Degenerative vascular disease
16. Osteoporosis
17. Cataracts
18. Abnormalities of mitochondria in one or more systems
19. Regional fibrosis
20. Abnormal amounts or distributions of adipose tissue
21. A miscellaneous group of syndromes with potential relevance to the pathobiology of aging

[a]From G. M. Martin (1977).   [b]Burnet (1974).

only an earlier time of onset but also an accelerated tempo and exaggerated severity of age-related pathology. Moreover, while the nature of the pathology may be indistinguishable from that of normal aging, organ involvement is almost never universal, but rather shows predilection for one or a few tissues.

3.2. A Specific Scoring System for Premature Aging

G. M. Martin (1977) conducted an exhaustive analysis of all disorders listed in the catalogue of McKusick (1975) on genetic phenotypes according to 21 selected criteria of aging (Table II). He concluded that 83 autosomal dominant, 70 autosomal recessive, and 9 X-linked recessive disorders have one or more regional, segmental, or more widespread features of accelerated biological aging. This total of 162 of the 2336 loci in McKusick's catalogue constitutes an overall 6.9%. Extrapolating from this value, on the assumption that there are 100,000 informational loci in the human genome, about 6900 loci could potentially modulate the aging phenotype. In reality, however, a much smaller proportion, perhaps a few dozen, might be more pertinent to aging. Martin also added the chromosomal disorders, which are "genetic" but not hereditary except in a few cases of balanced translocation trisomy. He evaluated them by determining how many of the 21 criteria were observed in each disorder (Table III). The anomalies of chromosome number, perhaps surprisingly, scored high and were included with other, more widely recognized "progeroid" syndromes. This analysis is clearly open to discussion but it provides a preliminary scaffolding from

Table III.   Rank Order of Premature Aging Syndromes Scored by
Criteria in Table II[a]

Number of times scored	Syndrome
14	Down syndrome
12	Werner syndrome
12	Cockayne syndrome
9	Progeria (Hutchinson–Gilford syndrome)
8	Ataxia–telangiectasia
8	Cervical lipodysplasia, familial
8	Seip syndrome, generalized lipodystrophy, hereditary type
8	Klinefelter syndrome
7	Turner syndrome
6	Myotonic dystrophy (Steinert disease)

[a]From G. M. Martin (1977).

which to view aging. Simultaneously, however, it underscores the complexity in evolving uniformly satisfactory criteria for aging. Remarkably, the entire list also appears within Table I.

The idea of deceleration or resistance to aging is also worth contemplating. G. M. Martin (1977) concluded that we cannot expect such a phenotype ("antigeria") to occur consequent to mutation at a single genetic locus. It seems clear, however, that vigorous longevity, or the converse, freedom from age-dependent pathology, does occur in certain select populations (Leaf, 1973). Perhaps persons with a relative paucity of detrimental genes are destined for vigorous longevity. Evidence for this proposal is adduced in Section 6.1.

The disorders listed in Tables I and III feature abnormalities in diverse tissues derived from various embryonic germ layers. Perhaps this explains why there is often a preponderant pathology restricted to one or a few organ systems that necessitates the term *segmental* aging (Martin, G. M.,

Table IV.   Number of Lesions Apparent at Autopsy in Relation to Age[a]

Number of subjects	Age group	Number of lesions	Average number of lesions per subject
100	65–69	571	5.71
100	70–74	639	6.39
100	75–79	757	7.57
100	80–84	842	8.42
40	90–99	498	12.45

[a]From Howell (1975). A group of 20 cases for every year of age from 65 to 84 and 40 nonagenarians were examined for gross ischemic, inflammatory, degenerative, and malignant changes.

1977). It must be recognized, however, that specific pathology and ultimate cause of death can be far removed, albeit causally related. For example, the primary features of Friedreich ataxia and Huntington disease are neurological deficits that ultimately lead to malnutrition, the propensity to infection, and premature death.

The remainder of this chapter will therefore be addressed to admittedly selected disorders that feature early and severe degenerative or malignant disease or both. It is conceded that few of these diseases will show all such features, but it must be understood that normal aging itself is rarely associated with the simultaneous appearance of several overt lesions in each person, even though the number of pathological foci apparent at autopsy increases progressively with age (Table IV). The situation is further complicated by the limited number of investigations carried out and, hence, the sparse data so far available. Some aspects of this survey, therefore, must inescapably be regarded as preliminary.

4. Description of Selected Disorders That Feature Premature Aging

4.1. Classic Progeroid Syndromes

4.1.1. The Hutchinson–Gilford Syndrome (Progeria)

a. Clinical Picture. J. Hutchinson (1886) first described what we now call progeria in a boy "with congenital absence of hair and mammary glands and atrophic condition of the skin and its appendages." Gilford (1897) was first to characterize the postmortem picture and subsequently propose the term *progeria*. A large number of reports in both the English and the foreign-language literature subsequently appeared defining clinico-pathological features and laboratory investigations (Paterson, D., 1922; Mostafa and Gabr, 1954; Keay *et al.*, 1955; Gabr *et al.*, 1960; Ghosh and Varma, 1964; Bhakoo *et al.*, 1965; Macleod, 1966; Ozonoff and Clemett, 1967; Rava, 1967; Giacomini and Rizzi, 1968; Margolin and Steinbach, 1968; Gardner and Majka, 1969; Kaiman *et al.*, 1969; Marcondes *et al.*, 1969; Wiedemann, 1969; Feingold and Kidd, 1971; Rosenbloom and Debusk, 1971; Kidd and Wilgram, 1972; Fleischmajer and Nedwich, 1973*a*; Ghosh and Berry, 1973; Grunebaum, 1973; Lenz and Majewski, 1974; Valdiserri and Stricchiola, 1974; Viegas *et al.*, 1974; Levine *et al.*, 1975; Welsh, 1975; Ishii, 1976; Piazzini *et al.*, 1976). An excellent review of 60 cases up to 1970 was also published (DeBusk, 1972).

The most striking clinical feature is severe growth retardation that first attracts attention between 6 and 12 months of age. Besides the dwarfism,

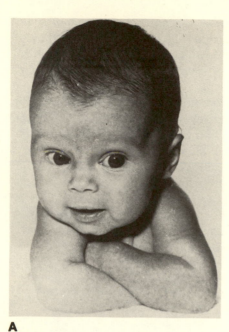

A

Fig. 1. Girl with progeria at 2 months of age with normal appearance (A), at 4 years 8 months showing characteristic craniofacial features (B), and lateral view at same age (C). Photographs provided through the courtesy of Dr. N. Rudd, Toronto Sick Children's Hospital, with permission of the parents.

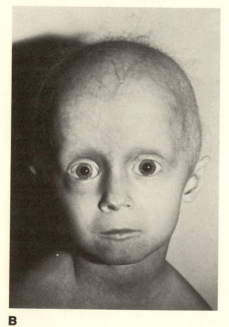

B

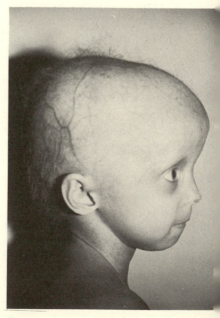

C

the picture invariably includes severe diminution of subcutaneous fat, a disproportionately large cranial/facial size ratio, a small chin, prominent scalp veins, scalp baldness, and prominent eyes (Fig. 1). Scleroderma is often prominent and sexual maturation is never attained, although psycho-motor development is almost always normal. Indeed, intelligence is said to be high as a rule. Also prominent are a number of hypoplastic, dysplastic, and degenerative skeletal abnormalities unique to progeria, and these abnormalities can be detected on both clinical and radiological examination (Reichel and Garcia-Bunuel, 1970; Reichel *et al.*, 1971*a,b*). Developmental anomalies appear as delayed eruption and crowding of deciduous and permanent teeth. There are also quantitative and qualitative anomalies of the chest cage (small ribs and clavicle) and skull (thin calvarium and delay in ossification of fontanels) as well as the mandible and long bones produc-ing the characteristic coxa valga deformity, "horse-riding" stance, and wide-based shuffling gait. While osteoporosis is a generalized problem in concordance with normal aging, degenerative osteoarthritis does not typi-cally occur.

Overt diabetes does not seem to be a feature of progeria although in the few cases tested, there is pronounced resistance to the hypoglycemia action of exogenous insulin (Villee *et al.*, 1969; Rosenbloom *et al.*, 1970). Basal metabolic rate is increased (Talbot *et al.*, 1945), as substantiated by higher glutamate oxidation by muscle mitochondria of two patients under both controlled ("state 4") and maximally functioning ("state 3") conditions (Villee *et al.*, 1969). Studies on bone metabolism in the same patients showed a markedly reduced turnover rate. There was also a high degree of cross-linkage in skin collagen (Villee *et al.*, 1969), as is found in tissues of elderly normals and diabetics (Hamlin *et al.*, 1975).

Hyperlipidemia was reported in one case (MacNamara *et al.*, 1970), but lipid abnormalities appear to be the exception rather than the rule. Progeric individuals do not become sexually mature due to gonadal hypo-plasia, but no other consistent abnormalities have been reported in the endocrines, including thyroid, parathyroid, pituitary, and adrenal glands (DeBusk, 1972).

b. Genetics. Despite the inclusion by McKusick (1975) of progeria in the autosomal recessive category, the hereditary picture is unclear at present. Pedigree analysis has revealed only a few cases of consanguinity, or two affected siblings in a family, compatible with recessive genetic transmission. Studies on cultured skin fibroblasts in three families (Danes, 1971), and on peripheral red blood cells in a fourth (Goldstein, S., and Moerman, 1976*a*), provide strong evidence for an autosomal recessive pattern of inheritance. On the other hand, after careful pedigree analysis, the vast majority of cases appear to be sporadic (DeBusk, 1972). Indeed, a recent survey supports the idea of a fresh dominant mutation related to paternal age (Jones *et al.,* 1975). It would therefore be wise at this juncture to consider progeria genetically heterogeneous despite the remarkably similar features of affected persons. Considerable precedent exists for such heterogeneity, not only in clinically overt disorders (see, for example, Neufeld *et al.,* 1975), but also as part of normal variation (Childs and Der Kaloustian, 1968).

c. *Age of Death and Pathology.* The most frequent causes of death relate to severe generalized atherosclerosis and thrombosis (DeBusk, 1972). These processes predominantly involve larger arteries such as the aorta and those of the cerebrovascular and coronary circulations. Most often, atheromatous lesions are typical of those found in adults with a mixture of lipid accumulation, fibrosis, and thrombus formation (Atkins, 1954). In some cases, however, vascular occlusion appears to be principally a consequence of a proliferative cellular reaction without much lipid. Generalized deposition of lipofuscin has been found, primarily in brain and heart (Reichel and Garcia-Bunuel, 1970), although a recent case showed no excessive evidence of this "age pigment" (Spence and Herman, 1973). There can also be patchy myocardial fibrosis that seems to be out of proportion to the degree of vascular occlusion (Reichel and Garcia-Bunuel, 1970). This finding strongly suggests primary cell death independent of ischemia (Goldstein, S., 1971*a*).

In 18 patients whose age at death was known (DeBusk, 1972), death occurred between 7 and 27.5 years, with a median age of 12 years and a mean of 13.4 years. Two of the cases died of extreme inanition and one of convulsions, but the immediate cause of death was unknown. Three cases died of congestive heart failure secondary to previous myocardial infarction from coronary atherosclerosis, while the remaining 12 patients died of acute myocardial infarction secondary to acute coronary thrombosis with underlying atherosclerosis. Unlike normal aging, malignancy was not apparent in any cases.

d. *Related Disorders.* Partial phenocopies of progeria have been described. The Hallermann–Streiff syndrome can be readily distinguished by its bilateral congenital cataracts and microphthalmia (Fraser and Friedmann, 1967; Hopkins and Horan, 1970), although the head and skin changes can suggest an incomplete form of progeria (Steele and Bass, 1970; Hutchinson, D., 1971; Hall *et al.,* 1974). Acrogeria is clearly different, since the process involves only skin of the extremities (Gottron, 1940), but one recently described phenocopy has more subtle differences and was termed *metageria* (Gilkes *et al.,* 1974). Two such subjects were noted to have certain craniofacial features of progeria early in childhood, but both eventually grew tall and developed overt diabetes mellitus. Additionally, they had normal secondary sex characteristics, and there was no loss or graying of hair until age 30, an unusual longevity for true progeria. Because only two cases were examined, the genetics of this syndrome could not be determined.

4.1.2. The Werner Syndrome

a. Clinical Picture. Werner (1904) first described this disorder in his doctoral thesis, "Cataract in combination with scleroderma." The initial report concerned four siblings, all of whom shared the findings of short stature, senile appearance, graying of hair beginning at age 20, and cataracts that appeared in the third decade (Fig. 2). Skin was prominently involved with tautness, atrophy, hyperkeratosis, and ulceration designated as scleroderma. These manifestations occurred primarily in the feet, but the hands were also affected to a lesser degree. Joint deformities were often associated with the skin problems, while muscle and connective tissue atrophy also appeared in the extremities.

In the first major review of the Werner syndrome, Thannhauser (1945) enunciated 12 principal characteristics for diagnosis: (1) shortness of stature with characteristic habitus; (2) premature graying of hair; (3) premature

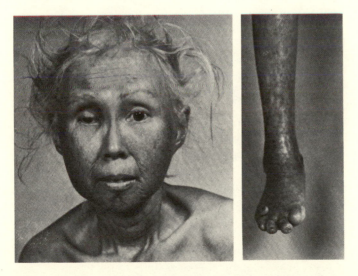

Fig. 2. A 48-year-old woman with the Werner syndrome. The generally senile appearance is evident. Bilateral cataracts were removed over a decade earlier, and the right eye, enucleated after an attack of acute glaucoma, was replaced by a prosthesis. The thinness of the feet, the hypopigmentation, and the smooth, shiny, tight skin are evident along with the chronic ulcerations over the ankles, the contractions of the toes, and the abnormal toenails. Reproduced from C. J. Epstein *et al.* (1966) with permission of the author and the Williams & Wilkins Co., Baltimore.

baldness; (4) scleropoikiloderma (hyperpigmentation and atrophy of the skin); (5) trophic leg ulcers; (6) juvenile cataracts; (7) hypogonadism; (8) diabetic tendency; (9) blood vessel calcification; (10) osteoporosis; (11) metastatic calcification; and (12) tendency to occur in brothers and sisters.

A number of reports on the Werner syndrome subsequently appeared (Boyd and Grant, 1959; McKusick, 1963; Kvale *et al.*, 1965; Tanenbaum, 1965; Murphy and Achkar, 1966; Gibbs, 1967; Burnett, 1968; Tibbetts *et al.*, 1968; Zucker-Franklin *et al.*, 1968; Gardner and Majka, 1969; Muller *et al.*, 1969; Payer, 1969; Schumacher *et al.*, 1969; Balci *et al.*, 1970; Bingham and Anderson, 1970; Frenkel, 1970; Rosen *et al.*, 1970; Degreef, 1971; Gsell and Haensch, 1971; Ferrari-Sacco *et al.*, 1972; Hoppe and Koritsch, 1972; Reynolds *et al.*, 1972; Wells, 1972; Bristow, 1973; Bullock and Howard, 1973; Faye *et al.*, 1973; Fleischmajer and Nedwich, 1973*b*; Kulenkamp *et al.*, 1973; Vandaele, 1973; Alberti *et al.*, 1974; Ishii and Hosoda, 1974, 1975; Larregue *et al.*, 1974; Lodi *et al.*, 1974; Richards, 1974; Wicks and Wall, 1974; Yasuhara *et al.*, 1974; Zackai *et al.*, 1974; Driban and Bertranou, 1975; Lelis, 1975; Simig and Fizelov, 1976). In a now classic review by C. J. Epstein *et al.* (1966), 125 definite cases of the Werner syndrome were identified. The disorder was clearly delineated, and important comparisons were made with both normal aging and other genetic disorders associated with premature aging.

The mean age of diagnosis was 38.7, with a range of 21–58 years, although in retrospect, many clinical features had presented much earlier. The most common initial sign appeared to be hair-graying at a mean age of 20 years, followed in order by skin changes (25.3 years), loss of hair (25.8 years), voice alteration (26.6 years), visual symptoms or cataract detection (30.0 years), skin ulcers (33.0 years), and diabetes (34.2 years).

In contrast to progeria, many Werner patients are fertile, although gonadal function generally appears to be reduced. In males, urinary 17-ketosteroid production tends to be low, with the expected reciprocal increase in the trophic hormone pituitary FSH. Similar findings on gonadal morphology as well as output of androgens and trophic hormones have been found in aging normal populations (Stearns *et al.*, 1974). Despite the same tendency to hypogonadism, most females are also able to reproduce. In 35 women, the range of ages at menarche was 9–20 years, with an average of 13.9 years, somewhat later than normal females. Menstrual flow, however, was frequently sparse and irregular; in 26 women, menstruation ceased between 18 and 45 years, with a mean of 33 years, significantly earlier than normal females. Although many Werner females never married, among those who did, many pregnancies and live normal births were recorded. Strikingly, a large proportion of other pregnancies ended either in spontaneous abortion, stillbirth, premature delivery, or death during delivery. Two of seven women tested had low estrogen assays, and in three who were no longer having menstrual periods, urinary excretion of FSH was normal. Since one would expect such females to have elevated FSH levels (Taymor *et al.*, 1968), it is likely that the pituitary–hypothalamic axis was unresponsive as part of a generalized tissue senescence (Goldstein, S., 1978*a,b*).

Diabetes mellitus was recognized in 55 of 125 cases (44.4%), 28 being male and 27 female. In general, diabetes was of the maturity-onset type, so that most patients could be managed by dietary restriction alone. When insulin was needed for management, or otherwise administered during investigation, responsiveness was frequently poor in terms of a sluggish hypoglycemic effect.

No consistent or striking abnormalities were found in serum lipids, although isolated abnormalities were found in cholesterol and lipoprotein levels. An interesting recent report found evidence of an increased urinary output of hyaluronic acid in five Japanese patients (Tokunaga *et al.*, 1975).

b. Genetics. Careful pedigree analysis in 21 sibships is compatible with autosomal recessive inheritance (Epstein, C. J., *et al.*, 1966). Very few exceptions to this general rule occur, in contrast to the case with progeria.

c. Age of Death and Pathology. The available data are sparse. In 23 of the 125 cases reported by C. J. Epstein *et al.* (1966), the age of death was ascertained to be 31–63 years, with a mean of 47 years. The two principal causes of death were malignancies and cardiovascular disease, either myocardial infarction or cerebrovascular accidents. The incidence of neo-plastic disease is high in the Werner syndrome, with anomalously high involvement of mesenchymal tissue (Epstein, C. J., *et al.*, 1966). Thus, sarcomas have been reported in adipose tissue, bone, nerve sheath, blood vessel, uterine wall, meninges, and connective tissue, and a case of acute myeloid leukemia was recently described (Tao *et al.*, 1971).

Pathology is widespread on postmortem examination, but the most striking changes involve the cardiovascular system. Atherosclerosis is almost always far advanced in severity beyond that of control age groups. The coronaries are common targets, with frequent production of myocar-dial infarction. Severe calcification of the aortic and mitral valve leaflets and rings is commonly seen, while myocardial tissue shows varying degrees of localized hypertrophy next to areas of atrophy and fibrosis. Lipofuscin pigment is not thought to be unusually abundant.

In keeping with the failure of gonadal endocrine secretions, the testes are strikingly atrophic. Seminiferous tubules are frequently hyalinized and those that remain intact are devoid of spermatogenic activity. Examina-tions of the ovaries were rarely noted in females, but one would expect accentuation of the normal atrophic postmenopausal picture.

4.1.3. The Cockayne Syndrome

a. Clinical Picture. Cockayne (1936) first described a brother and sister who became prototypes of this disorder. The characteristics accepted at present (Fig. 3) are dwarfism with loss of adipose tissue during infancy, precocious senile appearance, pigmentary retinal degeneration, optic atrophy, deafness, marble epitheses in some digits, mental retardation, and sensitivity to sunlight, resulting in photodermatitis. The oft-compared Neill–Dingwall syndrome (Neill and Dingwall, 1950) is likely one and the same disorder (McKusick, 1975).

Numerous reports have appeared in recent times to further delineate the nature of the Cockayne syndrome (MacDonald *et al.,* 1960; Paddison *et al.,* 1963; Norman and Tingey, 1966; Moossey, 1967; Roychoudhury and Banerjee, 1968; Coles, 1969; Rowlatt, 1969; Moosa and Dubowitz, 1970;

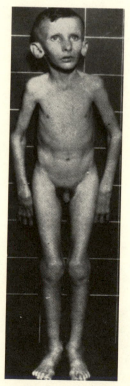

Fig. 3. A 14½-year-old boy with the Cockayne syndrome. Several of the features described in the text are evident. Reproduced from Blizzard (1965), courtesy of the author and Charles C. Thomas, Publishers, Springfield, Illinois.

Martin, J. J., *et al.*, 1971; Alton *et al.*, 1972; Riggs and Seibert, 1972; Brodrick and Dark, 1973; Pfeiffer and Backmann, 1973; Predescu *et al.*, 1973; Roy *et al.*, 1973; Ufermann *et al.*, 1973; Srivastava *et al.*, 1974; Hernandez *et al.*, 1975). Typical characteristics usually appear during the second year of life, with dwarfism, impaired vision, and widespread involvement of the nervous system. Microcephaly and mental retardation are constant features, while frequent concomitants are unsteady gait, tremor, weakness, and peripheral neuropathy. Visual deficits emanate from corneal and lenticular opacities as well as optic atrophy and retinitis pigmentosa. The liver is often enlarged, while the kidney can also be affected with albuminuria, glomerular hyalinization, tubular atrophy, and interstitial fibrosis (Ohno and Hiroaka, 1966). Unlike the case with progeria and the Werner syndrome, the mental deficit is progressive and ranges from moderate to severe, although normal intelligence has also been reported (Lanning and Simil, 1970).

Land and Nogrady (1969) emphasized the radiological findings in the skeleton in addition to the simple but severe osteoporosis. There is frequent squaring and notching of the short metacarpals, the phalanges, and the pelvis, with unfolding of the iliac crest.

Few endocrine studies have been carried out, but a few case studies have revealed low urinary 17-hydroxysteroids and 17-ketosteroids (Cotton *et al.*, 1970). Two patients had abnormally high blood glucose levels following an oral glucose load (Neill and Dingwall, 1950), with overt glycosuria reported in another instance (Spark, 1965). In one case report, hyperlipoproteinemia, hyperinsulinemia, and renal insufficiency with acidosis were found, but growth hormone levels were normal (Fujimoto *et al.*, 1969). Another recent case report also found hyperglycemia with elevated plasma insulin and inappropriately high growth hormone levels (Cotton *et al.*, 1970).

b. Genetics. Only 20 cases have been reported thus far, but it appears that this disorder is inherited as an autosomal recessive condition (McKusick, 1975).

c. Age of Death and Pathology. Little information is available on these aspects, but it would appear that the life span is appreciably shortened (Crome and Kanjilal, 1971). The most striking postmortem finding is calcification in the cerebral blood vessels, while the main arteries show normal or minimal arteriosclerosis for the chronological age. Calcification appears to be disseminated throughout the cerebral white matter, basal ganglia, and cerebellum, with concomitant hyalinization of the large and small blood vessels. While these vascular changes in the brain are characteristic of normal aging, there is no apparent evidence of the specific anatomical pathology of senile dementia as in the Down syndrome.

4.2. Numerical Chromosome Anomalies

4.2.1. The Down Syndrome

a. Clinical Picture. This disorder was first referred to in 1866 by Down (1866) as Mongolian idiocy. With an overall incidence of 1/660 newborns, it is the most common form of congenital malformation in man and hence the best documented (Penrose and Smith, 1966).

The typically affected person is easily recognizable by most laymen. Yet, in a number of cases, accurate clinical diagnosis is a specialized task requiring identification of a multitude of features. The general lack of muscle tone produces a tendency to keep the mouth open and protrude a typically furrowed tongue. There are also loose skin, hyperflexibility of joints, and malformations of soft and bony tissues. Craniofacial features that produce the typical "mongoloid" phenotype are most readily apparent (Fig. 4). In the eye, these features include oblique palpebral fissures, epicanthic folds, speckled irises (Brushfield spots), and fine lens opacities in 59% of cases. Fissured lips, small teeth, and a high-arched palate are also

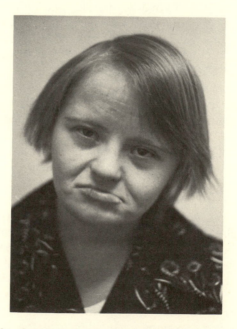

Fig. 4. A 26-year-old female with the Down syndrome. The patient shows many of the classic craniofacial features of this disorder along with an early senile appearance. Photograph courtesy of Dr. J. M. Berg, Surrey Place Centre, Toronto, with permission of the parents.

characteristic. Ears are prominent and frequently malformed, with small or absent lobes and a folded helix. The shape of the head is characteristic, with a round shape and flatness of the occiput, facial profile, and nasal bridge. There is also a thin cranium with late closure of fontanels. Excessive skin on the back of the neck is typical. The hands are characteristically involved and are short and broad, in part due to short fingers, especially the fifth, which is also curved. There is also a four-finger (simian) crease, and often, one flexion crease appears on the fifth finger due to a dysplastic middle phalanx. There is a high incidence of diabetes mellitus postulated to occur on an autoimmune basis (Burch and Milunsky, 1969). Thyroiditis leading to hypothyroidism is a frequent finding, probably consequent to an autoimmune etiology. That hypothyroidism *per se* is associated with altered lipid metabolism may explain the apparent increase in lipid abnormalities in the Down syndrome (Smith, G. F., and Berg, 1976).

b. Genetics. The Down syndrome is "genetic" in the pure sense because of excess chromosomal material, but is not inherited apart from cases of balanced translocations. Fortunately, the translocation group comprises only 3% of cases (Penrose and Smith, 1966). In over 90% of cases, the Down syndrome is caused by full trisomy of chromosome 21, which leads to the characteristic picture of growth deficiency and mental retardation.

As in the other disorders of premature aging, the etiology of the Down syndrome has not been elucidated. In Chapter 8, the relationship of parental aging to the Down syndrome and other chromosomal disorders is discussed. In the small fraction of cases in which the mother is herself trisomic, an affected conceptus will inevitably occur in half the pregnancies, but due to *in utero* lethality, premature births, and stillbirths, the risk in newborns is about 35% (Carr, 1975). Balanced translocation carrier and mosaic parents also run a high risk of producing affected children, but due to apparently stringent prenatal selection, the neonatal risk is closer to 10% (Smith, G. F., and Berg, 1976).

c. Age of Death and Pathology. Premature senility seems to be a prominent clinical feature, particularly affecting the CNS (Jervis, 1970; Malamud, 1972). Since patients are moderately to severely retarded to begin with, it might be thought difficult to assess intellectual deterioration. Nevertheless, a progressive decline in learning ability can be demonstrated in the Down syndrome (Dalton *et al.,* 1974). When post mortem was performed, prior intellectual deterioration could be correlated with three changes distinctive of senile dementia: senile plaques, Alzheimer's neurofibrillary degeneration, and Simcowitz's granulovacuolar degeneration of nerve cells (Crapper *et al.,* 1975).

Even after deaths from congenital cardiorespiratory malformations are excluded, there is still premature death in the remainder (Smith, G. F., and

Berg, 1976). A high incidence of malignant disease occurs, especially chronic myelogenous leukemia (Miller, R. W., 1970; Smith, G. F., and Berg, 1976).

4.2.2. The Turner Syndrome

a. Clinical Picture. In his classic paper, Turner (1938) reported a variety of morphological abnormalities occurring in association with gonadal dysgenesis. Engel and Forbes (1965) analyzed 48 cases and listed a number of features in addition to the classic morphological disturbances of stunted growth, webbed neck, cubitus valgus, and pectus excavatum (Fig. 5). There was lymphoedema, abnormally low hairline, low-set and malformed ears, strabismus, ptosis, and various irregularities in the skin creases, fingernails, and bones of the hands. During adolescence, a number of features that relate to the incomplete female genotype become manifest,

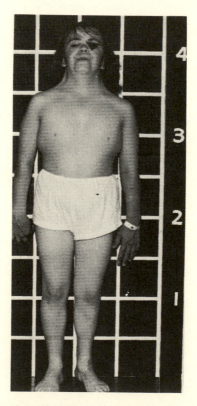

Fig. 5. A girl aged 14 years 10 months with Turner syndrome. Reproduced from D. W. Smith (1976) with permission of the author and publisher.

including amenorrhea, lack of breast development, infantile genitalia, and infertility. Of frequent occurrence during adulthood are hypertension, osteoporosis, and osteoarthritis. As in the progeroid syndromes, there is advanced thinning of the scalp hair, but early graying does not typically occur.

As would be expected with ovarian hypofunction and estrogen lack, the most obvious endocrine abnormality is elevation of plasma levels of FSH. Paradoxically, pituitary reserve is normal or increased in the Turner syndrome following injection of LHRH, the hypothalamic hormone that stimulates release of pituitary gonadotropins (Huang, K.-E., 1975).

Gastric achlorhydria and autoimmune thyroiditis are common (Engel and Forbes, 1965), and the incidence of diabetes mellitus also appears to be high, ranging from 16 to 61% in two separate surveys (Forbes and Engle, 1963; Van Campenhout *et al.*, 1973). Curiously, however, a third study of 57 subjects was unable to demonstrate a single instance of overt diabetes (Lindsten, 1963). The latter series, however, showed a delayed and diminished insulin response despite higher than normal blood glucose levels. Additionally, the fasting growth hormone level was elevated, and hyperglycemia induced a paradoxical increase in growth hormone levels (Lindsten *et al.*, 1967). In contrast, Nielsen *et al.* (1969) frequently found a brisk rise and sustained elevation in plasma insulin levels after glucose ingestion, in keeping with peripheral tissue unresponsiveness to insulin. More recently, however, Rasio *et al.* (1976) found that Turner individuals with overt diabetes had a delayed insulin release in response to a glucose load, but no gross alteration of tissue sensitivity to exogenous insulin. Output of growth hormone was blunted in response to hypoglycemia, but this blunting was not felt to contribute to the glucose intolerance.

Although arteriosclerosis and arcus senilis were commonly noted, serum cholesterol determinations in 25 short patients ranged from 156 to 327 mg/dl, with an average of 248 mg/dl, not strikingly abnormal (Engle and Forbes, 1965).

Serum uric acid levels in 17 short patients averaged 4.6 mg/dl (range 2.4–7.4), which is within the normal range of females rather than males (Engel and Forbes, 1965).

b. Genetics. The absent or rudimentary gonads found in this syndrome were first believed to be the result of an intrauterine accident until Ford *et al.* (1959) discovered that the entire clinical picture resulted from deletion of one of the sex chromosomes. In fact, the absence of one sex chromosome is so damaging to intrauterine development that about 98% of conceptuses with one sex chromosome are spontaneously aborted (Carr, 1975).

In large surveys of newborn females, 1 in 3000 have appreciable numbers of cells with a single X chromosome (Gerald, 1976). Almost all affected females have a 45, X karyotype, or a mixture of such cells with normal 46, XX female cells, i.e., mosaicism. In fact, mosaicism is so frequent in the Turner syndrome that three quarters of those ascertained in the newborn period are mosaic to varying degrees. Perhaps for technical reasons, one of the X chromosomes is occasionally missing from the metaphase plate. Thus, if sufficient cells are analyzed, XO mosaicism can become an almost universal finding, with obvious misleading effects on the incidence of this disorder. Further complexity is introduced by the wide range of clinical expression that can occur. Accurate diagnosis therefore requires demonstration of a deficiency of Barr-body-containing cells on buccal smear plus chromosome analysis that verifies the presence of a substantial number of 45, X cells (Gerald, 1976).

c. Age of Death and Pathology. There is clearly a reduced life span overall, and indeed, there is a compelling relationship to progeria. Atherosclerotic heart disease is common, even in those who have had estrogen replacement therapy from the teens (Engel and Forbes, 1965). Skin aging is also prominent. Unlike the case with progeria, there is a high incidence of neoplasia, as recorded in one series of 289 Turner subjects (Wertelecki *et al.,* 1970). The neoplasia occurs in nonovarian sites, particularly in nervous tissue.

4.3. Miscellaneous Inherited Syndromes

4.3.1. Ataxia–Telangiectasia (the Louis-Bar Syndrome)

a. Clinical Picture. Ataxia–telangiectasia, a rare disorder with predilection for the neurological, vascular, and lymphoid systems, was first documented in 1941 by Louis-Bar, (1941). Several reports subsequently appeared (Boder and Sedgwick, 1958; Korein *et al.,* 1961; Shuster *et al.,* 1966; Sourander *et al.,* 1966; Miller, M. E., and Chatten, 1967; Feigin *et al.,* 1970; Levin and Perlov, 1971; McFarlin *et al.,* 1972). Affected persons usually appear normal at birth, but growth deficiency appears during infancy or childhood, along with progressive cerebellar ataxia, which manifests initially as the inability to walk (Fig. 6). Somewhat later in infancy, there is evidence of oculocutaneous telangiectasia (chronic dilation of small blood vessels). Other neurological deficits are then expressed clinically as choreoathetosis, dysrhythmic speech, a dull, sad face, drooling, aberrant ocular movements, stooped posture, and occasional seizures. Postural instability progresses with time such that ambulation is no longer possible. Although mental deficiency is difficult to assess, it is a feature in about 50% of cases. It is noteworthy that psychometric tests in one case indicated a loss of previously established intellectual capacity, rather than a primary developmental lack (Reye and Mosman, 1960).

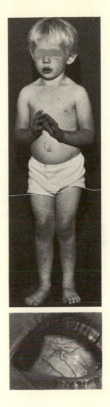

Fig. 6. A 9½-year-old boy with ataxia–telangiectasia. The patient shows unstable posture and short stature, but appears otherwise unremarkable in this photograph. The eye shows the characteristic tortuosity and dilatation of blood vessels in the conjunctiva. Reproduced from D. W. Smith (1976) with permission of the author and publisher.

Immunological abnormalities include hypoplasia of the thymus, markedly decreased levels of IgA (Peterson *et al.*, 1964, 1966; Strober *et al.*, 1968) and IgE (Ammann *et al.*, 1969), variable alterations in IgG and IgM, and impaired cellular immunity. Frequent bronchiectasis, recurrent sinopulmonary infections, and a high incidence of lymphoreticular neoplasia occur as a direct result of these immune deficiencies. Raised α-fetoprotein levels have been reported in several patients, which suggests defective differentiation of gut-associated endodermal organs such as liver and thymus (Waldmann and McIntire, 1972).

A peculiar form of diabetes mellitus is seen in a high proportion of cases and features massive output of insulin in response to a glucose challenge (Schalch *et al.*, 1970). This phenomenon suggests severe peripheral resistance to the effects of insulin.

Ataxia–telangiectasia is one of the chromosomal breakage disorders that include the Bloom syndrome, Fanconi anemia, and xeroderma pigmentosum (German, 1974). Thus, the pronounced radiosensitivity seen following conventional X-ray therapy for tumor treatment (Gotoff *et al.*, 1967; Morgan *et al.*, 1968; Cunliffe *et al.*, 1975) relates at the cellular level to multiple chromosomal breaks and rearrangements (Hecht *et al.*, 1966, 1973; Lisker and Cobo, 1970; Higurashi and Conen, 1973; Harnden, 1974; Cohen *et al.*, 1975; McCaw *et al.*, 1975; Oxford *et al.*, 1975; Rary *et al.*, 1975). The impaired responsiveness of DNA synthesis to phytohemagglutinin may also emanate from this problem (Hecht *et al.*, 1966), and all, in turn, may be a consequence of a defect in DNA repair that is now becoming evident (see Section 7.3).

b. Genetics. Pedigree analyses in 93 cases from 64 families clearly indicate that inheritance is autosomal recessive (Tadjoedin and Fraser, 1965). The possibility of heteroalleles at the ataxia–telangiectasia locus was suggested in certain patients (McKusick and Cross, 1966).

c. Age of Death and Pathology. Death usually occurs early as a consequence of lung infection, neurological deficit, or malignancy. Interestingly, one large sibship with 5 of 12 members affected had 2 cases of mucinous gastric adenocarcinoma in the second decade of life (Haerer *et al.*, 1969). A cerebellar tumor was also reported in another unrelated family (Shuster *et al.*, 1966).

4.3.2. The Rothmund–Thomson Syndrome

a. Clinical Picture. The German ophthalmologist Rothmund (1868) described five cases of cataracts and peculiar marblelike skin characterized by atrophy, pigmentation, and telangiectasia. Similar cases were described by Block and Stauffer (1929) and by Thomson (1936), who introduced the term *congenital poikiloderma.* Additional reports appeared (Cole *et al.*, 1945; Franceschetti, 1953; Sexton, 1954) until W. B. Taylor (1957), reviewing 45 cases from the literature, and following addition of one of his own, proposed that the earlier cases described by Rothmund and Thomson could be amalgamated and regarded as a single clinical entity. Many case reports subsequently appeared describing various features of this disorder (Siemens, 1963; Blinstrub *et al.*, 1964; Wahl and Ellis, 1965; Palmer, 1966; Silver, 1966; Maurer and Langford, 1967; Perlman *et al.*, 1967; Kraus *et al.*, 1970; Nissim, 1971; Oates *et al.*, 1971; Lewis, 1972; Zamith *et al.*, 1974; Diem, 1975; Kristensen, 1975; Sri-Skanda-Rajah-Sivayoham and Ratnaike, 1975; Bottomley and Box, 1976).

The disease usually begins during infancy between the third and sixth month of life, with an apparent female preponderance (Fig. 7). Over half the cases have juvenile cataracts, short stature, small hands and feet, hypoplastic to absent thumbs, and osteoporosis or areas of cystic or sclerotic change in the skeleton, or both. Ectodermal abnormalities include missing or sparse eyebrows and eyelashes, dystrophic nails, and defective teeth. In

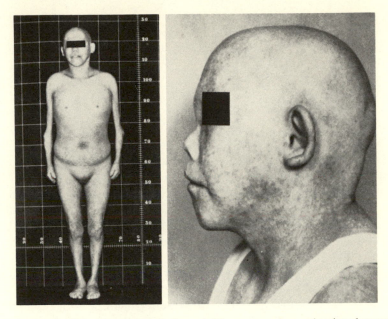

Fig. 7. A 32-year-old female with the Rothmund–Thomson syndrome showing characteristic body habitus, hair loss, skin changes, and abnormalities in the hands and feet. Reproduced from Werder *et al.* (1975) with permission of the author and Blackwell Scientific Publications Ltd.

most cases, there is increased sensitivity of the skin to sunlight. Cutaneous carcinomas have also been reported. Other physical signs include small saddle nose and small or missing teeth.

Werder *et al.* (1975) recently described two cases that are of interest from an endocrine standpoint. The first was a 36-year-old female with short stature and primary amenorrhea who did not develop secondary sexual characteristics. Following persistent hypercalcemia and increased levels of immunoreactive parathormone, a parathyroid adenoma was diagnosed and successfully removed at surgery. A 21-year-old male in the same report has small testes and high basal LH and FSH levels, as well as increased LH and FSH response to LHRH.

The overall incidence of diabetes mellitus in the Rothmund–Thomson syndrome cannot be evaluated because explicit mention of this feature has not been made in enough cases. In the two cases reported by Werder *et al.* (1975), however, both the response to exogenous insulin and the fasting blood glucose levels were normal.

b. Genetics. On analyzing 46 cases of the Rothmund–Thomson syndrome, W. B. Taylor (1957) concluded that this disorder was inherited as an autosomal recessive trait. McKusick (1975) concurs with this idea.

   c. Age of Death and Pathology. Few cases have been followed over
their life spans. Thus, although the prognosis for survival is appreciably
better than in progeria, the relative degree of life-span-shortening is still
unknown (see McKusick, 1975).

4.3.3. Diabetes Mellitus

   a. Clinical Picture. Diabetes mellitus is not usually associated with
known genetic syndromes (cf. Table I). As a rule, patients are within the
normal range of stature and have no morphologically distinct features
except for a high incidence of obesity (Renold *et al.,* 1972). Excess weight
is a frequent feature not only of the adult-onset form but also of juvenile-
onset diabetes (Ginsberg-Fellner and Knittle, 1973). The latter usually
depend on insulin therapy for survival, at least within a few years of onset
(Rosenbloom *et al.,* 1975; Lestradet *et al.,* 1976). The vast majority of
affected persons, however, have maturity-onset diabetes, a milder form
that is controllable with diet, weight reduction, and often the supplemental
help of oral hypoglycemic drugs. A certain proportion of cases will progress
in severity and eventually become insulin-dependent despite strict dietary
adherence and achievement of ideal weight (Fajans *et al.,* 1976).
   While the salient abnormality is a relative or absolute lack of insulin so
as to produce inappropriate hyperglycemia (Cahill, 1975), many other
hormones clearly play a role in the general imbalance (Johansen *et al.,*
1975; Unger, 1976; Felig *et al.,* 1976). Since hormones influence virtually
every aspect of the body's overall metabolism, it is now clear that carbohy-
drates are not uniquely involved, but rather that diabetes is associated with
widespread abnormalities in diverse metabolic pathways (Renold *et al.,*
1972.
   b. Genetics. The genetics of diabetes is not clear-cut. Although virtually every mode of inheritance from simple autosomal recessive to polygenic inheritance has been implicated, the true pattern of transmission
remains a mystery. It is becoming apparent that considerable heterogeneity
exists (Creutzfeldt *et al.,* 1975; Tattersall and Fajans, 1975; Zonana and
Rimoin, 1976). The recent discovery of frequent association with *HLA*
antigens A8 and BW15 may be of value in analyzing the patterns of
inheritance (Singal and Blajchman, 1973; Thomsen *et al.,* 1975; Nelson *et
al.,* 1975).
   c. Age of Death and Pathology. The advent of insulin therapy in the
1920's has prolonged life expectancy in the juvenile-onset forms and simultaneously allowed extended clinical observation on millions of patients.
Considerable controversy still exists on the question whether good control
of blood glucose levels delays or arrests the late complications (Cahill *et
al.,* 1976). Nevertheless, it is evident that diabetics have a significantly

decreased life span, particularly in the insulin-dependent group (Marks and Krall, 1971; Palumbo *et al.,* 1976). In all age groups, the proportion of vascular disease and consequently of mortality is higher with a long duration of diabetes than with a short duration. There is a heightened incidence of large-vessel atherosclerosis that, as in progeria and the Werner syndrome, is not unusual in morphology or distribution (Meissner and Legg, 1971). Diabetics, however, are often also afflicted with small-vessel disease, i.e., thickening of capillary basement membranes, which leads to luminal occlusion and localized tissue death (Vracko and Benditt, 1974). The patterns of presentation clearly depend on the tissue distribution leading, for example, to gangrene of the toes and feet if in the extremities, to renal failure and hypertension if in the kidneys, or to a combined hemorrhagic and proliferative picture progressing to blindness if in the retina.

Although the incidence of all malignancies in diabetes appeared to be higher in early surveys, this was recently contested (Marble and Ramos, 1971). There is little doubt, however, that cancer of the endometrium and pancreas is more common. The occurrence of autoimmune disorders is also increased in diabetics to frequencies usually observed in normal persons two or three decades older (Ungar *et al.,* 1968; Goldstein, D. E., *et al.,* 1970). In total, diabetics tend to have the earlier appearance and more severe progression of several diseases that are normally age-dependent (Goldstein, S., 1971*b*).

5. Comparison of Premature Aging Syndromes with Normal Biological Aging

Various pathological features of each syndrome described in the preceeding sections are unquestionably common to normal aging, but are often discordant in either frequency or severity. For example, the Werner syndrome epitomizes the difficulties inherent in the question whether these diseases constitute genuine models for the study of aging. Blood-vessel involvement occurs earlier and with greater severity in the Werner syndrome than in natural aging, but is qualitatively similar in character and distribution. On the other hand, the very high frequency of cataracts, atrophy, and ulceration of the distal extremities, severe testicular atrophy, and high incidence of mesenchymal neoplasia argue against a simple relationship between the two. Table V summarizes, as well as current clinical and autopsy reports allow, how the various syndromes show concordance or discordance with a common group of clinicopathological manifestations of normal aging.

Table V. Some Common Clinicopathological Features of Normal Aging

Syndrome	Short Stature[b]	Degenerative vascular disease	Hypertension	Epithelial malignancy	Auto-immunity	Hyperglycemia/insulin resistance	Osteoporosis
Progeria	++++	++++	+++	−	?	[d]	+++
Werner	+++	++++	+	[e]	?	+++	++++
Cockayne	+++	−	+++	+++	−	+++	+++
Down	+++	++	+	[g]	+++	+++	++
Turner	+++	+++	+++	+++	+++	+++	+++
Ataxia–telangiectasia	+++	−	?	++++	?	+++	?
Rothmund–Thomson	+++	+	?	+++	?	++	++
Diabetes mellitus	+	+++	+++	++	+++	++++	++

[a](+ to ++++) Slight to markedly increased frequency or severity or both; (?) unknown; (−) does not occur.
[b]In all cases, growth-stunting is primary rather than secondary.
[c]Primary apart from the Werner syndrome and diabetes. In diabetes, hypogonadism is secondary, in the Werner syndrome, it is primary and secondary combined.

6. Tissue Culture Approaches to Premature Aging

6.1. Studies on Cell Growth

Recent studies on cultured fibroblasts have provided considerable insight into the nature of the premature aging syndromes. Despite some dissenting views (Kohn, 1975; Schneider and Chase, 1976; Gershon and Gershon, 1976), cogent evidence has now been marshaled to support the validity of the fibroblast system as a model for aging (Hayflick, 1965; Cristofalo, 1972). An inverse correlation exists between the donor age and the replicative life span of cultured fibroblasts (Goldstein, S., et al., 1969; Martin, G. M., et al., 1970; Schneider and Mitsui, 1976; Goldstein et al., 1978). In sharp contrast to fibroblasts from age-matched controls, fibroblasts cultured from patients with progeria and the Werner syndrome have curtailed life spans or generally poor growth capacity or both (Goldstein, S., 1969; Martin, G. M., et al., 1970; Danes, 1971; Nienhaus et al., 1971; Spence and Herman, 1973; Holliday et al., 1974) (see also Fig. 8). Similar growth deficits have also been demonstrated in skin fibroblasts cultured from individuals with the Down syndrome (Schneider and Epstein, 1972; Segal and McCoy, 1974; Boué et al., 1975), other trisomies, the Turner syndrome (Boué et al., 1975), ataxia–telangiectasia (Hoar, 1975; Elmore and Swift, 1976b), Fanconi anemia (Elmore and Swift, 1976a), and Hun-

and Their Occurrence in the Syndromes of Premature Aging[a]

Senile dementia	Osteo-arthritis	Cataracts	Skin atrophy	Hair loss or graying or both	Hypogonadism[c]	Amyloid deposition	Lipofuscin deposition
−	?	−	++++	++++	++++	+	++
−	+++	++++	++++	++++	++++	+	++
f	+	++++	+++	+	+++	+	+++
++++	++	++++	++	+++	+++	+++	+++
+	+++	+++	+++	+++	++++	++	+
f	?	−	++	++	+++	?	?
f	+	++++	++++	++++	++++	?	?
+	++	+++	++	++	++	+++	++

[d]Not overt diabetes, but resistant to exogenous insulin.
[e]Mesenchymal malignancy increased.
[f]Other neurological deficits are present.
[g]Chronic myelogenous leukemia increased about 50-fold.

tington disease (Menkes and Stein, 1973). Although a recent study failed to confirm the latter observation, confluent density was found to be increased (Goetz et al., 1975). No reports have yet appeared on growth capacity in the Cockayne syndrome.

The diabetic genotype also seems to be detrimental to cell growth in vitro. Fibroblasts derived from the skin of otherwise normal subjects who are genetically predisposed to diabetes were shown to have reduced growth capacity compared with normal control cells (Goldstein, S., et al., 1969, 1975). These observations have now been confirmed in another group of such "prediabetics" as well as in overt diabetics (Goldstein, S., et al., 1974; Vracko and Benditt, 1975; Goldstein et al., 1978, and in prep.).

In total, therefore, it is becoming clear that physiological rather than chronological age is of paramount importance in determining the in vitro replicative life span (see Fig. 8). Fibroblasts cultured from a randomly chosen population give the expected inverse correlation between in vivo age and in vitro life span (Martin, G. M., et al., 1970), as do cultured cells from overt diabetics and prediabetics (Fig. 9). Cells from normal subjects selected according to stringent criteria perform differently (Fig. 9), however, and fail to show this inverse correlation. This unique population of normal subjects had negative family histories for diabetes and no evidence of metabolic disorders. Most important, they repeatedly showed normal glucose tolerance following challenge by administered glucose. Despite the

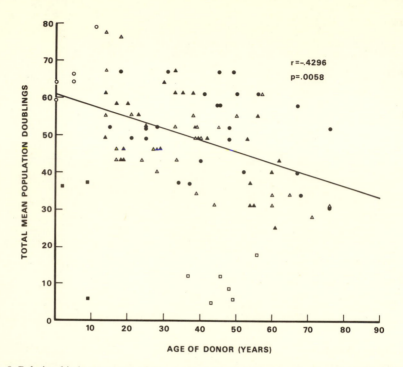

Fig. 8. Relationship between age of donor and replicative life span of cultured skin fibroblasts. The majority of the symbols represent a single comparative study of three groups of subjects: (●) 25 normal controls; (▲) 30 genetically prediabetic subjects: (△) 25 overt diabetic subjects. Additional symbols represent other cell strains interpolated to show the effect of accelerated physiological aging on the cellular life span *in vitro:* (■) progeria; (□) the Werner syndrome; (○) normal newborns and young controls. Modified from data of S. Goldstein *et al.* (1978), S. Goldstein (1969), G. M. Martin *et al.* (1970), and S. Goldstein and Moerman (1975a,b, 1976 a,b).

large statistical variance, they appear to be a genetically distinct group with slower rates of aging *in vivo* and *in vitro*. By carrying a minimum number of detrimental genes, perhaps they define one population at the polar extreme of a continuous distribution of aging rates that merges with "normal" aging and then the common forms of maturity-onset diabetes. The spectrum progresses through heterozygotes for the progeroid syndromes and other aging mutants, ending finally with the full-blown homozygous states for these disorders.

Limitations on Using Growth Deficits Alone as an Index of Aging. It would be fallacious to assume that replicative deficits need be the major criterion to validate cultured cells for aging studies. Indeed, the culture medium could as easily correct as well as elicit the expression of an intrinsic genetic lesion. Within clonally heterogeneous populations, hardy

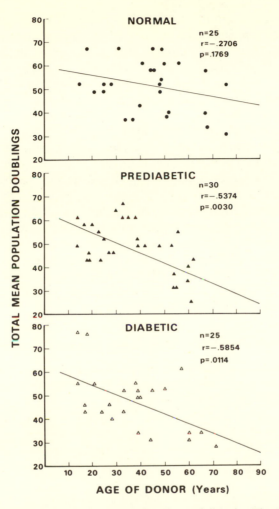

Fig. 9. Previous combined plot of normals, prediabetics, and diabetics (Fig. 8) segregated into three groups showing individual regression analyses. Note in normal subjects (top) that the correlation between fibroblast life span and age is not significant, and also that the slope of the regression line is flatter than in prediabetics (middle) and diabetics (bottom), indicating a general trend toward greater fibroblast longevity in middle age and beyond. Modified from data of S. Goldstein *et al.* (1978).

cells can assist more feeble cells by transmission of cellular factors through the medium (Fratantoni *et al.*, 1968), by exchange of cytoplasmic material (Cox, 1974), or by cellular hybridization (Ruddle and Creagan, 1975), although the latter process would be unlikely to occur at a rate high enough to correct a metabolic deficit. Other ambient conditions could clearly influence whether a specific phenotype is manifest or silent. For example, xeroderma pigmentosum cells maintained in subdued light achieve a normal life span *in vitro* (Goldstein, S., 1971*c*), but very minimal light or UV radiation rapidly kills the majority of cells and leads to rapid senescence of the survivors. In total, basal growth performance must be viewed in conjunction with a specific environmental perturbation to assess a given mutant *in vitro*.

It should also be emphasized that the cultured fibroblast represents only one of a myriad of cell types within the organism; therefore, biochemical mechanisms in fibroblasts cannot be generally extrapolated to all cells. Additionally, fibroblasts in culture preserve exquisite specificity regarding tissue, anatomical site, and gender, suggesting that a unique imprint has occurred *in vivo* (Hassell *et al.,* 1976; Griffin *et al.,* 1976; Kaufman *et al.,* 1977). Nevertheless, it appears that site-specific fibroblasts and parenchymal cells also have a finite life span that bears an inverse proportionality to donor age (Martin, G. M., *et al.,* 1970; Le Guilly *et al.,* 1973; Rheinwald and Green, 1975). It seems clear, therefore, that the study of cultures from subjects with specific aging disorders and carefully selected controls will be relevant to aging of the intact human organism.

6.2. Defective Molecules in Prematurely Aging Cells

The recently heightened interest in cellular aging has led to an explosive rise in new studies in various aging mutants, and it is evident that any survey must be considered tentative at this time. A variety of molecular defects have been found in cultured fibroblasts from prematurely aging donors, particularly in subjects with progeria and the Werner syndrome.

6.2.1. HLA Antigens

These surface-membrane antigens have proved valuable in fibroblast studies for two reasons: First, they provide inherited molecular markers to screen for age changes. Second, they are involved in self-recognition, and hence permit insights into the nature of immune disturbances accompanying normal and premature aging.

HLA phenotypes of three unrelated boys with progeria determined on circulating lymphocytes were not unusual, inasmuch as these antigens are frequently seen in normal populations (Singal and Goldstein, 1973; Goldstein, S., *et al.,* 1975; Goldstein, S., and Moerman, 1976*b*). Many more subjects with progeria would have to be examined before one could conclude that progeria correlates with specific *HLA* antigens, as is now the case with several disorders (Bach and van Rood, 1976).

When autologous skin fibroblasts were examined for concordance with lymphocytes, no antigens could be detected by the conventional cytotoxicity test (Singal and Goldstein, 1973). This test is only a screening assay with limited sensitivity, and so experiments were repeated using the quantitative microabsorption assay (Singal and Goldstein, 1973). Results obtained with two different anti-HLA2 sera are shown in Fig. 10. With either serum, there was no diminution of antibody activity following absorption with 10^4–10^7

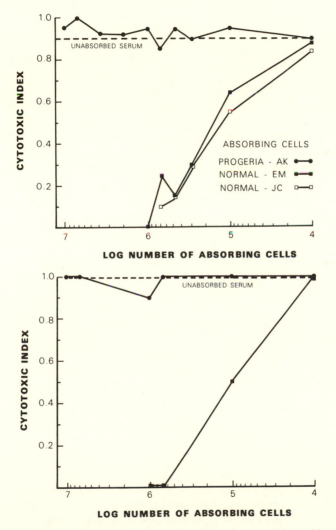

Fig. 10. Absorption of anti-HLA-A2 serum by fibroblasts from a subject with progeria and from normal controls. Normal lymphocytes served as target cells for assay of residual cytotoxic activity following absorption with fibroblasts. (---)Activity of unabsorbed serum. The two graphs represent absorption with two separate anti-HLA-A2 sera with virtually identical results. Reproduced from Singal and Goldstein (1973) with permission of the authors and Rockefeller University Press.

progeric fibroblasts. On the other hand, 10^6 fibroblasts from two HLA-A2-positive controls absorbed virtually all specific antibody. Taking the 50% level of the cytotoxicity index as a reference point, antigen expression can be quantified. Thus, the progeric fibroblasts had at least 100 times less HLA-A2 antigen detectable on their cell surface than control cells.

The possibility that specific substances were masking the antigens was also investigated. Cells were treated first with collagenase, neuraminidase (Goldstein, S., *et al.,* 1975), or hyaluronidase (Goldstein, S., and Singal, unpublished) to digest putatively masking collagen, excess sialation, or hyaluronic acid, respectively, but HLA-A2 expression was not even partially restored.

Other antigens on fibroblasts of this progeria subject were also tested by the quantitative absorption technique (Goldstein, S., *et al.,* 1975; Goldstein, S., and Moerman, 1976*b*). In contrast to HLA-A2, HLA-A9 expression was reduced about threefold, but only at late stages of passage, prior to senescence. HLA-B14, on the other hand, was reduced threefold at early passage, with no further progression to termination of the culture. More recent experiments (Goldstein, S., and Singal, in prep.) on a new progeria subject also revealed a partial reduction in HLA-A1 and HLA-A8 expression at late stages of passage. It is important to emphasize that mass cultures of normal control fibroblasts showed no significant reduction in antigen expression throughout the culture life span (Goldstein, S., *et al.,* 1975; Goldstein, S., and Moerman, 1976*b*), as was also reported by Brautbar *et al.* (1973) in several human strains.

Werner syndrome fibroblasts also showed defects in *HLA* expression (Goldstein, S., and Singal, 1974). In the single case so far examined, there was severe reduction in HLA-A2 and partial reduction in HLA-A9 of more than 50- and 5-fold, respectively.

6.2.2. Increased Heat Lability of Cytoplasmic Enzymes

Progeria and Werner syndrome fibroblasts also have an increased subfraction of heat-labile enzymes. The enzymes examined were glucose-6-phosphate dehydrogenase (G-6-PD), 6-phosphogluconate dehydrogenase (6-PGD), and hypoxanthine-guanine phosphoribosyltransferase (HGPRT). The first two represent sequential enzymes in the hexose monophosphate shunt, while the third is a scavenger enzyme in purine metabolism. G-6-PD and HGPRT are both X-linked, and therefore single-gene determined, while 6-PGD was recently assigned to autosome number 1. Progeria fibroblasts (Fig. 11) showed an increased heat-labile fraction in all three enzymes. This increase obtains even in comparison with control fibroblasts at late passage, when a small but significant increase in enzyme heat lability also occurs. Werner syndrome fibroblasts showed an even larger increase in the heat-labile fraction of all three enzymes (Goldstein, S., and Singal,

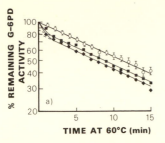

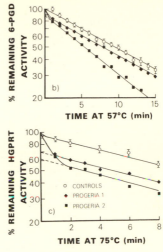

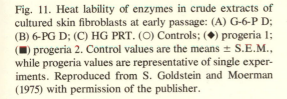

Fig. 11. Heat lability of enzymes in crude extracts of cultured skin fibroblasts at early passage: (A) G-6-P D; (B) 6-PG D; (C) HG PRT. (O) Controls; (◆) progeria 1; (■) progeria 2. Control values are the means ± S.E.M., while progeria values are representative of single experiments. Reproduced from S. Goldstein and Moerman (1975) with permission of the publisher.

1974; Goldstein, S., and Moerman, 1975*b*, 1976*b*), and similar results on G-6-PD were reported in a second Werner patient (Holliday *et al.*, 1974).

Additional data on enzyme heat lability in progeria and Werner cells are of interest (Goldstein, S., and Moerman, 1976*b*). There was a significant inverse correlation between specific activity and percentage heat lability of each enzyme, and a direct correlation between the percentage thermolabilities of paired enzymes. These phenomena suggest that a single mechanism may operate simultaneously on all three enzymes.

Comparisons with Enzyme Aging in Other Biological Systems. The circulating human erythrocyte normally has a life span of 120 days, and also shows deterioration of enzymes including G-6-PD and HGPRT (see Goldstein, S., and Moerman, 1976*b*). Since erythrocytes lose their ribosomal apparatus soon after release into the circulation, however, enzyme alterations can be ascribed, not to the synthesis of new isoenzymes or to errors in synthesis, but rather to postsynthetic modifications, partial denaturation, or a combination of both (Goldstein, S., and Moerman, 1976*b*). In other nonmitotic systems such as aging mouse muscle and liver, as well as in lower forms (Reiss and Gershon, 1976; Rothstein, 1977), enzymatic alterations similar to those of the erythrocyte have been demonstrated and identical mechanisms invoked. Werner fibroblasts, with their severely impaired growth capacity (Martin, G. M., *et al.*, 1970, 1974; Holliday *et al.*, 1974), might be comparable to these nonmitotic systems. Progeric fibroblasts are clearly different, however, since they grow as well as controls at a time when significantly increased thermolability exists in all three enzymes. On this basis, as well as the unique clinical and genetic pictures, it appears that the underlying defect will turn out to be substantially different in these two disorders.

6.2.3. Insulin Receptors

The function of insulin receptors is also altered in premature aging (Rosenbloom *et al.*, 1976). Fibroblasts from patients with progeria and the Rothmund–Thomson syndrome needed a higher concentration of native insulin to displace 50% of the specifically bound [^{125}I]insulin (Fig. 12). There was also a significant direct correlation with donor age in the control group. Aging of the insulin-binding system therefore appears as increased affinity for insulin at levels corresponding to peak physiological concentrations *in vivo* (Rosenbloom *et al.*, 1976). This implies that more insulin needs to bind to aged cells to achieve the same hormonal response that can be effected in younger cells with less insulin.

Whether the aging defect relates to the presence of a structural defect in the receptor is unclear. A generalized impairment in the fluidity of the plasma membrane is a possibility, and could also account for the defects in *HLA* expression. A problem could also reside in the cyclic nucleotide systems (Haslam and Goldstein, 1974), or could result from a lethargy in activating key intracellular events due to defective enzymes that exercise feedback control on the insulin receptor. The data on enzyme heat lability are consistent with this notion.

6.2.4. A Tissue Factor That Promotes Clotting

Skin cultures from progeria and Werner subjects have high levels of a tissue factor (TF) that promotes coagulation (Fig. 13). Slow growth of these prematurely aging cells could not account for the findings, because control fibroblasts assayed during their senescent phase still had far less TF activity. When cells were disrupted by sonication, TF activity increased fivefold in all strains. Differences between controls and premature aging cells, however, were maintained. That they were suggests that the higher level of TF in progeria and Werner cells relates primarily to increased content rather than to increased availability. It was also determined that fibroblast TF was specific for the extrinsic clotting mechanism, i.e., activation via factor VII, rather than through factor VIII and the intrinsic mechanism.

The mechanism whereby TF activity becomes elevated in prematurely aging cells is unknown. Another question is how an increased amount of TF in skin fibroblasts relates to the severe disease of blood-vessel walls seen in progeria and the Werner syndrome. There is evidence that the cultured skin fibroblast may originate from vascular cells such as endothelium or pericytes (Franks, 1972). Moreover, plasma membranes of intimal and medial cells have been found to be rich in TF antigen in large blood vessels and also in their vasa vasorum (Zeldis *et al.*, 1972). TF is particularly abundant in the vicinity of atherosclerotic plaques, where it encompasses cholesterol

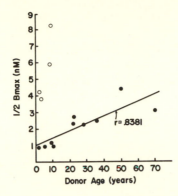

Fig. 12. Concentration of native insulin required to displace 50% of the [¹²⁵I]insulin specifically bound to cultured fibroblasts as a function of donor age. Symbols are mean values of three or more experiments with replicate dishes of cells incubated at 20°C in medium containing 1 nM [¹²⁵I]insulin or added native insulin at 1.0, 2.5, 5.0, 10, 25, 50, or 100 nM. (●) Normal donors; (○) precociously aged donors (bottom three symbols are children with progeria; the top symbol, a child with the Rothmund–Thomson syndrome). Reproduced from Rosenbloom *et al.* (1976) with permission of the authors and publisher. Copyright 1976 by the American Association for the Advancement of Science.

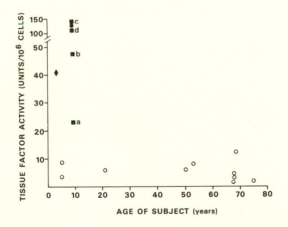

Fig. 13. Tissue factor activity of cultured fibroblasts as a function of donor age. Platelet-poor citrated human plasma from healthy donors was mixed with suspensions of early-passage fibroblasts at various dilutions, then recalcified and incubated (Zacharski and McIntyre, 1973). Clotting times were recorded, and the procoagulant activity of fibroblasts was compared with that of rabbit brain thromboplastin as a standard. Tissue factor activity of fibroblasts is expressed in arbitrary units compared with the standard. (■, ●, ◆) Progeria; (▲) Werner's syndrome; (○) normal controls.(a–d) Single subject with progeria using individual cultures initiated from skin of various anatomical sites: (a) anterior forearm; (b) anterior thigh; (c,d) bilateral calves. (●) Strain originated from skin over the lumbar area; all other cultures originated from skin of the anterior forearm. Values are the means of 3–14 experiments, except for (b–d), which represent single observations. Reproduced from S. Goldstein and Niewiarowski (1976) with permission of the authors and MacMillan Journals Limited.

crystals. In this way, TF could initiate coagulation, not merely as a consequence of plaque disruption, but also after minimal cellular damage.

7. Significance of Biochemical Defects in Prematurely Aging Fibroblasts

There are several possibilities for the multiplicity of altered proteins in prematurely aging cells based on errors at any of the three levels of genetic information flow—DNA, RNA, and protein turnover.

7.1. Defects in Protein Turnover

Orgel (1973) postulated that aging is related to a change in the accuracy of protein synthesis, with the production of a mixture of normal and abnormal proteins. The latter fraction would be heterogeneous, since errors would be a random collection of amino acid substitutions. Indeed, changes in the primary sequence of amino acids have usually been associated with increased thermolability of human G-6-PD, HGPRT, and several enzymes in lower forms (see Goldstein, S., and Moerman, 1976*b*). These changes, however, represent examples of homogeneously altered proteins in which the entire population of molecules is heat-labile. Orgel's notion, therefore, would explain why electrophoretic studies on progeria and Werner cells, whether run on starch (Goldstein, S., and Moerman, 1975*a,b*) or polyacrylamide gels (Goldstein, S., and Moerman, in prep.), have all been negative so far, since it predicts that the altered proteins would be dispersed in many positions in the gel.

It is also possible that a defect exists in proteolysis, a normal cellular mechanism that selectively degrades proteins either incorrectly synthesized or in other ways altered with time (Goldstein *et al.,* 1976). In fact, since both processes are probably linked, defects might coexist in both limbs of protein turnover such that progeria and Werner cells first generate, then tolerate, more defective proteins than normal cells. Recent work, in fact, suggests that degradation of a certain class of proteins may be altered in progeric and Werner cells (Goldstein, S., *et al.,* 1976).

7.2. Defects in RNA Turnover

It is evident that errors in RNA metabolism could also decrease the fidelity of protein synthesis. Information is accumulating about RNA synthesis, processing, and transport from the nucleus to the cytoplasm in permanent lines (Perry, 1976), but less is known about the mechanisms that degrade RNA species and the half-life of each RNA in the cytoplasm.

Relatively little data exist on RNA metabolism in human fibroblasts, and virtually nothing on premature aging. It is evident that abnormalities in the critical RNA polymerase(s) or in subsequent intranuclear cleavage or transport enzymes could change the quality and quantity of messenger produced.

There are preliminary suggestions that RNA metabolism may be amiss in late-passage WI-38 cells. Beginning at the template, transcription of chromatin seems to be reduced (Ryan and Cristofalo, 1975; Stein and Stein, 1976). This finding, however, must be reconciled with the findings that all species of RNA increase significantly at late passage, both per cell and per unit DNA, and in parallel with protein content (Ryan and Cristofalo, 1975; Schneider and Shorr, 1975). These observations point to a problem in RNA and protein turnover in aging normal cells. Further studies are now needed on the various aging mutants to see whether RNA metabolism is a primary source of defects in these disorders.

7.3. Defects in DNA Repair

This subject is dealt with in greater detail in Chapter 3, but some pertinent details warrant mention in this context. Progeric fibroblasts were shown to be deficient in the capacity to ligate broken DNA strands following γ-radiation (Epstein, J., *et al.*, 1973, 1974), but this finding has been controversial (Regan and Setlow, 1974; Bradley *et al.*, 1976; Rainbow and Howes, 1977). In any case, progeria cells apparently retain the ability to perform normal UV repair (Fig. 14) (Cleaver, 1970). Cockayne fibroblasts (Schmickel *et al.*, 1975) and those from Fanconi anemia (Poon *et al.*, 1974; Remsen and Cerutti, 1976) and the Rothmund–Thomson syndrome (Cleaver, 1970) also appear to be normal in UV (excision) repair, but are deficient in γ-repair. In total, this may relate to the different enzymes involved in each form of repair, or to the qualitatively different changes brought about by each form of radiation, or to both. Evidence for this idea was recently obtained in ataxia–telangiectasia fibroblasts, which seem to lack the full complement of functional γ-endonucleases (Vincent *et al.*, 1975; Paterson, M. C., *et al.*, 1976). Thus, ataxia fibroblasts have normal sensitivity to UV light and excision of UV photoproducts, but are killed more readily than normal cells by γ-radiation (Taylor, A. M. R., *et al.*, 1975).

The deficiency in DNA repair following γ-radiation of ataxia–telangiectasia cells would offer a direct explanation for the high incidence of chromosomal breaks and sensitivity to mutagens (Hoar and Sargent, 1976). Clinically, it could account for the radiosensitivity, degenerative phenomena, high incidence of malignancy, and premature death of affected persons. In progeria, a ligase deficiency could explain most of the abnormal

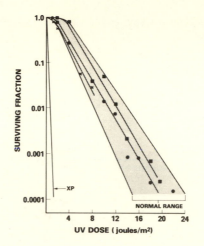

Fig. 14. Survival of progeria cells following UV irradiation. AK (●) is the classic progeria strain showing assorted defects in Figs. 10–13. KH (X) is the atypical progeroid strain first reported to be defective for γ-repair by J. Epstein *et al.* (1973) and Little *et al.* (1975); these cells grew poorly, so that only a partial survival curve could be obtained. S.J. (■) had not been studied before. Survival of two XP strains is shown for reference. These are the 20- and 21-year-old siblings with 10–20% of normal UV repair in Table II of Cleaver (1970) and in S. Goldstein (1971*c*). The range for several normal strains at early and late passage is shown as the shaded portion. From S. Goldstein (1971*c*) and previously unpublished data.

proteins via multiple somatic mutations. In fact, this very picture was described in *Escherichia coli* by Morse and Pauling (1975). It must be recognized, however, that defective enzymes for DNA repair may also be a consequence of a more primary disturbance in protein turnover. The reversion to normal γ-repair capability of progeria fibroblasts following simian-virus-40 transformation (Little *et al.*, 1975) is in accord with this idea.

The other chromosomal breakage–high malignancy syndromes such as Fanconi anemia (Finkelberg, 1976), xeroderma pigmentosum (Cleaver and Bootsma, 1975), and the Bloom syndrome (German, 1974) may also have specific defects in DNA repair. While the Bloom syndrome has increased baseline rates of sister chromatid exchange (Chaganti *et al.*, 1974), the others apparently do not (Galloway and Evans, 1975; Latt *et al.*, 1975; Kato and Stich, 1976). This dichotomy may relate, at least in part, to an error-prone postreplication repair system that depends on recombinational events between daughter strands of DNA.

New information on various forms and steps of DNA repair is appearing rapidly (Cleaver *et al.*, 1975; Hart and Trosko, 1976; Lieberman, 1976). Accordingly, judgment on the precise nature of the defects in DNA repair of certain aging mutants must be tempered with this in mind.

7.4. Defects in DNA Replication

While abnormalities in repair enzymes that conserve the original information encoded within DNA are clearly important, so are the various DNA polymerase molecules involved in semiconservative replication. A recent report by Linn *et al.* (1976) indicates that the fidelity of such DNA polymerase(s) may decline during *in vitro* aging of MRC-5 fibroblasts. Such "mutator" DNA polymerase molecules could obviously have widespread repercussions throughout the cell. Although defective DNA polymerases could conceivably be the primary defect in some of the aging mutants, it is again possible that such molecules may simply arise consequent to errors in protein synthesis.

8. Conclusions and Future Directions

Whether the syndromes of premature aging represent acceleration of normal aging remains a moot point. In fact, it might be more palatable if these syndromes were regarded as restricted caricatures of normal aging. Yet it is clear that if we conformed to rigidly defined criteria imposed by biomedical purists, we would squander precious opportunities to exploit these rare syndromes for what they can teach us about fundamental mechanisms of aging and attendant pathology. Academic debates at this current stage of limited knowledge should not impede investigations: any relatively discrete clinical entity that is reminiscent of aging in some features and—far more important—is determined by a single gene merits intensive study.

The fundamental aging process is most likely determined by a genetic program similar or perhaps identical to that which controls development. Both programs can therefore clearly be modified by specific inherited defects and by environmental agents. The specific phenotypic result will depend, however, on the relationship between the exact time that genes are expressed in a given tissue or clone and the time that a specific environmental agent impinges on them. Thus, it seems likely that the same gene or environmental agent that produces one phenotype early in life, e.g., malformations *in utero,* can produce age-dependent degeneration or malignancy later in life. Accordingly, although aging manifests in all cells with time, it proceeds cell by cell along an uneven front. Indeed, mounting evidence now suggests a clonal origin for various age-dependent disorders (Benditt and Benditt, 1973; Friedman and Fialkow, 1976; Nowell, 1976).

The aging process will probably turn out to be a diverse panorama in molecular terms. We must appreciate, therefore, that the nature of aging may be unique to each organism and even to each cell. What seems clear is that there is a limited number of choices available to a cell once it ages and enters the "final common pathway" to degenerative and neoplastic disorders. This limitation implies that a substantial fraction of senescent cells are not removed by lysis or phagocytosis *in vitro* but persist to form a potential pathological nidus. Thus, for example, if *HLA* antigens were altered in such cells, they could predispose to the autoimmune phenomena that increase rapidly with age (Good and Yunis, 1974). This would also explain why the exhausted pancreatic islets of many insulin-dependent diabetics are often infiltrated by autoaggressive lymphocytes both in humans (see Goldstein, S., 1971*b;* Huang, S. -W., and Maclaren, 1976) and in experimental animals (Like and Rossini, 1976).

If aged cells remained within the vascular wall with an elevated content of TF activity, they could initiate atherothrombotic events. On the other hand, aging cells with a higher content of defective molecules and deranged homeostatic mechanisms could be more susceptible to redirection by oncogenic agents such as chemicals, endogenous RNA viruses, or exogenous DNA viruses, i.e., malignant transformation. In any case, the questions posed should galvanize new research activity.

The tissue culture approach offers three major advantages that are worth repeating: (1) It circumvents ethical constraints rightfully imposed on direct human experimentation using viruses, drugs, radiation, and even hormones and nutrients in quantitative extremes. (2) It allows us to study cell populations in a controlled environment several generations removed from the neurohumoral influence of the donor, so that the principal experimental variable is the genetic endowment of cells. (3) It enables direct studies on aging in humans, rather than in lower forms. It then dictates, however, that further correlations be sought between *in vivo* and *in vitro* phenomena for validation. Numerous benefits would nevertheless accrue from these exercises, perhaps tantamount to "cellular epidemiology" in illuminating the way to more precise questions in cellular systems.

This approach will perforce involve a concerted effort between classic pathologists and physiologists and cellular and molecular biologists, but only in this way can we span the immense spectrum between total-organism aging and underlying molecular events. The goals of studying a diversity of inherited syndromes that exhibit accelerated aging should be clearly stated: (1) a better understanding of how specific genetic defects modulate the normal process of aging and its pathological concomitants; (2) a more rational approach to genetic counseling, early diagnosis, specific treatment, and rapid amelioration of the physical, emotional, and financial load imposed by these syndromes on patients, their families, and society.

Acknowledgments

The author's work is supported by grants from the Medical Research Council of Canada, the Canadian Diabetic Association Foundation Fund, and the Ontario Heart Foundation.

References

Alberti, K. G., Young, J. D., and Hockaday, T. O., 1974, Werner's syndrome: Metabolic observations, *Proc. R. Soc. Med.* **67**:36–38.

Alton, D. J., McDonald, P., and Reilly, B. J., 1972, Cockayne's syndrome: A report of three cases, *Radiology* **102**:403–406.

Ammann, A. J., Cain, W. A., Ishizaka, K., Hong, R., and Good, R. A., 1969, Immunoglobulin E deficiency in ataxia–telangiectasia, *N. Engl. J. Med.* **281**:469–472.

Andres, W., Pozefsky, T., Swerdloff, R. S., and Tobin, J. D., 1975, Effect of aging on carbohydrate metabolism, *Adv. Metab. Disord. Suppl.* **1**:349–355.

Atkins, L., 1954, Progeria: Report of a case with post-mortem findings, *N. Engl. J. Med.* **250**:1065–1069.

Bach, F. H., and van Rood, J. J., 1976, The major histocompatibility complex: Genetics and biology, *N. Engl. J. Med.* **295**:806–813, 872–878, 927–936.

Balci, S., Say, B., and Kinik, E., 1970, Werner's syndrome, *Turk. J. Pediatr.* **12**:89–97.

Benditt, E. P., and Benditt, J. M., 1973, Evidence for a monoclonal origin of human atherosclerotic plaques, *Proc. Natl. Acad. Sci. U.S.A.* **70**:1753–1756.

Bhakoo, O. N., Garg, S. K., and Sehgal, V. N., 1965, Progeria with unusual ocular manifestations: Report of a case with a review of the literature, *Indian Pediatr.* **2**:164–169.

Bingham, H. G., and Anderson, P. G., 1970, Coverage of cutaneous ulcers in Werner's syndrome, *Acta Derm.-Venereol.* **50**:237–239.

Blinstrub, R. W., Lehman, R., and Steinberg, T. H., 1964, Poikiloderma congenitale: Report of two cases, *Arch. Dermatol.* **89**:659–664.

Blizzard, R. M., 1965, Dwarfism, in: *Diagnosis and Treatment of Endocrine Disorders in Childhood and Adolescence* (L. Wilkins, ed.), pp. 160–194, Charles C. Thomas, Springfield, Illinois.

Block, B., and Stauffer, H., 1929, Skin diseases of endocrine system (dyshormonal dermatoses): Poikiloderma-like changes in connection with underdevelopment of the sexual glands and dystrophia adiposogenitalis, *Arch. Dermatol. Syphilol.* **19**:22–34.

Boder, E., and Sedgwick, R. P., 1958, Ataxia–telangiectasia: A familial syndrome of progressive cerebellar ataxia, oculocutaneous telangiectasia and frequent pulmonary infection, *Pediatrics* **21**:526–554.

Bottomley, W. K., and Box, J. M., 1976, Dental anomalies in the Rothmund–Thomson syndrome: Report of a case, *Oral Surg.* **41**:321–326.

Boué, A., Boué, J., Cure, S., Deluchat, C., and Perraudin, N., 1975, *In vitro* cultivation of cells from aneuploid human embryos: Initiation of cell lines and longevity of the culture, *In Vitro* **11**:409–413.

Boyd, M. W. J., and Grant, A. P., 1959, Werner's syndrome (progeria of the adult): Further pathological and biochemical observations, *Br. Med. J.* **2**:920–925.

Bradley, M. O., Erickson, L. C., and Kohn, K. W., 1976, Normal DNA strand rejoining and absence of DNA crosslinking in progeroid and aging human cells, *Mutat. Res.* **37**:279–292.

Brautbar, C., Pellegrino, M. A., Ferrone, S., Reisfeld, R. A., Payne, R., and Hayflick, L., 1973, Fate of *HL-A* antigens in aging cultured human diploid cell strains. II. Quantitative absorption studies, *Exp. Cell Res.* **78**:367–375.

Bristow, J. H., 1973, Werner's syndrome: Clinical features and cataract surgery, *S. Afr. Med. J.* **47**:566–569.

Brodrick, J. D., and Dark, A. J., 1973, Corneal dystrophy in Cockayne's syndrome, *Br. J. Opthalmol.* **57**:391–399.

Bullock, J. D., and Howard, R. O., 1973, Werner's syndrome, *Arch. Ophthalmol.* **90**:53–56.

Burch, P. R. J., and Milunsky, A., 1969, Early-onset diabetes mellitus in general and Down's syndrome populations: Genetics, etiology, and pathogenesis, *Lancet* **1**:554–558.

Burnet, F. M., 1974, *Intrinsic Mutagenesis: A Genetic Approach to Aging,* John Wiley & Sons, New York.

Burnett, J. W., 1968, Werner's syndrome, *South. Med. J.* **61:**207–209.

Cahill, G. F., 1975, Disorders of carbohydrate metabolism, in: *Textbook of Medicine* (P. B. Beeson and W. McDermott, eds.), pp. 1599–1619, W. B. Saunders Co., Philadelphia.

Cahill, G. F., Etzwiler, D. D., and Freinkel, N., 1976, "Control" and diabetes, *N. Engl. J. Med.* **294:**1004–1005.

Carr, D. H., 1975, Cytogenetics and the pathologist, *Pathobiol. Annu.* **10:**93–144.

Chaganti, R. S. K., Schonberg, S., and German, J., 1974, A manyfold increase in sister chromatid exchanges in Bloom's syndrome lymphocytes, *Proc. Natl. Acad. Sci. U.S.A.* **71:**4508–4512.

Childs, B., and Der Kaloustian, V. M., 1968, Genetic heterogeneity, *N. Engl. J. Med.* **279:**1205–1212, 1267–1279.

Cleaver, J. E., 1970, DNA damage and repair in light-sensitive human skin disease, *J. Invest. Dermatol.* **54:**181–195.

Cleaver, J. E., and Bootsma, D., 1975, Xeroderma pigmentosum: Biochemical and genetic characteristics, *Annu. Rev. Genet.* **9:**19–38.

Cleaver, J. E., Bootsma, D., and Friedberg, E., 1975, Human diseases with genetically altered DNA repair processes, *Genetics* **79:**215–225.

Cockayne, E. A., 1936, Dwarfism with retinal atrophy and deafness, *Arch. Dis. Child.* **11:** 1–8.

Cohen, M. M., Shaham, M., Dagan, J., Shmueli, E., and Kohn, G., 1975, Cytogenetic investigations in families with ataxia–telangiectasia, *Cytogenet. Cell Genet.* **15:**338–356.

Cole, H. N., Giffen, H. K., Simmons, J. T., and Stroud, G. M., III, 1945, Congenital cataracts in sisters with congential ectoderma dysplasia, *J. Am. Med. Assoc.* **129:**723–728.

Coles, W. H., 1969, Ocular manifestations of Cockayne's syndrome, *Am. J. Ophthalmol.* **67:**762–764.

Comfort, A., 1964, *Ageing: The Biology of Senescence,* Holt, Rinehart & Winston, New York.

Comfort, A., 1969, Test-battery to measure ageing-rate in man, *Lancet* **2:**1411–1415.

Cotton, R. B., Keats, T. E., and McCoy, E. E., 1970, Abnormal blood glucose regulation in Cockayne's syndrome, *Pediatrics* **46:**54–60.

Cox, R. P., 1974, *Cell Communication,* John Wiley & Sons, New York.

Crapper, D. R., Dalton, A. J., Skopitz, M., Scott, J. W., and Hachinski, V. C., 1975, Alzheimer degeneration in Down syndrome: Electrophysiologic alterations and histopathologic findings, *Arch. Neurol.* **33:**618–623.

Creutzfeldt, W., Kobberling, J., and Neel, J. V. (eds.), 1975, *The Genetics of Diabetes Mellitus,* Springer-Verlag, New York.

Cristofalo, V. J., 1972, Animal cell cultures as a model system for the study of aging, *Adv. Gerontol. Res.* **4:**45–79.

Crome, L., and Kanjilal, G. C., 1971, Cockayne's syndrome: Case report, *J. Neurol. Neurosurg. Psychiatry* **34:**171–178.

Cunliffe, P. N., Mann, J. R., Cameron, A. H., Roberts, K. D., and Ward, H. W. C., 1975, Radiosensitivity in ataxia telangiectasia, *Br. J. Radiol.* **48:**374–376.

Dalton, A. J., Crapper, D. R., and Schlotterer, G. R., 1974, Alzheimer's disease in Down's syndrome: Visual retention deficits, *Cortex* **10:**366–377.

Danes, B. S., 1971, Progeria: A cell culture study on aging, *J. Clin. Invest.* **50:**2000–2003.

DeBusk, F. L., 1972, The Hutchinson–Gilford progeria syndrome: Report of four cases and review of the literature, *J. Pediatr.* **80**(Part 2):695–724.

Degreef, H., 1971, The Werner syndrome, *Dermatologica* **142:**45–49.

Diem, E., 1975, The Rothmund–Thomson syndrome: A case report, *Hautarzt* **26:**425–429.

Down, J. L. H., 1866, Observations on ethnic classification of idiots, *Clin. Lect. Rep. London Hosp.* **3:**259–262.

Driban, N. E., and Bertranou, E. G., 1975, Adult progeria (Werner's syndrome), *Med. Cutanea* **3**:213–222.

Elmore, E., and Swift, M., 1976*a*, Growth of cultured cells from patients with Fanconi's anemia, *J. Cell. Physiol.* **87**:229–234.

Elmore, E., and Swift, M., 1976*b*, Growth of cultured cells from patients with ataxia–telangiectasia, *J. Cell. Physiol.* **89**:429–432.

Engle, E., and Forbes, A. P. 1965, Cytogenetic and clinical findings in 48 patients with congenitally defective or absent ovaries, *Medicine (Baltimore)* **44**:135–164.

Epstein, C. J., Martin, G. M., Schultz, A. L., and Motulsky, A. G., 1966, Werner's syndrome: A review of its symptomatology, natural history, pathologic features, genetics and relationship to the natural aging process, *Medicine (Baltimore)* **45**:177–221.

Epstein, J., Williams, J. R., and Little, J. B., 1973, Deficient DNA repair in human progeroid cells, *Proc. Natl. Acad. Sci. U.S.A.* **70**:977–981.

Epstein, J., Williams, J. R., and Little, J. B., 1974, Rate of DNA repair in progeric and normal human fibroblasts, *Biochem. Biophys. Res. Commun.* **59**:850–856.

Fajans, S. S., Floyd, J. C., Tattersall, R. B., Williamson, J. R., Pek, S., and Taylor C. I., 1976, The various faces of diabetes in the young, *Arch. Intern. Med.* **136**:194–202.

Faye, I., Ruscher, H., Marchand, J. P., Bloc, G., and Toure, M. F., 1973, A case of Werner's syndrome, *Bull. Soc. Med. Afr. Noire Lang. Fr.* **18**:564–566.

Feigin, R. D., Vietti, T. J., Wyatt, R. G., Kaufman, D. G., and Smith, C. H., 1970, Ataxia telangiectasia with granulocytopenia, *J. Pediatr.* **77**:431–438.

Feingold, M., and Kidd, R., 1971, Progeria and scleroderma in infancy, *Am. J. Dis. Child.* **122**:61–62.

Felig, P., Wahren, J., Sherwin, R., and Hendler, R., 1976, Insulin, glucagon, and somatostatin in normal physiology and diabetes mellitus, *Diabetes* **25**:1091–1099.

Ferrari-Sacco, A., Carolei, P., Emanuele, B., Marasso, A., and Marengo, G., 1972, Etiopatho-genetic, clinical and anatomo-histological notes on a very rare form of congenital anomaly (Werner's syndrome or Rothmund–Thomson syndrome) associated with pulmonary tuberculosis, *Minerva Med.* **63**:2563–2573.

Finkelberg, R., 1976, Studies on cells from patients with Fanconi's anemia, Ph.D. thesis, University of Toronto.

Fleischmajer, R., and Nedwich, A., 1973*a*, Progeria (Hutchinson–Gilford), *Arch. Dermatol.* **107**:253–258.

Fleischmajer, R., and Nedwich, A., 1973*b*, Werner's syndrome, *Am. J. Med.* **54**:111–118.

Forbes, A. P., and Engel, E., 1963, The high incidence of diabetes mellitus in 41 patients with gonadal dysgenesis and their close relatives, *Metabolism* **12**:428–439.

Ford, C. E., Kones, K. W., Polani, P. E., DeAlmeida, J. C., and Briggs, J. H., 1959, A sex chromosome anomaly in a case of gonadal dysgenesis (Turner's syndrome) *Lancet* **1**:711.

Franceschetti, A., 1953, Les dysplasies ectodermiques et les syndromes hereditaires apparantes, *Dermatologica* **106**:129–156.

Franks, L. M., 1972, The ultrastructure of tissue culture cells, *Symp. Biol. Hung.* **14**:31–35.

Fraser, G. R., and Friedmann, A. I., 1967, *The Causes of Blindness in Childhood: A Study of 776 Children with Severe Visual Handicaps,* Johns Hopkins University Press, Baltimore.

Fratontoni, J. C., Hall, C. W., and Neufeld, E. F., 1968, Hurler and Hunter syndromes: Mutual correction of the defect in cultured fibroblasts, *Science* **162**:570–572.

Frenkel, G., 1970, Mucosal atrophy with special reference to the Werner syndrome, *Dtsch. Zahnaerztl. Z.* **25**:1026–1029.

Friedman, J. M., and Fialkow, P. J., 1976, Cell marker studies of human tumorigenesis, *Transplant. Rev.* **28**:17–33.

Fujimoto, W. Y., Green, M. L., and Seegmiller, J. E., 1969, Cockayne's syndrome: Report of a case with hyperlipoproteinemia, hyperinsulinemia, renal disease, and normal growth hormone, *J. Pediatr.* **75**:881–884.

Gabr, M., Hashem, N., Hashem, F., Fahmi, A., and Safouh, M., 1960, Progeria, a pathologic study, *J. Pediatr.* **57**:70–77.

Galloway, S. M., and Evans, H. J., 1975, Sister chromatid exchange in human chromosomes from normal individuals and patients with ataxia telangiectasia, *Cytogenet. Cell Genet.* **15**:17–29.

Gardner, D. G., and Majka, M., 1969, The early formation of irregular secondary dentine in progeria, *Oral Surg. Oral Med. and Oral Pathol.* **28**:877–884.

Gerald, P. S., 1976, Current concepts in genetics—Sex chromosome disorders, *N. Engl. J. Med.* **294**:706–708.

German, J., 1974, *Chromosomes and Cancer,* John Wiley & Sons, New York.

Gershon, D., and Gershon, H., 1976, An evaluation of the "error catastrophe" theory of ageing in the light of recent experimental results, *Gerontology* **22**:212–219.

Ghosh, S., and Berry, A. M., 1973, Progeria—A follow up of 8 years, *Indian Pediatr.* **10**:45.

Ghosh, S., and Varma, K. P. S., 1964, Progeria: Report of a case with review of the literature, *Indian Pediatr.* **1**:146–155.

Giacomini, F., and Rizzi, B., 1968, Considerations on the osteogenic healing process in a case of true progeria, *Arch. Ortop.* **81**:379–389.

Gibbs, D. D., 1967, Werner's syndrome (progeria of the adult), *Proc. R. Soc. Med.* **60**:135–136.

Gilford, H., 1897, On the condition of mixed premature and immature development, *Trans. Med.-Chir. Soc. Edinburgh* **80**:17–45.

Gilkes, J. J., Sharvill, D. E., and Wells, R. S., 1974, The premature ageing syndromes: Report of eight cases and description of a new entity named metageria, *Br. J. Dermatol.* **91**:243–262.

Ginsberg-Fellner, F., and Knittle, J. L., 1973, Adipose tissue cellularity and metabolism in newly diagnosed juvenile diabetics, *Diabetes* **22**:528–536.

Goetz, I., Roberts, E., and Comings, D. E., 1975, Fibroblasts in Huntington's disease, *N. Engl. J. Med.* **293**:1225–1227.

Gold, P., 1971, Antigenic reversion in human cancer, *Annu. Rev. Med.* **22**:85–94.

Goldstein, D. E., Drash, A., Gibbs, J., and Blizzard, R. M., 1970, Diabetes mellitus: The incidence of circulating antibodies against thyroid, gastric and adrenal tissue, *J. Pediatr.* **77**:304–306.

Goldstein, S., 1969, Lifespan of cultured cells in progeria, *Lancet* **1**:424.

Goldstein, S., 1971*a,* The biology of aging, *N. Engl. J. Med.* **285**:1120–1129.

Goldstein, S., 1971*b,* On the pathogenesis of diabetes mellitus and its relationship to biological aging, *Humangenetik* **12**:83.

Goldstein, S., 1971*c,* The role of DNA repair in aging of cultured fibroblasts from Xeroderma pigmentosum and normals, *Proc. Soc. Exp. Biol. Med.* **137**:730–734.

Goldstein, S., 1978*a,* Senescence. I. Hormones and aging, in: *Metabolic Basis of Endrocrinology* (Degroot, Martins, Potts, Nelson, Winegrad, Odell, Steinberger, and Cahill, eds.), Grune and Stratton, New York (in press).

Goldstein, S., 1978*b,* Senescence. II. General and cellular aging, in: *Metabolic Basis of Endocrinology* (Degroot, Martins, Potts, Nelson, Winegrad, Odell, Steinberger, and Cahill, eds.), Grune and Stratton, New York (in press).

Goldstein, S., and Moerman, E., 1975*a,* Heat-labile enzymes in skin fibroblasts from subjects with progeria, *N. Engl. J. Med.* **292**:1305–1309.

Goldstein, S., and Moerman, E. J., 1975*b,* Heat-labile enzymes in Werner's syndrome fibroblasts, *Nature (London)* **255**:159.

Goldstein, S., and Moerman, E. J., 1976*a,* The Hutchinson–Gilford (progeria) syndrome: Heat-lability of enzymes, in red blood cells in a family, *Clin. Res.* **24**:668A.

Goldstein, S., and Moerman, E. J., 1976*b*, Defective proteins in normal and abnormal human fibroblasts during aging *in vitro, Interdiscip. Top. Gerontol.* **10:**24–43.

Goldstein, S., and Niewiarowski, S., 1976, Increased procoagulant activity in cultured fibroblasts from progeria and Werner's syndromes of premature ageing, *Nature (London)* **260:**711–713.

Goldstein, S., and Singal, D. P., 1974, Alteration of fibroblast gene products *in vitro* from a subject with Werner's syndrome, *Nature (London)* **251:**719–721.

Goldstein, S., and Trieman, G., 1975, Glucose consumption by early and late-passage diploid human fibroblasts during growth and stationary phase, *Experientia* **31:**177–180.

Goldstein, S., Littlefield, J. W., and Soeldner, J. S., 1969, Diabetes mellitus and aging: Diminished plating efficiency of cultured human fibroblasts, *Proc. Natl. Acad. Sci. U.S.A.* **64:**155–160.

Goldstein, S., Moerman, E. J., Soeldner, J. S., Gleason, R. E., and Barnett, D. M., 1974, Diabetes mellitus and prediabetes: Decreased replicative capacity of cultured fibroblasts, *J. Clin. Invest.* **53:**27a–27b.

Goldstein, S., Niewiarowski, S., and Singal, D. P., 1975, Pathological implications of cell aging *in vitro, Fed. Proc. Fed. Am. Soc. Exp. Biol.* **34:**56–63.

Goldstein, S., Stotland, D., and Cordeiro, R. A. J., 1976, Decreased proteolysis and increased amino acid efflux in aging human fibroblasts. *Mech. Ageing Dev.* **5:**221–233.

Goldstein, S., Moerman, E. J., Soeldner, J. S., Gleason, R. E., and Barnett, D. M., 1978, Chronologic age and physiologic status: Effect on replicative lifespan of cultured human fibroblasts from diabetic, prediabetic and normal donors, *Science* (in press).

Good, R. A., and Yunis, E., 1974, Association of autoimmunity, immunodeficiency and aging in man, rabbits and mice, *Fed. Proc. Fed. Am. Soc. Exp. Biol.* **33:**2040–2050.

Gotoff, S. P., Amirmokri, E., and Liebner, E. J., 1967, Ataxia telangiectasia, neoplasia, untoward response to X-irradiation, and tuberous sclerosis, *Am. J. Dis. Child.* **114:**617–625.

Gottron, H., 1940, Familiare akrogerie, *Arch. Dermatol. Syphilol.* **181:**571–583.

Greene, M. L., Glueck, C. J., Fujimoto, W. Y., and Seegmiller, J. E., 1970, Benign symmetric lipomatosis (Launois–Bensaude adenolipomatosis) with gout and hyperlipoproteinemia, *Am. J. Med.* **48:**239–246.

Griffin, J. E., Punyashthiti, K., and Wilson, J. D., 1976, Dihydrotestosterone binding by cultured human fibroblasts: Comparison of cells from control subjects and from patients with hereditary male pseudohermaphroditism due to androgen resistance, *J. Clin. Invest.* **57:**1342–1351.

Grunebaum, M., 1973, Progeria, *Postgrad. Med.* **53:**221–222.

Gsell, O., and Haensch, G., 1971, Werner's syndrome: A case report on premature aging, *Schweiz. Med. Wochenschr.* **101:**418–421.

Haerer, A. F., Jackson, J. F., and Evers, C. G., 1969, Ataxia–telangiectasia with gastric adenocarcinoma, *J. Am. Med. Assoc.* **210:**1884–1887.

Hall, B. D., Berg, B. O., Rudolph, R. S., and Epstein, C. J., 1974, Pseudoprogeria–Hallermann–Streiff (PHS) syndrome, *Birth Defects: Orig. Artic. Ser.* **10:**137–146.

Hamlin, C. R., Kohn, R. R., and Luschin, J. H., 1975, Apparent accelerated aging of human collagen in diabetes mellitus, *Diabetes* **24:**902–904.

Harnden, D. G., 1974, Ataxia telangiectasia syndrome: Cytogenetic and cancer aspects, in: *Chromosomes and Cancer* (J. German, ed.), pp. 619–636, John Wiley & Sons, New York.

Hart, R. W., and Trosko, J. E., 1976, DNA repair processes in mammals, *Interdiscip. Top. Gerontol.* **9:**134–167.

Haslam, R. J., and Goldstein, S., 1974, Adenosine $3':5'$-cyclic monophosphate in young and senescent human fibroblasts during growth and stationary phase *in vitro:* Effects of prostaglandin E_1 and of adrenaline, *Biochem. J.* **144:**253–263.

Hassell, T. M., Page, R. C., Narayanan, S., and Cooper, C. G., 1976, Diphenylhydantoin (Dilantin) gingival hyperplasia: Drug-induced abnormality of connective tissue, *Proc. Natl. Acad. Sci. U.S.A.* **73**:2909–2912.

Hayflick, L., 1965, The limited *in vitro* lifetime of human diploid cell strains, *Exp. Cell Res.* **37**:614–636.

Hecht, F., Koler, R. D., Rigas, D. A., Dahnke, G. S., Case, M. P., Tisdale, V., and Miller, R. W., 1966, Leukemia and lymphocytes in ataxia–telangiectasia, *Lancet* **2**:1193.

Hecht, F., McCaw, B. K., and Koler, R. D., 1973, Ataxia–telangiectasia–Clonal growth of translocation lymphocytes, *N. Engl. J. Med.* **289**:286–291.

Hernandez, A. L., DeLeon, B., Garcia de la Puenti, S., and Del Castillo, V., 1975, Ultrastructural renal lesions in the Cockayne syndrome: A case report, *Rev. Invest. Clin.* **27**:153–158.

Higurashi, M., and Conen, P. E., 1973, *In vitro* chromosomal radiosensitivity in chromosomal breakage syndromes, *Cancer* **32**:380–383.

Hoar, D. I., 1975, Phenotypic manifestations of ataxia–telangiectasia, *Lancet* **2**:1048.

Hoar, D. I., and Sargent, P., 1976, Chemical mutagen hypersensitivity in ataxia–telangiectasia, *Nature (London)* **261**:590–592.

Holliday, R., Porterfield, J. S., and Gibbs, D. D., 1974, Premature ageing and occurrence of altered enzyme in Werner's syndrome fibroblasts, *Nature (London)* **248**:762–763.

Hopkins, D. J., and Horan, E. C., 1970, Glaucoma in the Hallermann–Streiff syndrome, *Br. J. Ophthalmol.* **54**:416–422.

Hoppe, W., and Koritsch, H. D., 1972, Another case of meningioma in a patient with Werner's syndrome, *Psychiatr. Neurol. Med. Psychol.* **24**:611–617.

Howell, T. H., 1975, *Old Age,* p. 115, H. K. Lewis, London.

Huang, K.-E., 1975, Pituitary response to synthetic luteinizing hormone-releasing hormone in patients with Turner's syndrome, *J. Clin. Endocrinol. Metab.* **41**:771–776.

Huang, S.-W., and Maclaren, N. K., 1976, Insulin-dependent diabetes: A disease of autoaggression, *Science* **192**:64–66.

Hutchinson, D., 1971, Oral manifestations of oculomandibulodyscephaly with hypotrichosis (Hallermann–Streiff syndrome), *Oral Surg. Oral Med. Oral Pathol.* **31**:234–244.

Hutchinson, J., 1886, Congenital absence of hair and mammary glands, *Trans. Med.-Chir. Soc. Edinburgh* **69**:473–477.

Ishii, T., 1976, Progeria: Autopsy report of one case, with a review of pathologic findings reported in the literature, *J. Am. Geriatr. Soc.* **24**:193–202.

Ishii, T., and Hosoda, Y., 1974, Autopsy of Werner's syndrome, *Jpn. J. Geriatr.* **11**:408–415.

Ishii, T., and Hosoda, Y., 1975, Werner's syndrome: Autopsy report of one case, with a review of pathologic findings reported in the literature, *J. Am. Geriatr. Soc.* **23**:145–154.

Jervis, G. A., 1970, Premature senility in Down's syndrome, *Ann. N. Y. Acad. Sci.* **171**:559–561.

Johansen, K. Soeldner, J. S., Gleason, R. E., Gottlieb, M. S., Park, B. N., Kaufmann, R. L., and Tan, M. H., 1975, Serum insulin and growth hormone response patterns in monozygotic twin siblings of patients with juvenile-onset diabetes, *N. Engl. J. Med.* **293**:57–61.

Jones, K. L., Smith, D. W., Harvey, M. A., Hall, B. D., and Quan, L., 1975, Older paternal age and fresh gene mutation: Data on additional disorders, *J. Pediatr.* **86**:84–88.

Kaiman, H., Lambie, R. W., and Metzl, 1969, Progeria: Case description, *Clin. Pediatr. (Philadelphia)* **8**:411–415.

Kato, H., and Stich, H. F., 1976, Sister chromatid exchanges in aging and repair-deficient human fibroblasts, *Nature (London)* **260**:447–448.

Kaufman, M., Straisfeld, C., and Pinsky, L., 1977, Expression of androgen-responsive properties in human skin fibroblast strains of genital and nongenital origin, *Somat. Cell Genet.* **3**:17–25.

Keay, A. J., Oliver, M. F., and Boyd, G. S., 1955, Progeria and atherosclerosis, *Arch. Dis. Child.* **30**:410–414.

Kidd, R. L., and Wilgram, G. F., 1972, Morphea and progeria, *Arch. Dermatol.* **105**:770–771.

Kohn, R. R., 1975, Aging and cell division, *Science* **188**:203–204.

Korein, J., Steinman, P. A., and Senz, E. H., 1961, Ataxia–telangiectasia: Report of a case and review of the literature, *Arch. Neurol.* **4**:272–280.

Kraus, B. S., Gottlieb, M. A., and Meliton, H. R., 1970, The dentition in Rothmund's syndrome, *J. Am. Dent. Assoc.* **81**:895–915.

Kristensen, J. K., 1975, Poikiloderma congenitale—An early case of Rothmund–Thomson's syndrome, *Acta Derm.-Venereol.* **55**:316–318.

Kulenkamp, D., Scholz-Kordan, D., Passarge, E., Rudiger, H. W., and Ruprecht, K. W., 1973, Werner's syndrome: A hereditable disorder of multiple organ systems, *Andrologie* **5**:299–310.

Kvale, P. A., Rutt, W. M., Birk, R. E., and Eyler, W. R., 1965, Werner's syndrome, *Henry Ford Hosp. Med. J.* **13**:411–420.

Land, V. J., and Nogrady, M. B., 1969, Cockayne's syndrome, *J. Can. Assoc. Radiol.* **20**:194–203.

Lanning, M., and Simil, A. S., 1970, Cockayne's syndrome: Report of a case with normal intelligence, *Z. Kinderheilkd.* **109**:70–75.

Larregue, M., Cathelineau, G., Binet, O., Lhullier, N., Timsit, E., and Graciansky, P. De, 1974, Werner's syndrome and hyperinsulinic diabetes, *Ann. Dermatol. Syphiligr.* **101**:135–144.

Latt, S. A., Stetten, G. M., Juergens, L. A., Buchanan, G. R., and Gerald, P. S., 1975, Induction by alklyating agents of sister chromatid exchanges and chromatid breaks in Fanconi's anemia, *Proc. Natl. Acad. Sci. U.S.A.* **72**:4066–4070.

Leaf, A., 1973, Unusual longevity: The common denominator, *Hosp. Pract.* **8**:79–86.

Le Guilly, Y., Simon, M., Lenoir, P., and Bourel, M., 1973, Long-term culture of human adult liver cells: Morphological changes related to *in vitro* senescence and effect of donor's age on growth potential, *Gerontologia* **19**:303–313.

Lelis, I. I., 1975, Progeria of adults (Werner's syndrome) *Ter. Arkh.* **47**(1):99–102.

Lenz, W. D., and Majewski, F., 1974, A generalized disorder of the connective tissues with progeria, choanal atresia, symphalangism, hypoplasia of dentine and craniodiaphyseal hypostosis, *Birth Defects: Orig. Artic. Ser.* **10**:133–136.

Lestradet, H., Deschamps, I., and Giron, B., 1976, Insulin and free fatty acid levels during oral glucose tolerance tests and their relation to age in 70 healthy children, *Diabetes* **25**:505–508.

Levin, S., and Perlov, S., 1971, Ataxia–telangiectasia in Israel, with observations on its relationship to malignant disease, *Isr. J. Med. Sci.* **7**:1535–1541.

Levine, M. D., Alexander, E., and Rimoin, D. L., 1975, Progeroid syndrome, *Birth Defects: Orig. Artic. Ser.* **11**:308–309.

Lewis, M. B., 1972, Rothmund–Thomson syndrome and fibrocystic disease, *Australas. J. Dermatol.* **13**:105–106.

Lieberman, M. W., 1976, Approaches to the analysis of fidelity of DNA repair in mammalian cells, *Int. Rev. Cytol.* **45**:1–23.

Like, A. A., and Rossini, A. A., 1976, Streptozotocin-induced pancreatic insulitis: A new model of diabetes mellitus, *Science* **193**:415–417.

Lindeman, R. D., 1975, Age changes in renal function, in: *The Physiology and Pathology of Human Aging* (R. Goldman and M. Rockstein, eds.), pp. 19–38, Academic Press, New York.

Lindsten, J., 1963, in: *The Nature and Origin of X Chromosome Aberrations in Turner's Syndrome* (Almquist and Wiksell, eds.), Stockholm.

Lindsten, J., Cerasi, E., Luft, R., and Hultquist, G., 1967, The occurrence of abnormal insulin and growth hormone (HGH) responses to sustained hyperglycaemia in a disease with sex chromosome aberrations (Turner's syndrome): Including a histological study of the pancreas in two such patients, *Acta Endocrinol. (Copenhagen)* **56**:107–131.

Linn, S., Kairis, M., and Holliday, R., 1976, Decreased fidelity of DNA polymerase activity isolated from aging human fibroblasts, *Proc. Natl. Acad. Sci. U.S.A.* **73**:2818–2822.

Lisker, R., and Cobo, A., 1970, Chromosome breakage in ataxia–telangiectasia, *Lancet* **1**: 618.

Little, J. B., Epstein, J., and Williams, J. R., 1975, Repair of DNA strand breaks in progeric fibroblasts and aging human diploid cells, *Basic Life Sci.* **58**:793–800.

Lodi, A., Ravaglia, G., Grigioni, F., Ravaioli, R., and Gritti, F., 1974, Endocrine and morphological aspects of Werner's syndrome, *J. Clin. Med.* **55**:652–674.

Louis-Bar, D., 1941, Sur un syndrome progressif comprenant des télangiectasies capillaires cutanées et conjonctivales, à disposition naevoïde et des troubles cérébelleux, *Confin. Neurol.* **4**:32–42.

MacDonald, W. B., Fitch, K. D., and Lewis, I. C., 1960, Cockayne's syndrome: A heredo-familial disorder of growth and development, *Pediatrics* **25**:997–1007.

Macleod, W., 1966, Progeria, *Br. J. Radiol.* **39**:224–226.

MacNamara, B. G., Farn, K. T., Mitra, A. K., Lloyd, J. K., and Fosbrooke, A. S., 1970, Progeria: Case report with long-term studies of serum lipids, *Arch. Dis. Child.* **45**:553–560.

Malamud, N., 1972, Neuropathology of organic brain syndromes associated with aging, in: *Aging and the Brain* (C. M. Gaitz, ed.), pp. 63–87, Plenum Press, New York.

Marble, A., and Ramos, E., 1971, Cancer and diabetes, in: *Joslin's Diabetes Mellitus* (A. Marble, P. White, R. F. Bradley, and L. P. Krall, eds.), pp. 695–700, Lea & Febiger, Philadelphia.

Marcondes, E., Campos, J. V., Barbieri, D., Quarentei, G., and Cavallo, A., 1969, Progeria: Case report with progressive systemic sclerotic manifestations since birth, *Rev. Hosp. Clin. Fac. Med. Univ. Sao Paulo* **24**:147–154.

Margolin, F. R., and Steinbach, H. L., 1968, Progeria: Hutchinson–Gilford syndrome, *Am. J. Roentgenol. Radium Ther. Nucl. Med.* **103**:173–178.

Marks, H. H., and Krall, L. P., 1971, Onset, course, prognosis and mortality in diabetes mellitus, in: *Joslin's Diabetes Mellitus* (A. Marble, P. White, R. F. Bradley, and L. P. Krall, eds.), pp. 209–254, Lea & Febiger, Philadelphia.

Martin, G. M., 1977, Genetic syndromes in man with potential relevance to the pathobiology of aging, in: *Genetic Effects on Aging, Birth Defects: Orig. Artic. Ser.* (D. Bergsma and D. E. Harrison, eds.) The National Foundation–March of Dimes, New York (in press).

Martin, G. M., Sprague, C. A., and Epstein, C. J., 1970, Replicative life-span of cultivated human cells: Effects of donor's age, tissue, and genotype, *Lab. Invest.* **23**:86–92.

Martin, G. M., Sprague, C. A., Norwood, T. H., and Pendergrass, W. R., 1974, Clonal selection, attenuation and differentiation in an *in vitro* model of hyperplasia, *Am. J. Pathol.* **74**:137–154.

Martin, J. J., Deberot, R., Philippart, M., Van Acker, K. J., and Hooft, C., 1971, Peculiar dysmorphic syndrome with orthochromatic leucodystrophy: Discussion of its relationship with Cockayne's syndrome and Pelizaeus–Merzbacher's disease, *Acta Neuropathol.* **18**:224–233.

Maurer, R. M., and Langford, O. L., 1967, Rothmund's syndrome: A cause of resorption of phalangeal tufts and dystrophic calcification, *Radiology* **89**:706–708.

McCaw, B. K., Hecht, F., Harnden, D. G., and Teplitz, R. L., 1975, Somatic rearrangement of chromosome 14 in human lymphocytes, *Proc. Natl. Acad. Sci. U.S.A.* **72**:2071–2075.

McFarlin, D. W., Strober, W., and Waldmann, T. A., 1972, Ataxia telangiectasia, *Medicine (Baltimore)* **51**:281–314.

McKusick, V. A., 1963, Medical genetics, 1962, *J. Chronic Dis.* **16:**457–634.

McKusick, V. A., 1975, *Mendelian Inheritance in Man—Catalogs of Autosomal Dominant, Autosomal Recessive and X-Linked Phenotypes,* Johns Hopkins University Press, Baltimore.

McKusick, V. A., and Cross, H. E., 1966, Ataxia–telangiectasia and Swiss-type agammaglobulinemia: Two genetic disorders of the immune mechanism in related Amish sibships, *J. Am. Med. Assoc.* **195:**739–745.

Meissner, W. A., and Legg, M. A., 1971, The pathology of diabetes, in: *Joslin's Diabetes Mellitus* (A. Marble, P. White, R. F. Bradley, and L. P. Krall, eds.), pp. 157–190, Lea & Febiger, Philadelphia.

Menkes, J. H., and Stein, N., 1973, Fibroblast cultures in Huntington's disease, *N. Engl. J. Med.* **288:**856–857.

Miller, M. E., and Chatten, J., 1967, Ovarian changes in ataxia telangiectasia, *Acta Paediatr. Scand.* **56:**559–561.

Miller, R. W., 1970, Neoplasia and Down's syndrome, *Ann. N. Y. Acad. Sci.* **171:**637–644.

Moosa, A., and Dubowitz, V., 1970, Peripheral neuropathy in Cockayne's syndrome, *Arch. Dis. Child.* **45:**674–677.

Moossey, J., 1967, The neuropathology of Cockayne's syndrome, *J. Neuropathol. Exp. Neurol.* **26:**654–660.

Morgan, J. L., Holcomb, T. M., and Morrissey, R. W., 1968, Radiation reaction in ataxia telangiectasia, *Am. J. Dis. Child.* **116:**577–558.

Morse, L. S., and Pauling, C., 1975, Induction of error-prone repair as a consequence of DNA ligase deficiency in *E. coli, Proc. Natl. Acad. Sci. U.S.A.* **72:**4645–4649.

Mostafa, A. H., and Gabr, M., 1954, Heredity in progeria: With follow-up of two affected sisters, *Arch. Pediatr.* **71:**163–172.

Muller, J., Kunkov, A. A., and Kepertov, A. A., 1969, Werner's syndrome: Case report, *Wien. Z. Inn. Med. Ihre Grenzgeb.* **50:**112–116.

Murphy, R., and Achkar, E. J., 1966, Werner's syndrome, *Lahey Clin. Found. Bull.* **15:**1–7.

Neill, C. A., and Dingwall, M. M., 1950, A syndrome resembling progeria: A review of two cases, *Arch. Dis. Child.* **25:**213–223.

Nelson, P. G., Pyke, D. A., Cudworth, A. G., Woodrow, J. C., and Batchelor, J. R., 1975, Histocompatibility antigens in diabetic identical twins, *Lancet* **2:**193–194.

Neufeld, E. F., Lim, T. W., and Shapiro, L. J., 1975, Inherited disorders of lysosomal metabolism, *Annu. Rev. Biochem.* **44:**357–376.

Nielsen, J., Johansen, K., and Yde, H., 1969, The frequency of diabetes mellitus in patients with Turner's syndrome and pure gonadal dysgenesis, *Acta Endocrinol. (Copenhagen)* **62:**251–269.

Nienhaus, A. J., De Jong, B., and Kate, L. P. Ten, 1971, Fibroblast culture in Werner's syndrome, *Humangenetik* **13:**244–246.

Nissim, J. E., 1971, Rothmund syndrome, *Birth Defects: Orig. Artic. Ser.* **7:**294–295.

Norman, R. M., and Tingey, A. H., 1966, Syndrome of micrencephaly, strio-cerebellar calcifications and leucodystrophy, *J. Neurol. Neurosurg. Psychiatry* **29:**157–163.

Nowell, P. C., 1976, The clonal evolution of tumor cell populations: Acquired genetic lability permits stepwise selection of variant sublines and underlies tumor progression, *Science* **194:**23–28.

Oates, R. K., Lewis, M. B., and Walker-Smith, J. A., 1971, The Rothmund–Thomson syndrome: Case report of an unusual syndrome, *Aust. Paediatr. J.* **7:**103–107.

Ohno, T., and Hiroaka, M., 1966, Renal lesions in Cockayne's syndrome, *Tohoku J. Exp. Med.* **89:**151–166.

Orgel, L. E., 1973, Ageing of clones of mammalian cells, *Nature (London)* **243:**441–445.

Oxford, J. M., Harnden, D. G., Parrington, J. M., and Delhanty, J. D., 1975, Specific chromosome aberrations in ataxia telangiectasia, *J. Med. Genet.* **12:**251–262.

Ozonoff, M. B., and Clemett, A. R., 1967, Progressive osteolysis in progeria, *Am. J. Roentgenol. Radium Ther. Nucl. Med.* **100**:75–79.

Paddison, R. M., Moossy, J., Derbes, V. J., and Kloepfer, H. W., 1963, Cockayne's syndrome: A report of five new cases with biochemical, chromosomal, dermatologic, genetic and neuropathologic observations, *Dermatol. Trop. Ecol. Geogr.* **2**:195–203.

Palmer, G., 1966, Rothmund–Thomson syndrome, *Australas. J. Dermatol.* **8**:253–254.

Palumbo, P. J., Elveback, L. R., Chu, C.-P., Connolly, D. C., and Kurland, L. T., 1976, Diabetes mellitus: Incidence, prevalence, survivorship, and causes of death in Rochester, Minnesota, 1945–1970, *Diabetes* **25**:566–573.

Paterson, D., 1922, Case of progeria, *Proc. R. Soc. Med.* **16**:42.

Paterson, M. C., Smith, B. P., Lohman, P. H. M., Anderson, A. K., and Fishman, L., 1976, Defective excision repair of γ-ray-damaged DNA in human (ataxia telangiectasia) fibroblasts, *Nature (London)* **260**:444–447.

Payer, G., 1969, Two cases of Werner's syndrome, *Klin. Monatsbl. Augenheilkd.* **155**:901–904.

Penrose, L. S., and Smith, G. F., 1966, *Down's Anomaly,* Churchill, London.

Perlman, H. H., Luscombe, H. A., and Rosenberg, P. E., 1967, Poikiloderma congenitale of Thomson–Rothmund vs. localized linear scleroderma, *Arch. Dermatol.* **96**:593–594.

Perry, R. P., 1976, Processing of RNA, *Annu. Rev. Biochem.* **45**:605–630.

Peterson, R. D. A., Kelly, W. D., and Good, R. A., 1964, Ataxia–telangiectasia: Its association with a defective thymus, immunological-deficiency disease and malignancy, *Lancet* **1**:1189–1193.

Peterson, R. D. A., Cooper, M. D., and Good, R. A., 1966, Lymphoid tissue abnormalities associated with ataxia–telangiectasia, *Am. J. Med.* **41**:342–359.

Pfeiffer, R. A., and Backmann, K. D., 1973, An atypical case of Cockayne's syndrome, *Clin. Genet.* **4**:28–32.

Piazzini, M., Conti, C., Guazzelli, R., and Bigozzi, U., 1976, On a rare case of progeria in brother and sister, *Acta Med. Auxol.* **8**:75–79.

Poon, P. K., O'Brien, R. L., and Parker, J. W., 1974, Defective DNA repair in Fanconi's anaemia, *Nature (London)* **250**:223–225.

Predescu, V., Christodorescu, D., Coltoiu, A., Costiner, E., Hagiopol, V., and Alexianu, M., 1973, Cockayne's syndrome, *Arch. Fr. Pediatr.* **30**:527–532.

Rainbow, A. J., and Howes, M., 1977, Decreased repair of gamma ray damaged DNA in progeria, *Biochem. Biophys. Res. Commun.* **77**:714–719.

Rary, J. M., Bender, M. A., and Kelly, T. E., 1975, A 14/14 marker chromosome lymphocyte clone in ataxia telangiectasia, *J. Hered.* **66**:33–35.

Rasio, E., Antaki, A., and Van Campenhout, J., 1976, Diabetes mellitus in gonadal dysgenesis: Studies of insulin and growth hormone secretion, *Eur. J. Clin. Invest.* **6**:59–66.

Rava, G., 1967, Su un nucleo familiare di progeria, *Minerva Med.* **58**:1502–1509.

Regan, J. D., and Setlow, R. B., 1974, DNA repair in human progeroid cells, *Biochem. Biophys. Res. Common.* **59**:858–864.

Reichel, W., and Garcia-Bunuel, R., 1970, Pathologic findings in progeria: Myocardial fibrosis and lipofuscin pigment, *Am. J. Clin. Pathol.* **53**:243–253.

Reichel, W., Garcia-Bunuel, R., and Dilallo, J., 1971*a,* Progeria and Werner's syndrome as models for the study of normal human aging, *J. Am. Geriatr. Soc.* **19**:369–375.

Reichel, W., Bailey, J. A., Zigel, S., Garcia-Bunuel, R., and Knox, G., 1971*b,* Radiological findings in progeria, *J. Am. Geriatr. Soc.* **19**:657–674.

Reiss, U., and Gershon, D., 1976, Rat liver superoxide dismutase: Purification and age-related modifications, *Eur. J. Biochem.* **63**:617–623.

Remsen, J. F., and Cerutti, P. A., 1976, Deficiency of gamma-ray excision repair in skin fibroblasts from Fanconi's anemia, *Proc. Natl. Acad. Sci. U.S.A.* **73**:2419–2423.

Renold, A. E., Stauffacher, W., and Cahill, G. F. Jr., 1972, Diabetes mellitus, in: *The Metabolic Bases of Inherited Disease* (J. B. Stanbury, J. B. Wyngaarden, and D. S. Fredrickson, eds.), pp. 83–118, McGraw-Hill, New York.

Reye, C., and Mosman, N. S. W., 1960, Ataxia–telangiectasia, *Am. J. Dis. Child.* **99:**238–247.

Reynolds, C., O'Duffy, J. D., and Sams, W., 1972, Werner's syndrome: Case report of a variant, *Minn. Med.* **55:**917–921.

Rheinwald, J. G., and Green, H., 1975, Serial cultivation of strains of human epidermal keratinocytes: The formation of keratinizing colonies from single cells, *Cell* **6:**331–337.

Richards, D., 1974, Werner's syndrome, *Proc. R. Soc. Med.* **67:**721–722.

Riggs, W., and Seibert, J., 1972, Cockayne's syndrome: Roentgen findings, *Am. J. Roentgenol. Radium Ther. Nucl. Med.* **116:**623–633.

Rosen, R. S., Cimini, R., and Coblentz, D., 1970, Werner's syndrome, *Br. J. Radiol.* **43:**193–198.

Rosenbloom, A. L., and Debusk, F. L., 1971, Progeria of Hutchinson–Gilford: A caricature of aging, *Am. Heart J.* **83:**287–289.

Rosenbloom, A. L., Karacan, I. J., and DeBusk, F. L., 1970, Sleep characteristics and endocrine response in progeria, *J. Pediatr.* **77:**692–695.

Rosenbloom, A. L., Wheeler, L., Bianchi, R., Chin, F. T., Tiwary, C. M., and Grgic, A., 1975, Age-adjusted analysis of insulin responses during normal and abnormal glucose tolerance tests in children and adolescents, *Diabetes* **24:**820–828.

Rosenbloom, A. L., Goldstein, S., and Yip, C. C., 1976, Insulin binding to cultured human fibroblasts increases with normal and precocious aging, *Science* **193:**412–415.

Rothmund, A., 1868, Über Kataracten in Verbindung mit einer eigenthümlichen Haut Degeneration, *Graefe. Arch. Ophthalmol.* **14:**159–182.

Rothstein, M., 1977, Recent developments in the age-related alteration of enzymes: A review, *Mech. Ageing Dev.* **6:**241–257.

Rowe, J. W., Andres, R., Tobin, J. D., Norris, A. H., and Shock, N. W., 1976, The effect of age on creatinine clearance in man: A cross-sectional and longitudinal study, *J. Gerontol.* **31:**155–163.

Rowlatt, U., 1969, Cockayne's syndrome: Report of case with necropsy findings, *Acta Neuropathol.* **14:**52–61.

Roy, S., Srivastava, R. N., Gupta, P. C., and Mayekar, G., 1973, Ultrastructure of peripheral nerve in Cockayne's syndrome, *Acta Neuropathol.* **24:**345–349.

Roychoudhury, D. S., and Banerjee, A. K., 1968, Heredofamilial study of Weber–Cockayne disease, *Bull. Calcutta Sch. Trop. Med.* **16:**12–13.

Rubin, P., and Casarett, G. W., 1968, *Clinical Radiation Pathology,* pp. 881–893, W. B. Saunders Co., Philadelphia.

Ruddle, F. H., and Creagan, R. P., 1975, Parasexual approaches to the genetics of man, *Annu. Rev. Genet.* **9:**407–486.

Ryan, J. M., and Cristofalo, V. J., 1975, Chromatin template activity during aging *in vitro,* *Exp. Cell Res.* **90:**456–458.

Saunders, J. W., and Fallon, J. F., 1966, Cell death in morphogenesis, in: *Major Problems in Developmental Biology* (M. Locke, ed.), pp. 289–314, Academic Press, New York.

Schalch, D. S., McFarlin, D., and Barlow, M. H., 1970, An unusual form of diabetes mellitus in ataxia telangiectasia, *N. Engl. J. Med.* **282:**1396–1402.

Schmickel, R. D., Chu, E. H. Y., and Trosko, J., 1975, The definition of a cellular defect in two patients with Cockayne syndrome, *Pediatr. Res.* **9:**317 (abstract).

Schneider, E. L., and Chase, G. A., 1976, Relationship between age of donor and *in vitro* life span of human diploid fibroblasts, *Interdiscip. Top. Gerontol.* **10:**62–69.

Schneider, E. L., and Epstein, C. J., 1972, Replication rate and lifespan of cultured fibroblasts in Down's syndrome, *Proc. Soc. Exp. Biol. Med.* **141:**1092–1096.

Schneider, E. L., and Mitsui, Y., 1976, The relationship between *in vitro* cellular aging and *in vivo* human age, *Proc. Natl. Acad. Sci. U.S.A.* **73:**3584–3588.

Schneider, E. L., and Shorr, S. S., 1975, Alteration in cellular RNA's during the *in vitro* lifespan of cultured human diploid fibroblasts, *Cell* **6:**179–184.

Schumacher, K., Rodermund, O. E., and Doepfmer, R., 1969, Werner's syndrome: Contribution to symptomatology and etiology, *Arch. Klin. Med.* **216:**116–147.

Segal, D. J., and McCoy, E. E., 1974, Studies on Down's syndrome in tissue culture. I. Growth rates and protein contents of fibroblast cultures, *J. Cell. Physiol.* **83:**85–90.

Sexton, G. B., 1954, Thomson's syndrome (poikiloderma congenitale), *Can. Med. Assoc. J.* **70:**662–665.

Shuster, J., Hart, Z., Stimson, C. W., Brough, A. J., and Poulik, M. D., 1966, Ataxia–telangiectasia with cerebellar tumor, *Pediatrics* **37:**776–786.

Siemens, H. W., 1963, The lens, in: *Genetics and Ophthalmology* (P. J. Waardenburg, A. Franceschetti, and D. Klein, eds.), p. 896, Charles C. Thomas, Springfield, Illinois.

Silver, H. K., 1966, Rothmund–Thomson syndrome: An oculocutaneous disorder, *Am. J. Dis. Child.* **111:**182—190.

Simig, I., and Fizelov, A. E., 1976, Werner's syndrome, *Cesk. Oftalmol.* **32:**45–49.

Singal, D. P., and Blajchman, M. A., 1973, Histocompatibility (*HL-A*) antigens, lymphocytotoxic antibodies and tissue antibodies in patients with diabetes mellitus, *Diabetes* **22:**429–432.

Singal, D. P., and Goldstein, S., 1973, Absence of detectable *HL-A* antigens on cultured fibroblasts in progeria, *J. Clin. Invest.* **52:**2259–2263.

Smith, D. W., 1976, Ataxia–telangiectasia syndrome in: *Recognizable Patterns of Human Malformation*, pp. 102–103, W. B. Saunders Co., Philadelphia.

Smith, G. F., and Berg, J. M., 1976, *Down's Anomaly*, pp. 239–246, Churchill Livingstone, Edinburgh.

Sourander, P., Bonnevier, J. O., and Olsson, Y., 1966, A case of ataxia telangiectasia with lesions in the spinal cord, *Acta Neurol. Scand.* **42:**354–366.

Spark, H., 1965, Cachetic dwarfism resembling the Cockayne–Neill type, *J. Pediatr.* **66:**41–47.

Spence, A. M., and Herman, M. M., 1973, Critical re-examination of the premature aging concept in progeria: A light and electron microscopic study, *Mech. Ageing Dev.* **2:**211–227.

Sri-Skanda-Rajah-Sivayoham, I., and Ratnaike, V. T., 1975, Rothmund–Thomson syndrome in an Oriental patient, *Ann. Ophthalmol.* **7:** 417–420.

Srivastava, R. N., Gupta, P. C., Mayekar, G., and Roy, S., 1974, Cockayne's syndrome in two sisters, *Acta Paediatr. Scand.* **63:**461–464.

Stearns, E. L., MacDonnell, J. A., Kaufman, B. J., Padua, R., Lucman, T. S., Winter, J. S. D., and Faiman, C., 1974, Declining testicular function with age, *Am. J. Med.* **57:**761–766.

Steele, R. W., and Bass, J. W., 1970, Hallermann–Streiff syndrome: Clinical and prognostic considerations, *Am. J. Dis. Child.* **120:**462–465.

Stein, G. S., and Stein, J. L., 1976, *In vitro* studies of transcription as a function of age in mammalian cells, *Interdiscip. Top. Gerontol.* **10:**83–99.

Strober, W., Wochner, R. D., Barlow, M. H., McFarlin, D. E., and Waldmann, T. A., 1968, Immunoglobulin metabolism in ataxia telangiectasia, *J. Clin. Invest.* **47:**1905–1915.

Tadjoedin, M. K., and Fraser, F. C., 1965, Heredity of ataxia telangiectasia (Louis-Bar syndrome), *Am. J. Dis. Child.* **110:**64–68.

Talbot, N. B., Butler, A. M., Pratt, E. L., MacLachlan, E. A., and Tannheimer, J., 1945, Progeria: Clinical, metabolic and pathologic studies on a patient, *Am. J. Dis. Child.* **69:**267–279.

Tanenbaum, M. H., 1965, Werner's syndrome: Progeria of the adult, *Arch. Intern. Med.* **116**:499–504.

Tao, L. C., Stecker, E., and Gardner, H. A., 1971, Werner's syndrome and acute myeloid leukemia, *Can. Med. Assoc. J.* **105**:951–953.

Tattersall, R. B., and Fajans, S. S., 1975, A difference between the inheritance of classical juvenile-onset and maturity-onset type of diabetes of young people, *Diabetes* **24**:44–53.

Taylor, A. M. R., Harnden, D. G., Arlett, C. F., Harcourt, S. A., Lehmann, A. R., Stevens, S., and Bridges, B. A., 1975, Ataxia telangiectasia: A human mutation with abnormal radiation sensitivity, *Nature (London)* **258**:427–429.

Taylor, W. B., 1957, Rothmund's syndrome—Thomson's syndrome, *Arch. Dermatol.* **75**:236–244.

Taymor, M. L., Toshihiro, A., and Pheteplace, C., 1968, Serum levels of FSH and LH by radioimmunoassay, in: *Gonadotropins 1968, Proceedings of the Workshop Conference—Vista Hermosa, More., Mexico* (Rosemberg, ed.), pp. 349–365, Geron-X, California.

Thannhauser, S. J., 1945, Werner's syndrome (progeria of the adult) and Rothmund's syndrome: Two types of closely related heredofamilial atrophic dermatosis with juvenile cataracts and endocrine features: A critical study with five new cases, *Ann. Intern. Med.* **23**:559.

Thomsen, M., Platz, P., Ortved Andersen, O., Christy, M., Lyngsoe, J., Nerup, J., Rasmussen, K., Ryder, L. P., Staub Nelsen, L., and Svejgaard, A., 1975, MLC typing in juvenile diabetes mellitus and idiopathic Addison's disease, *Transplant. Rev.* **22**:125–147.

Thomson, M. S., 1936, Poikiloderma congenitale, *Br. J. Dermatol.* **48**:221–234.

Tibbetts, P. G., Rose, H. D., and Kersting, D. W., 1968, Werner's syndrome, *Wis. Med. J.* **67**:550–557.

Tokunaga, M., Futami, T., Wakamatsu, E., Endo, M., and Yosizawa, Z., 1975, Werner's syndrome as "hyaluronuria," *Clin. Chim. Acta* **62**:89–96.

Turner, H. H., 1938, A syndrome of infantilism, congenital webbed neck and cubitus valgus, *Endocrinology* **23**:566–574.

Ufermann, K., Heege-Dohr, R., and Kosenow, W., 1973, Ocular manifestation in Cockayne's syndrome, *Klin. Monatsbl. Augenheilkd.* **162**:655–658.

Ungar, B., Stocks, A. E., Martin, F. I. R., Whittingham, S., and Mackay, I. R., 1968, Intrinsic factor antibody, parietal-cell antibody, and latent pernicious anemia in diabetes mellitus, *Lancet* **2**:415–418.

Unger, R. H., 1976, Diabetes and the alpha cell, *Diabetes* **25**:136–151.

Valdiserri, L., and Stricchiola, G., 1974, Hutchinson–Gilford progeria in a 14-year-old adolescent, *Chir. Organi Mov.* **61**:291–300.

Van Campenhout, J., Antaki, A., and Rasio, E., 1973, Diabetes mellitus and thyroid autoimmunity in gonadal dysgenesis, *Fertil. Steril.* **24**:1–9.

Vandaele, R., 1973, Werner's syndrome: Familial ulcerous scleroderma with cataract and diabetes, *Arch. Belg. Dermatol. Syphiligr.* **29**:251–254.

Viegas, J., Souza, P. L., and Salzano, F. M., 1974, Progeria in twins, *J. Med. Genet.* **11**:384–386.

Villee, D. B., Nichols, G., Jr., and Talbot, N. B., 1969, Metabolic studies in two boys with classical progeria, *Pediatrics* **43**:207–216.

Vincent, R. A., Sheridan, R. B., and Huang, P. C., 1975, DNA strand breakage repair in ataxia telangiectasia fibroblast-like cells, *Mutat. Res.* **33**:357–366.

Vracko, R., and Benditt, E. P., 1974, Manifestations of diabetes mellitus: Their possible relationships to an underlying cell defect, *Am. J. Pathol.* **75**:204–223.

Vracko, R., and Benditt, E. P., 1975, Restricted replicative life-span of diabetic fibroblasts *in vitro:* Its relation to microangiopathy, *Fed. Proc. Fed. Am. Soc. Exp. Biol.* **34:**68–70.

Wahl, J. W., and Ellis, P. P., 1965, Rothmund–Thomson syndrome, *Am. J. Ophthalmol.* **60:**722–726.

Walburg, H. E., 1975, Radiation-induced life shortening and premature aging, *Adv. Radiat. Biol.* **5:**145–179.

Waldmann, T. A., and McIntire, K. R., 1972, Serum-alpha-fetoprotein levels in patients with ataxia–telangiectasia, *Lancet* **2:**1112–1115.

Wells, R. S., 1972, Werner's syndrome: Acrogeria, *Proc. R. Soc. Med.* **65:**525–526.

Welsh, O., 1975, Study of a family with a new progeroid syndrome, *Birth Defects: Orig. Artic. Ser.* **11:**25–38.

Werder, E. A., Murset, G., Illig, R., and Prader, A., 1975, Hypogonadism and parathyroid adenoma in congenital poikiloderma (Rothmund–Thomson syndrome), *Clin. Endocrinol.* (Oxford) **4:**75–82.

Werner, O., 1904, *Über Katarakt in Verbindung mit Sklerodermie* (doctoral dissertation, Kiel University), Schmidt and Klaunig, Kiel, Germany.

Wertelecki, W., Fraumeni, J. F., and Mulvihill, J. J., 1970, Non-gonadal neoplasia in Turner's syndrome, *Cancer* **26:**485–488.

Wicks, A. C., and Wall, D. W., 1974, Werner's syndrome: A case report in a Rhodesian African, *Cent. Afr. J. Med.* **20:**251–254.

Wiedemann, H. R., 1969, Some progeroid cases and their diagnostic classification, *Z. Kinderheilkd.* **107:**91–106.

Yasuhara, M., Kiyokane, K., Sakai, T., Oiwa, T., and Hashi, N., 1974, A case of Werner's syndrome, *Jpn. J. Hum. Genet.* **19:**86–87.

Zacharski, L. R., and McIntyre, O. R., 1973, Tissue factor (thromboplastin, Factor III) synthesis by cultured cells, *J. Med.* **4:**118–131.

Zackai, A. H., Weber, D., and Noth, R., 1974, Cardiac findings in Werner's syndrome, *Geriatrics* **29:**141–148.

Zamith, V. A., Campos, J. V., and Chizzotti, M. T., 1974, Rothmund's syndrome: Serum and urine aminogram—Study of a family, *Rev. Bras. Pesqui. Med. Biol.* **7:**23–27.

Zeldis, S. M., Nemerson, Y., Pitlick, F. A., and Lentz, T. L., 1972, Tissue factor (thromboplastin): Localization to plasma membranes by peroxidase-conjugated antibodies, *Science* **175:**766–768.

Zonana, J., and Rimoin, D. L., 1976, Current concepts in genetics: Inheritance of diabetes mellitus, *N. Engl. J. Med.* **295:**603–605.

Zucker-Franklin, D., Rifkin, H., and Jacobson, H. G., 1968, Werner's syndrome: An analysis of ten cases, *Geriatrics* **23:**123–135.

Chapter 8

Parental-Age Effects: Increased Frequencies of Genetically Abnormal Offspring

David Kram and Edward L. Schneider

1. Introduction

In the previous chapters, the authors have discussed at length the effect of genotype on aging. In this chapter, we will focus on the effect of aging on human genotype—the increased risk faced by the older parent of having a child with a genetic disorder. This increased risk of genetically abnormal offspring with parental aging represents a sizable socioeconomical as well as clinical problem. The magnitude of this problem is reflected in the cost of one parental-age-related disorder, the Down syndrome. If the number of annual Down syndrome births (approximately 8000) is multiplied by the average life expectancy of a newborn with the Down syndrome (30 years) and by the average cost of specialized care for these persons ($5000 per year is a modest estimate), the staggering annual cost of 1.2 billion dollars is obtained (Swanson, 1970). In addition to the economic burden, one must consider the emotional and psychological problems that occur in a family with a Down syndrome child. The high frequency of parental-age-related disorders is also seen in institutions for the mentally retarded, where Down syndrome patients may comprise as much as one third of the entire patient population.

David Kram and Edward L. Schneider • Laboratory of Cellular and Comparative Physiology, Gerontology Research Center, National Institute on Aging, National Institutes of Health, Public Health Service, U.S. Department of Health, Education and Welfare, Baltimore, Maryland 21224

The frequency of the chromosomal disorders associated with advanced parental age is approximately 1 in 200 live births, and these disorders rank among the most common genetic diseases. This figure is conservative, however, in terms of genetically abnormal conceptions related to advanced parental age. With reproductive aging, the frequency of spontaneous abortions rises to as high as 4% (Mariona, 1975). In an extensive study of spontaneous abortuses, Boué and Boué (1973) demonstrated that approximately 60% of these aborted fetuses possessed abnormal chromosome complements. Most of these abnormal chromosomal complements appear to be related to parental age. Thus, if these percentages are multiplied, as many as 24% of the fetuses in pregnant older women may be chromosomally abnormal.

Despite this high frequency of genetic disorders associated with advanced parental age, little is known about the mechanisms responsible for the production of genetically abnormal offspring. In this chapter, we will discuss a number of the clinical disorders associated with advanced parental age. The bulk of the chapter, however, will focus on the etiological considerations for these important parental-age-related events. Emphasis will also be placed on the positive steps that can be taken to reduce the risk faced by the older parent of having a genetically abnormal offspring.

2. Maternal- vs. Paternal-Age Effects

It is important to distinguish maternal- from paternal-age-related disorders, since they appear to have diverse etiologies. All the maternal-age-related genetic disorders involve possession of an extra chromosome. In contrast, most conditions associated with advanced paternal age appear to be inherited in an autosomal dominant manner, which would indicate a single gene abnormality or single gene mutation.

For many years, disorders such as the Down syndrome were thought to be due to advanced parental age. It was not until 1933 that Penrose (1933) demonstrated, on a statistical basis, that maternal age was the dominant factor, and that paternal age was elevated only secondarily, since older mothers tend to have older spouses. Many subsequent analyses of parental age related to Down syndrome births have confirmed this observation (Cohen, B. L., and Lilienfeld, 1970). One representative technique utilized to discriminate between maternal- and paternal-age effects is presented in Tables I and II. When the ages of mothers of Down syndrome newborns were matched with those of mothers of normal offspring, no significant difference was observed in paternal age, except perhaps in one age cohort (Table I). The overall age differences, however, were not significant. If paternal age is controlled and maternal age analyzed (Table II), a statistically significant elevation in maternal age is clearly seen.

Table I. Matched-Pair Analysis of Paternal Age with Maternal Age
Controlled (Paired t Test)[a]

Maternal-age group	Number of fathers	Mean differences[b]	t	P
15–19	6	0	0	NS
20–24	34	0	0	NS
25–29	30	− 0.07	0.07	NS
30–34	46	− 3.07	3.79	< 0.001
35–39	62	+ 0.45	0.66	NS
40+	37	+ 1.1	1.05	NS
All cases	215	− 0.34	0.79	NS

[a]From B. L. Cohen and Lilienfeld (1970, p. 325, Table 6).
[b]Down paternal age minus control paternal age.

Developments in the field of human cytogenetics have led to further insight into the effects of maternal vs. paternal aging on genetic disorders such as the Down syndrome (see Chapter 2). Shortly after Tijo and Levan (1956) reported that the human chromosome complement contained 46 chromosomes, Lejeune *et al.* (1959) reported that cells from children with the Down syndrome had 47 chromosomes and possessed an extra small acrocentric chromosome, number 21 (Fig. 1). Early cytogenetic analyses were crude, and specific chromosomes were difficult to identify. The advent of new chromosome-staining techniques, however, which produced the karyotype seen in Fig. 1, now permits identification of all the individual human chromosomes based on their characteristic banding patterns. These new techniques also revealed that several human chromosomes possess polymorphic regions that are inherited in a Mendelian manner (Schedl, 1971). Since mutations and crossing over in these polymorphic regions are rare (Craig-Holmes *et al.*, 1975), they can be utilized to determine which of

Table II. Matched-Pair Analysis of Maternal Age with Paternal Age
Controlled (Paired t Test)[a]

Paternal-age group	Number of mothers	Mean differences[b]	t	P
20–24	22	− 0.09	0.14	NS
25–29	40	+ 0.73	1.03	NS
30–34	41	+ 3.4	3.09	< 0.01
35–39	53	+ 2.3	6.28	< 0.001
40–44	39	+ 4.9	6.20	< 0.001
45+	20	+ 0.8	0.53	NS
All cases	215	2.3	6.05	< 0.001

[a]From B. L. Cohen and Lilienfeld (1970, p. 325, Table 5).
[b]Down maternal age minus control maternal age.

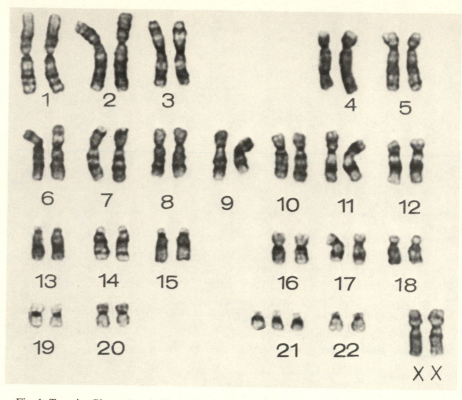

Fig. 1. Trypsin–Giemsa banded karyotype of a metaphase cell from a female patient with the Down syndrome. Note that this child has three number 21 chromosomes in place of the normal pair. Courtesy of Helen Lawce, University of California Medical Center, San Francisco, California.

the two homologous chromosomes of an offspring was derived from the mother or the father. This determination can be accomplished, however, only when distinctive polymorphic banding is present.

To illustrate how these banding techniques are able to determine the parental origin of the extra 21 chromosome in a Down syndrome child, we have prepared several schematized examples (Figs. 2–4). In Fig. 2, the mother's karyotype has two polymorphic 21 chromosomes, one possessing a prominent distal band on the long chromosome arm and the other having a prominent satellited band on the short arm. After segregation of daughter chromatids at the first and second meiotic divisions and fertilization by a sperm containing a paternal 21 chromosome (along with the remaining 22 chromosomes in the gamete), a normal offspring will be produced possessing one or the other of these distinctive maternal 21 chromosomes.

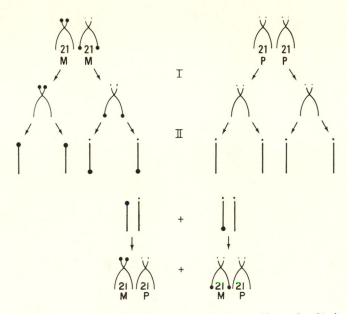

Fig. 2. Schema illustrating segregation of two maternal polymorphic number 21 chromosomes during normal meiotic division.

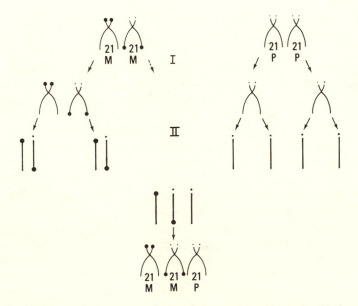

Fig. 3. Schema illustrating segregation of two maternal polymorphic number 21 chromosomes with nondisjunction occurring during the first maternal meiotic division.

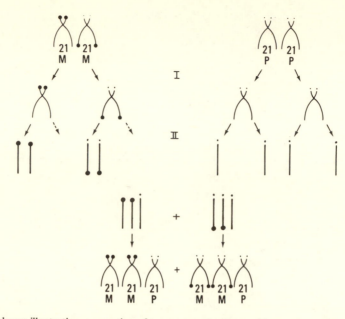

Fig. 4. Schema illustrating segregation of two maternal polymorphic number 21 chromosomes with nondisjunction occurring at the second maternal meiotic division.

Nondisjunction for chromosome 21 at the first or second maternal meiotic division results in the formation of a Down syndrome zygote. In Fig. 3, nondisjunction at the first maternal meiotic division is illustrated. In this case, all four chromatids derived from the 21st chromosomal pair segregate to one daughter cell. A second maternal meiotic division then results in the formation of an oocyte that possesses each of the two distinguishable maternal chromosomes. When this oocyte is fertilized with a normal gamete, the resultant Down syndrome zygote has three 21 chromosomes, including each of the two maternally identifiable 21 chromosomes.

Nondisjunction at the second maternal meiotic division is illustrated in Fig. 4. After a normal first meiotic division, both identical chromatids segregate to the daughter oocytes at the second meiotic division. Fertilization of these oocytes by a normal sperm containing one chromatid 21 results in a Down syndrome zygote that possesses two identical maternal chromosomes.

In addition to demonstrating how maternal (or paternal) nondisjunction can result in the creation of a chromosomally abnormal offspring, these figures illustrate how insight into the mechanisms of chromosomal nondisjunction can be acquired. Since the first meiotic division is completed just prior to ovulation, nondisjunction during the first maternal meiotic division would implicate mechanisms operating at the ovarian level. Alternatively, nondisjunction at the second maternal meiotic division would point toward pathology occurring between ovulation and fertilization, since the second meiotic division is completed after the latter process.

In Table III, we have summarized the evidence accumulated to date from Down syndrome children whose chromosomes could be assigned to either a maternal or a paternal origin. To obtain a representative survey, we have not included individual case reports. Of the 243 Down syndrome children examined, 54 had chromosomal polymorphisms that permitted assignment. Of these 54 cases, the majority (36) possess two maternal chromosomes. Surprisingly, 33% of the cases indicate a paternal origin for the additional 21 chromosome. Analysis of the maternal and paternal ages in some of these cases was most interesting (Wagenbichler *et al.,* 1976). When the additional chromosome was maternally derived, maternal age was significantly elevated above control population levels. In those cases in which the additional chromosome was derived from the father, however, paternal age was not significantly increased. These studies would indicate that the majority of Down syndrome births that result from chromosomal nondisjunction are related to maternal aging. A considerable number of these births, however, are probably of paternal origin and are independent of age effects. In the majority (19/36) of the cases of maternal origin of the additional chromosome, nondisjunction occurred during the first meiotic division. There is a considerable bias, however, in analyzing the frequency of first vs. second meiotic division errors. If the parent has only one identifiable polymorphic chromosome 21, nondisjunction at the second meiotic division could be detected, while first-meiotic-division nondisjunction would be missed. In an extensive mathematical analysis of these data, Langenbeck *et al.* (1976) concluded that maternal first-meiotic-division nondisjunction events were probably 5–10 times more frequent than second-meiotic-division nondisjunction occurrences. This evidence acquired from chromosomal studies would therefore point toward an ovarian etiology for maternal-age-related aneuploidy. The cases of second-maternal-meiotic nondisjunction indicate, however, that multiple etiological mechanisms may be operative. Further studies on larger populations will be required to confirm these findings.

Although the vast majority of Down syndrome and other maternal-age-related chromosomal disorders appear to involve possession of an additional chromosome, a small percentage of these patients (approximately 5% in the Down syndrome) have 46 chromosomes, with an additional 21 chromosome translocated onto another chromosome. These translocations usually involve the other acrocentric chromosomes (13, 14, 15, 21, and 22). Clinically, these patients are identical to those possessing 47 chromosomes.

Table III. Determination of Maternal vs. Paternal Origin of the Extra Chromosome 21 in the Down Syndrome

Reference	Total cases examined	Informative cases	Maternal nondisjunction[a]			Paternal nondisjunction[a]		
			1st MD	2nd MD	Undet.	1st MD	2nd MD	Undet.
Lieznerski and Lindsten (1972)	6	1	1	0	0	0	0	0
G. F. Smith and Sachdeva (1973)	20	0	0	0	0	0	0	0
J. A. Robinson (1973)	12	4	4	0	0	0	0	0
Bott et al. (1975)	59	7	0	3	0	0	4	0
Giraud et al. (1975)	32	2	1	1	0	0	0	0
Hara and Sasaki (1975)	36	6	1	2	2	0	1	0
Mikkelsen et al. (1976)	40	16	5	4	2	2	2	1
Wagenbichler et al. (1976)	38	18	7	2	1	4	3	1
TOTALS:	243	54	19	12	5	6	10	2

[a](MD) Meiotic division.

That the translocation results in extra chromosomal dose for only the long arms of the involved chromosome (in contrast to complete trisomy) would suggest that the short arms of these chromosomes do not contribute to the clinical manifestation of these disorders.

Finally, some patients with the Down syndrome (approximately 1%) and many with the sex chromosome trisomies (XXX and XXY) are chromosomal mosaics and possess two or more distinct chromosome complements. These patients can display a wide variety of clinical manifestations, depending on the proportion of normal to abnormal chromosome complements.

Neither maternal nor paternal ages appear to be elevated in the Down syndrome births related to translocations and mosaicism. That they do not is not surprising, since neither translocations nor mosaicism results from meiotic-division abnormalities.

3. Maternal-Age-Related Disorders

The most frequent maternal-age-related disorder is the Down syndrome. This condition was first described by Dr. Langdon Down (1866). Because of the distinctive facial features of these children, he called this disorder "Mongolian idiocy." Unfortunately, the term "mongolism" has persisted and has been extensively used. Since this disease has been observed in all racial groups (Lilienfeld, 1969), however, the *Down syndrome* is a more appropriate name for this entity.

The clinical diagnosis in most cases of the Down syndrome is relatively simple. These infants are brachycephalic (i.e., they have skulls that are shortened on the anterior–posterior axis) and have epicanthic folds, flattened nasal bridges, small chins, low-set ears, and outward slanting eyes (Fig. 5). Examination of the hands of these children reveals characteristic anomalies and dermatoglyphic patterns that further facilitate diagnosis. Marked physical, as well as mental, retardation is also observed. Few of these children attain 5 feet in height, and only rare cases have been reported with normal intelligence. Many do not survive infancy due to severe congenital malformations of the cardiovascular systems (Rowe and Uchida, 1961).

Down syndrome patients also have many features that resemble accelerated aging, including an increased frequency of neoplasms (Miller, 1970), altered immune competence (Hsia *et al.*, 1971), and an early onset of senile dementia (Burger and Vogel, 1973). In fact, postmortem examination of brain tissue from Down syndrome patients in their 30's reveals findings very similar to those usually seen in persons in their seventh and eighth decades (Burger and Vogel, 1973). This aspect of the Down syndrome is discussed in detail in Chapter 7.

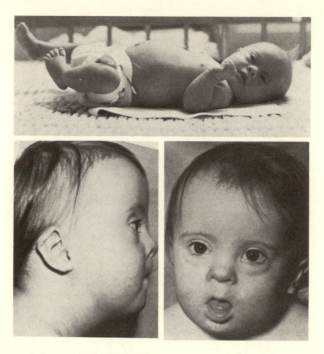

Fig. 5. Two young infants with the Down syndrome. These photographs illustrate some of the common features of this syndrome, including flattening of the nasal bridge, low-set ears, small chin, upslanting of the eye fissures, and a tendency toward tongue protrusion. Top photograph reproduced from D. W. Smith and Wilson (1973); bottom photographs reproduced from D. W. Smith (1970).

The risk of having a Down syndrome offspring increases with maternal age from 1 in 2300 at age 20 to 1 in 45 after age 45 (Table IV). Other studies have produced figures as high as 1 in 20 after age 45 (Zellweger and Simpson, 1973). It is this high risk that makes prenatal diagnosis advisable for the older pregnant woman.

There are two other common autosomal trisomies: the Edwards syndrome (Edwards, J. H., *et al.*, 1960), which involves chromosome 18, and the Patau syndrome (Patau *et al.*, 1960), which involves chromosome 13. Both these syndromes involve severe mental and physical retardation, and these infants rarely survive the first year of life. As with the Down syndrome, both these conditions show a dramatically increased frequency with maternal aging (Magenis *et al.*, 1968).

Two sex-chromosome conditions are associated with advanced maternal age: the Klinefelter syndrome, XXY, and the Triplo-X syndrome, XXX (Zuppinger *et al.*, 1967). In contrast to the autosomal trisomies, the sex-chromosome trisomies have relatively few clinical findings. The Klinefelter

Table IV. Risk of Down
Syndrome Births as a
Function of Maternal Age[a]

Maternal-age range	Risk
< 20	1/2300
20–24	1/1600
25–29	1/1200
30–34	1/870
35–39	1/290
40–44	1/100
> 45	1/45

[a]From Collman and Stoller (1962).

syndrome is usually diagnosed at puberty, when the affected males do not develop the normal secondary sexual characteristics (Klinefelter *et al.,* 1942). In addition, they appear eunuchoid in body build and have mild mental retardation. The majority of Triplo-X females are asymptomatic, and the diagnosis is usually fortuitous. The mildness of these sex-chromosome trisomies is probably related to the inactivation of the additional X chromosome during early fetal development—the Lyon hypothesis (Lyon, 1961).

The only common chromosome monosomy, the Turner syndrome (XO), does not appear to be related to increased maternal age (Boyer *et al.,* 1961). Studies of the origin of the X chromosome in these patients indicate that in the majority of these cases, the chromosome is of maternal origin (Race and Sanger, 1969). This finding is consistent with paternal nondisjunction, and could explain the lack of a maternal-age effect.

4. Paternal-Age-Related Disorders

Penrose, the British geneticist who played an important role in delineating the maternal-age effect in the Down syndrome, was also the first to propose that advanced paternal age could be related to an increased frequency of the human genetic disorder achondroplasia (Penrose, 1955).

Until recently, only a handful of human genetic diseases had been reported to be related to increased paternal age (Table V). These disorders included achondroplasia and three other autosomal dominant disorders, the Apert syndrome, the Marfan syndrome, and fibrodysplasia ossificans progressiva. There was some controversy over three other disorders: bilateral retinoblastoma (Tunte, 1972), hemophilia (Herrmann, 1962), and Duch-

Table V.   Syndromes Associated with Advanced Paternal Age

Syndrome	Paternal-age association described by:
Apert syndrome	Blank (1960), Erickson and Cohen (1974)
Marfan syndrome	Lynas (1958), Murdoch *et al.* (1972), C. A. B. Smith (1972)
Achondroplasia	Penrose (1955), Murdoch *et al.* (1970)
Fibrodysplasia ossificans progessiva	Tunte *et al.* (1967)
Basal cell nevus syndrome	Jones *et al.* (1975)
Waardenburg syndrome	Jones *et al.* (1975)
Crouzon syndrome	Jones *et al.* (1975)
Oculo-dental-digital syndrome	Jones *et al.* (1975)
Treacher–Collins syndrome	Jones *et al.* (1975)
Progeria	Jones *et al.* (1975)
Acrodystosis	Jones *et al.* (1975)
Bilateral retinoblastoma	Tunte (1972)

ene's muscular dystrophy (Hutton and Thompson, 1970). In the last two disorders, which are inherited as X-linked recessive traits, grandpaternal age was examined, since the mutation first occurs in the mother of the affected male. These observations in hemophilia and Duchene's muscular dystrophy have been challenged, however, by more recent reports (Barrai *et al.,* 1968; Pellie *et al.,* 1973). Recently, Jones *et al.* (1975) looked at a variety of genetic disorders with autosomal dominant, X-linked, and undetermined inheritance. In the first group, the majority of the conditions examined revealed increased paternal age (Table V). There were also two conditions in the latter group that revealed significantly elevated paternal age: progeria and acrodysostosis. This study would suggest that advanced paternal age may be involved in many autosomal-dominant-inherited disorders. It will certainly be of interest to see whether future studies confirm these observations.

In contrast to maternal-age-related disorders, these paternal-age-related conditions have received relatively little attention because of their low frequencies. Achondroplasia, a form of dwarfism, is the most common of these disorders, with an incidence of 1 in 50,000 live births, and is approximately 100 times less frequent than the Down syndrome.

As in the maternal-age effect, there has been considerable speculation as to the cause of paternal-age-related disorders. Some of the proposed etiological considerations include accumulated exposure to mutagenic chemical agents, increased susceptibility of aged spermatogonia to mutation, and normal aging of spermatogonia leading to errors in DNA replication or in the repair of DNA damage or in both.

Unfortunately, there are few experimental models available for studying the paternal-age effect. Several difficulties make the pursuit of this problem impractical. First, the low frequency of these disorders, even at late paternal ages, indicates that large numbers of experimental animals would be needed. Second, these disorders feature different clinical presentations and lack a unifying feature such as chromosomal abnormality that permits investigation of the maternal-age-related disorders.

Since these disorders are not amenable to prevention by prenatal diagnosis, it is vital that research be initiated at delineating the mechanisms for the paternal-age effect, and that an effort be made to identify those fathers at risk for genetically abnormal offspring.

5. Proposed Etiological Agents

In this section, we will critically examine some of the proposed etiological agents for the maternal-age-related increase in chromosomal disorders.

5.1. Radiation

Several epidemiological and experimental studies have focused on the relationship between radiation and chromosomally abnormal offspring. Natural exposure to environmental radiation has been estimated to be approximately 5 rads during the 30-year female reproductive life span (Glass and Ritterhoff, 1961). The advent of diagnostic as well as therapeutic X-irradiation has increased the radiation exposure of women during the childbearing years. Older mothers, therefore, would have more cumulative exposure to these radiation sources. In addition, the older mother is more likely to have medical conditions such as cholecystitis (gallbladder infections) that require extensive abdominal radiation exposure.

5.1.1. Epidemiological Studies

While maternal exposure to X-irradiation appears to play a significant role in the production of Down syndrome offspring, retrospective studies indicate that paternal exposure does not appear to be a contributing factor (Cohen, B. L., and Lilienfeld, 1970; Searle and Beechey, 1974; Uchida and Curtis, 1961). The results of one extensive study are presented in Table VI. Note that mothers of Down syndrome patients received seven times more exposure than control mothers to a combination of diagnostic, fluoroscopic, and therapeutic radiation. There have also been retrospective studies, however, that did not find that there was a significantly greater amount of radiation exposure among mothers of Down syndrome patients (Carter *et al.*, 1961; Lunn, 1959; Marmol *et al.*, 1969).

Table VI.   Summary of Maternal Radiation Exposure Prior to Birth of
Index Child[a]

Radiation exposure	Mothers of:	
	Mongols (%)	Controls (%)
No radiation	50.0	59.9
Radiation		
Diagnostic only	24.0	27.1
Fluoroscopic only	4.8	3.4
Therapeutic only	3.3	1.4
Diagnostic and fluoroscopic	6.7	3.9
Diagnostic and therapeutic	3.4	2.9
Fluoroscopic and therapeutic	1.0	0.5
Diagnostic, fluoroscopic, and therapeutic	6.3	0.9
Unknown	3.7	4.2

[a]From B. L. Cohen and Lilienfeld (1970, p. 322, Table 1).

A retrospective study by Alberman and his co-workers demonstrated
that the time interval between radiation exposure and conception may be a
critical factor in the production of Down syndrome offspring. When the
average radiation dosage to gonadal tissues of 465 mothers of Down
syndrome patients was compared with that of controls, a significant
increase in exposure to radiation was found in the group that had received
X rays 10 or more years prior to conception (Alberman *et al.*, 1972). Age-
related comparisons of gonadal exposure to radiation revealed that older
(30–39 years of age) control mothers had received twice as much exposure
as the younger controls (30 years of age). In contrast to this modest
increase, an eightfold increase was noted between age groups for mothers
of Down syndrome patients. This last report also indicated that the size and
frequency of the radiation doses were less important than the total accumulated exposure.

Although prospective studies are more difficult to design and more
time-consuming, they permit a clearer epidemiological examination of the
effect of irradiation. In one extensive prospective study, Uchida *et al.*
(1968) compared the frequency of Down syndrome births in 861 mothers
who received abdominal X-irradiation prior to pregnancy with an equal
number of age-matched controls who were irradiated during pregnancy.
Eight pregnancies resulted in the birth of Down syndrome offspring in the
former group, while only one case occurred in the latter group.

In contrast to these findings, Stevenson *et al.* (1970) found no significant increase in the frequency of Down syndrome births in more than 1000
mothers given abdominal X-irradiation before pregnancy. These conflicting

observations may reflect differences in the quantity or quality of radiation exposure. Certainly, more studies are needed to define the role of maternal X-irradiation in the production of Down syndrome offspring.

In a recent study, the incidence of Down syndrome and severe mental retardation (SMR) was examined in a region of Kerala, South India, that has high background radiation (1500–3000 mrads yr^{-1}). Frequencies of these disorders were compared with those observed in a similar region in Kerala with normal background radiation (100 mrads yr^{-1}). In young mothers (ages 20–29) who lived in the high-radiation region, the incidence of Down syndrome offspring was 1/862 and this frequency rose to 1/81 for women between 30 and 39 years of age. These values were considerably higher than those obtained in these age groups from population studies. (Table IV). No cases of Down syndrome were found in the control population. The incidence of SMR was also five times higher in the high-radiation region (Kochupillai *et al.*, 1976).

5.1.2. Experimental Studies

Experimental studies with a variety of animal models have demonstrated a dose-dependent relationship between radiation exposure and the production of chromosomally abnormal offspring. When *Drosophila* females were subjected to X-irradiation, a striking increase in the frequency of sex-chromosome nondisjunction was noted with increasing age (Uchida, 1962).

At the mammalian level, maternal X-irradiation exposure can also produce increased frequencies of chromosomally abnormal oocytes. When the time period between oocyte irradiation and subsequent examination was increased from 1 to 3 weeks, a rise in the frequency of multivalents and fragments resulted. This observation suggests that less mature oocytes were more sensitive to X-irradiation. A reduced number of chiasmata was also reported in oocytes of females receiving X rays (Searle and Beechey, 1974). This reduced chiasma frequency has been implicated in the formation of univalents, resulting in the production of trisomic zygotes.

In the male, spontaneous sex chromosome nondisjunction occurs in mouse spermatocytes with a very low frequency (Ohno *et al.* 1959). Exposure of male mice to X-irradiation produced both autosomal and sex-chromosome nondisjunction (Szemere and Chandley, 1975). Early spermatogonia were found to be less sensitive, while spermatocytes in the preleptotene stage showed the highest rates of nondisjunction. When these irradiated males were mated with normal females, however, no aneuploid embryos were detected at day 9 of gestation. This finding suggests strong selection against aneuploid sperm, and perhaps explains the lack of a paternal-age effect in the production of chromosomally abnormal offspring.

5.2. Chemicals

Although many drugs and chemicals are capable of producing profound chromosomal damage, the large number of compounds and their diverse metabolic effects make their study difficult. For more effective examination, compounds have been classified according to their mechanisms of action (i.e., drugs that alkylate, bind, or intercollate into DNA, cross-link, rupture lysosomes, or inhibit DNA repair) (Cohen, M. M., 1970). Although there are exceptions, the groups of compounds that have been found to induce the most cytogenetic damage are the mutagens, teratogens, and carcinogens. Observations have also indicated that either chronic or acute exposure to specific chemicals may lead to the production of abnormal offspring.

Because of the difficulties outlined above, relatively few epidemiological studies have been conducted on the effects of drugs on the production of genetically abnormal offspring. Rapaport (1956) reported a two- to threefold increase in the frequency of Down syndrome births in a community that utilized fluoridated water. Investigators have objected to the methodology used in this study (Dunning, 1965), however, especially the failure to compare maternal ages in test and control communities. Two subsequent studies found similar frequencies of Down syndrome births in communities with and without water fluoridation (Berry, 1958; Needleman *et al.*, 1974).

Experimental studies in laboratory animals have shown that many chemical compounds are capable of affecting germ cells in both sexes. When male rats were treated with methadone prior to mating, increased neonatal mortality was found (Smith, D. J., and Joffe, 1975). Mercury compounds have been found to disrupt meiosis in mouse ova cultures *in vitro* (Jagiello and Lin, 1973). The drugs 2,3,5-triethyleneimonobenzoquinone-1,4,-cyclophosphamide and methotrexate, when administered to mice shortly before ovulation, produced chromosomal aberrations and aneuploidy in metaphase II oocytes. The fertilization of such oocytes could lead to monosomic and trisomic fetuses. It is not clear, however, whether chronic exposures to these drugs would produce similar effects (Rohrborn and Hansmann, 1971).

The synthetic estrogen diethylstilbestrol diphosphate (DES) has been shown to produce aneuploidy when administered to female mice at 8.5 days of gestation (Chrisman, 1974). This steroid has been used clinically as a means of inducing abortion shortly before or at the time of implantation; it has also been used as a measure for preventing abortions in women who have low endogenous estrogen levels. Because DES has been shown to produce aneuploidy in embryonic cells in a dose-dependent manner, the use of exogenous steroids during pregnancy should be approached with caution.

The types of studies that would be most instructive would involve testing old and young animals for susceptibility to various drugs. Chamberlain and Kasahara (1971) found that when old and young female rats were treated with 6-aminonicotinamide, a higher incidence of fetal death was noted in the older animals. When embryos were checked on day 21 of gestation, an increase in eye defects was noted for these embryos derived from the older animals. These studies would suggest that drugs may play a role in the maternal- as well as the paternal-age effect. Older patients planning on having further offspring should therefore avoid any unnecessary drug or chemical exposure.

5.3. Autoimmunity

Autoantibodies have been proposed as possible etiological factors in the production of genetically abnormal offspring. Most studies have been directed at establishing correlations between the presence of maternal thyroid autoantibodies and the frequencies of offspring with particular types of aneuploidy. Although several studies have demonstrated strong positive correlations (Burgio *et al.,* 1966; Engel, 1967; Fialkow, 1966; Fialkow *et al.,* 1971; Vanhaelst *et al.,* 1970), others have found none (Day and Wright, 1964; Furguson-Smith *et al.,* 1966; Wren *et al.,* 1967).

Nielsen (1972) summarized the data from several of these studies. Although no clear trend could be established for mothers of children with sex-chromosome aneuploidy, a significant increase in autoantibodies was observed in patients with the Down syndrome as well as in their mothers.

Fialkow (1966), in an extensive study, examined a group of 148 mothers of Down syndrome patients for thyroid antibodies. Of this group, 28% were seropositive, compared with 14% of controls. These observations were later confirmed in an expanded study of patients living at home as well as in institutions (Fialkow *et al.,* 1971). While increased frequencies of thyroid antibodies were found both in patients with the Down syndrome and in their mothers, no correlation was found between the incidence of paternal thyroid antibodies and Down syndrome offspring.

Because thyroid diseases were found to precede the index pregnancy, the possibility that thyroid antibodies developed as a result of the pregnancy with a Down syndrome child was unlikely. Frequencies of thyroid disease and autoantibodies were also higher in siblings of Down syndrome patients and in maternal first-degree relatives than in controls (Fialkow *et al.,* 1971). These observations suggest that development of thyroid antibodies and the subsequent increased risk of fostering a Down syndrome child may have a genetic basis.

While the frequency of thyroid autoantibodies remained constant at about 30% in all age groups of mothers of Down syndrome patients, the frequencies of autoantibodies in the control population increased with

Table VII.   Thyroid Autoantibodies in Mothers of Down Syndrome Children
Compared with Control Females[a]

Age range (at time of testing)	Mothers of Down patients			Control females			χ^2	P
	Number tested	Positive		Number tested	Positive			
		N	%		N	%		
20–32	52	14	27	52	2	4	8.9	<0.005
33–45	58	18	31	58	8	14	4.0	<0.05
46–60	38	10	26	38	11	29	0.066	<0.8
TOTALS								
In all age groups (20–60)	148	42	28	148	21	14	8.0	>0.005
In childbearing age groups (20–45)	110	32	29	110	10	9	13.0	<0.001

[a]From Fialkow (1966, p. 93, Table 4).

advancing maternal age (Table VII); only in the oldest age control group
were autoantibody levels comparable to those in mothers of Down syndrome patients. The high incidence of thyroid antibodies in young mothers
of Down syndrome children and in mothers of Down syndrome mosaics
(patients who possess both normal and trisomic-21 cells) led Fialkow to
conclude that thyroid autoimmunity may be more involved in postzygotic
chromosomal abnormalities than in maternal-age-dependent meiotic
nondisjunction.

Other studies by Dallaire and Lebouf (1973) showed that autoantibodies in mothers of Down syndrome patients are not restricted to the thyroid
(Table VIII). The observation that antibodies against ovarian tissue were
eight times more frequent in mothers of Down patients than in controls
lends further support to the hypothesis that autoimmunity may lead to
chromosomal nondisjunction.

Table VIII.   Autoantibodies Against Several Tissues in Sera from Mothers of
Down Syndrome Patients and from Controls[a]

Human tissue	Sera (N)	Positivity (%)		P
		Down syndrome	Controls	
Thyrotoxic	101	52.5	12.2	0.0005
Ovary	83	24.7	3.1	0.0005
Liver	92	27.2	4.8	0.0005
Placenta	67	20.9	0	0.0005
Thyroid	66	34.8	22.7	0.20
Kidney	89	29.2	4.4	0.0005

[a]From Dallaire and Leboeuf (1973, p. 334, Table 2).

The mechanisms by which autoantibodies may be able to produce aneuploidy are unknown. Failkow (1966) tested extracts of lymphocytes from patients with Hashimoto's thyroiditis for the production of hyperploidy in allogenic fibroblast cultures. Such extracts were found to increase hyperploidy in a dose-related manner in mitotic cells. In another study, chromosomal aberrations were measured in cultured lymphocytes obtained from patients with various autoimmune diseases and from an equal number of matched controls (Israsena *et al.*, 1967). No significant differences in aneuploidy, breaks, or rearrangements were noted for the two groups. The importance of these latter observations is diminished, however, by the failure to use homologous serum for cell culture. Clearly, further studies are required to determine whether autoantibodies may affect meiosis or embryonic chromosomal complements or both.

5.4. Infectious Agents

The suggestion that infectious agents may play an important etiological role in the production of aneuploid offspring has come from both epidemiological and experimental studies. Epidemiological studies have demonstrated geographic and temporal clusterings of births of children with autosomal and sex-chromosome abnormalities (Collman and Stoller, 1962; Harlap, 1974; Heindrichs *et al.*, 1963). Collmann and Stoller (1962) found that the incidence of Down syndrome births in Victoria, Australia, appeared to cycle over the 15-year period 1942–1957 (Fig. 6). High frequencies were noted at 5-year intervals, with urban peaks preceding those in rural areas. Significant clustering of these births was also noted for certain geographical areas. These observations led Stoller and Collman (1965) to suggest that an infectious agent may be responsible for the Down syndrome.

In contrast to these observations, Leck (1966) found no annual variation or clustering of Down syndrome births in Birmingham, England, between 1953 and 1964. Kogan *et al.* (1967) were also unable to find any clustering of Down syndrome births in Seattle and King's County between 1952 and 1964. The latter authors questioned the findings, statistical methods, and interpretations of Collman and Stoller, and concluded that the annual fluctuations observed by these authors could have been due to chance alone.

Other studies, however, have supported Collman and Stoller's observations. The frequencies of births of 18-trisomy and 21-trisomy in South Dakota from 1954 to 1963 revealed clusterings of index births during 1954–1956, 1958–1960, and 1961–1963 (Heindrichs *et al.*, 1963). Because these two autosomal trisomies appeared in the same cluster group, a common etiological factor was suggested.

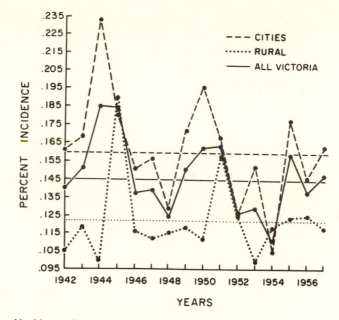

Fig. 6. Annual incidence of the Down syndrome in Victoria, Australia, 1942–1957. Reproduced from Collman and Stoller (1962).

Both long-term and seasonal cycling were observed in a study of the incidence of Down syndrome births in Jerusalem between 1964 and 1970 (Harlap, 1974). A 6-month cycle for Down syndrome births was noted for every year with the exception of 1966. Periods of highest risk were for births occurring during the spring and autumn. A long-term cycle of about 10 years' duration was also predicted in this study.

Seasonal clustering for certain sex-chromosome aneuploidies (47, XXY; 47, XYY; 47, XXX; and 45, XO) have also been reported (Neilsen *et al.*, 1973; Robinson, A., and Puck, 1967). The highest frequencies were noted for the summer months, but could not be correlated with seasonal incidence of infectious diseases.

Since viruses (Nichols, 1970) as well as mycoplasmas (Schneider *et al.*, 1974) have been shown to induce chromosomal aberrations, they are the most likely candidates for the proposed infectious agents. Both agents, however, induce considerably more chromosomal aberrations than aneuploidy. Since an increase in fetal aneuploidy rather than fetal chromosomal aberrations is observed with maternal aging, it is unlikely that these microorganisms are the chief etiological agents. There remains, however, the possibility that they may be contributing factors in the maternal-age effect.

5.5. Genetic Predisposition

Genes that regulate chromosome behavior during meiosis were reported in *Drosophila* (Sandler *et al.*, 1968). Mutants have been described that result in irregular segregation and nondisjunction of autosomal and sex chromosomes during the first meiotic division. A mutation that results in high rates of second-meiotic-division nondisjunction was also described.

These observations, together with reports in man of familial occurrence of aneuploidy, suggested that a genetic factor may predispose to mammalian chromosomal nondisjunction. Hauschka *et al.* (1962) reported a family in which a Down syndrome child was born to a man who was shown to have an XYY chromosome complement. Broustet *et al.* (1975) reported a case of Turner syndrome (XO) and Down syndrome in a sibship of four. Such isolated observations have prompted carefully controlled studies designed to determine whether familial predisposition toward nondisjunction could be statistically demonstrated. Bell and Cripps (1974) examined siblings of 30 subjects having sex-chromosome aneuploidies. Among the 51 siblings examined, one XXY brother and one XYY brother were discovered. Although this finding represented an observed incidence of sex-chromosome aneuploidy above the expected frequency, the difference was not statistically significant ($p = 0.06$).

In these studies, one must be careful to exclude subjects with translocations. A parent having a balanced chromosomal translocation can produce gametes deficient in a single chromosome or containing an extra one. Offspring have clinical signs identical with aneuploid offspring resulting from nondisjunction. The inheritance of translocations, however, is not related to parental age. An example is a family studied by Dallaire and Fraser (1964) in which the father carried a 21/21 translocation. Since his gametes had either no or two chromosomes 21, five of five children had the Down syndrome. (Monosomy 21 appears to have limited viability.) Clearly, data derived from this family would result in an overestimate of familial nondisjunction.

In a large study, 312 siblings of 642 patients with the Down syndrome were examined (Carter and Evans, 1961). Frequencies of abnormal sibs born before and after the birth of the index child were examined in relation to maternal age. These data suggest that the risk of giving birth to a second child with the Down syndrome is higher than the random risk for a particular age group. When Hamerton *et al.* (1961) analyzed the karyotypes of nine of these affected children, however, three were found to be carrying translocations or isochromosomes involving chromosome 21. These difficulties did not allow a definitive conclusion to be made as to whether an inherited predisposition for nondisjunction existed for chromosome 21.

In a detailed study on the incidence of the Down syndrome in an inbred Amish community, Juberg and Davis (1970) could find no evidence for genetic control of nondisjunction. Futhermore, the relatively constant frequency of Down syndrome births in different countries (Lilienfeld, 1969) does not support a strong genetic influence.

The current prenatal diagnostic studies may contribute to our understanding of the role of genetic predisposition. Many mothers of Down syndrome children have undergone this procedure to avoid having a second affected offspring. The results of prenatal diagnosis of these women should provide a prospective analysis of genetic predispostion toward chromosomal nondisjunction.

5.6. Preovulatory Overripeness

The alterations that occur in the hypothalamic–pituitary–ovarian axis as women near the time of menopause are discussed in detail in previous chapters. These changes in menstrual cycles often result in the delayed release of oocytes. Both epidemiological and experimental studies have shown that the preovulatory aging of oocytes in the aging female reproductive system can lead to reduced fertility, increased incidence of spontaneous abortions, and genetically abnormal offspring.

5.6.1. Epidemiological Studies

Jongbloet (1975) noted that increased numbers of conceptions occurred during the spring and autumn months. He attributed this observation to seasonal changes in fecundity resulting from an alternating pattern of ovulatory and anovulatory cycles. He predicted that such periods of changing cycles would produce periods of increased risk for preovulatory aging of oocytes, and thus increased frequency of genetically abnormal offspring. High frequencies of births of chromosomally abnormal offspring might therefore be expected at the beginning and end of the winter and the summer. Data on seasonal variations of births of children with the Down, Klinefelter, and Turner syndromes have followed his predictions.

Hertig (1967) analyzed fertilized ova from women with known dates of coitus. Of those ova that were ovulated on or before day 14 of the menstrual cycle, 8% were abnormal, while 57% of those ovulated after day 14 were abnormal. This observation further supports preovulatory aging as an etiological factor in the production of abnormal offspring.

5.6.2. Experimental Studies

Xenopus has proved to be a good model in which to study the effects of preovulatory overripeness, since animals maintained in the laboratory ovulate only in response to exogenous gonadotropins. *Xenopus* eggs can therefore be aged for specific periods of time. Larvae spawned after an extended anovulatory period displayed a variety of congenital malformations, including acephaly, microcephaly, cyclopia, and spina bifida (Mikamo and Hamaguchi, 1975). In addition to these congenital anomalies, a high incidence of trisomy, monosomy, and mosaicism was reported in larvae spawned by females that had not ovulated for several months (Witschi and Laguens, 1963).

In rats, ovulation can be delayed by pentobarbital injection. This technique delays the normal proestrus peaks of LH, FSH, and estrogen and results in ovarian retention of the mature oocytes for an extra 2 days. During this 48-hr period, the oocyte remains in meiotic arrest, while follicular growth continues (Freeman *et al.*, 1970). Butcher *et al.* (1969) demonstrated that such a delay leads to decreased implantation, increased embryonic abnormalities, and increased embryonic death. Chromosome counts performed in 390 rat embryos derived from pentobarbital-treated mothers and 410 controls revealed a threefold increase in aneuploid fetuses in the former group. These aneuploidies included trisomies and polyploidy as well as mosaicism (Butcher and Fugo, 1967). The prolonged estrus cycles that frequently occur as a function of aging in the rat might also result in similar developmental abnormalities. Female rats that conceived after a prolonged (6-day) estrus cycle had fewer implantations and a greater number of abnormal embryos than age-matched females with normal (4-day) estrus cycles. These observations indicate that both spontaneous and induced delays in ovulation can lead to increased frequencies of developmental anomalies.

5.7. Postovulatory Aging

Increasing the time between ovulation and insemination results in decreased rates of fertilization and increased numbers of abnormal embryos. This observation has led to the suggestion that postovulatory aging of oocytes may be an etiological factor in the production of genetically abnormal offspring in aging women because of decreased frequency of coitus.

5.7.1. Animal Models

Fetilization of amphibian eggs after retention *in utero* resulted in spina bifida, caudal duplication, microcephaly, and acephaly, as well as other abnormalities (Witschi, 1952). The frequencies of these anomalies were directly related to the length of retention of eggs in the uterus.

Female rabbits normally ovulate in response to coitus; this mechanism insures that eggs are fertilized within 2 or 3 hr after ovulation. Shaver and Carr (1967) induced ovulation in rabbits by injection of human chorionic gonadotropin and allowed matings to occur at timed intervals after injection. Separation of ovulation and mating by more than 10 hr resulted in a decrease in the number of blastocysts that could be recovered on day 6 of development. Karyotypes of blastocyst cells revealed that chromosomal abnormalities were most frequent in the groups delayed 8–9 hr, the most common abnormality being triploidy (Shaver and Carr, 1967). In a follow-up study, the sex-chromosome complement of ten triploid blastocysts was analyzed; seven were XXY and three were XXX. The lack of XYY chromosome complements led the authors to conclude that digyny (failure of oocyte cell division) was the most likely cause of the triploid chromosomal complements (Shaver and Carr, 1969).

In another study of delayed insemination in rabbits, Austin (1967) examined frequencies of hypodiploidy in embryonic cells. Of the blastocyst cells from the delayed-insemination group, 63% were hypodiploid, as compared with 26% for control cells. Again, an increase in triploidy was noted in the group subjected to delayed insemination. Decreased fertility and increased polyploidy and aneuploidy were also found in hamster embryos when fertilization was delayed for 3 hr. Again, triploidy was the most common anomaly and apparently resulted from digyny.

Studies of delayed fertilization in the mouse have produced controversial results. Gates and Beatty (1954) and Branden and Austin (1954) found no increase in triploid embryos when fertilization was delayed, while Vickers (1969) found that a 7- to 13-hr delay in fertilization produced a ninefold increase in triploidy.

Rodman (1971) examined oocytes recovered from mouse oviducts after superovulation. The condition of the cumulus mass and location in the oviduct were used to evaluate the age of the egg. He found an increase in the occurrence of chromatid nondisjunction in older eggs, and concluded that fertilization of these oocytes could result in aneuploid offspring. Other investigators, however, have found an increased frequency of parthenogenesis but no increase in triploid or aneuploid embryos derived from fertilized "aged" oocytes (oocytes that had an 11- to 15-hr delay in fertilization).

5.7.2. Human Studies

The human oocyte remains in the prophase of the first meiotic division until just prior to ovulation. At this time, the first meiotic division is completed and the second meiotic division is initiated. The second division is completed only after fertilization. German (1968) suggested that the increase in genetically abnormal offspring observed in older mothers may be related to the decreased frequency of sexual activity in older couples.

Since the lifetime of sperm in the female is approximately 48 hr, the decreased sexual activity with age and with duration of marriage might produce more frequent delayed fertilization of oocytes in older women. When the duration of marriage before the delivery of a Down syndrome child was analyzed for young (18–34) and old (35–47) mothers, significant differences were found; the mean duration of marriage in the young group was 4.94 years, vs. 12.08 years in the older group (German, 1968). Thus, these data might support German's hypothesis. Other investigators have criticized this hypothesis, however, pointing out that the rise in the incidence of the Down syndrome follows an exponential curve, rather than the type of curve German's hypothesis generated (James, 1968). Furthermore, mathematical analysis of available data has shown that delayed fertilization cannot be the sole etiological factor in the Down syndrome (James, 1968; Matsunaga and Maruyama, 1969). Nevertheless, these criticisms do not exclude the possibility that postovulatory oocyte aging may be a contributing factor to the maternal-age effect.

In an extensive study, Guerrero and Rojas (1975) measured the probability of abortion as a function of the day in the menstrual cycle on which fertilization occurred. The shift in basal body temperature was used to estimate the time of ovulation. Abortions that resulted from inseminations occurring before the temperature shift were attributed to aging sperm, while those occurring after the shift were attributed to aging ova. The highest probability of abortion (24% of inseminations) occurred on the third day after temperature shift, indicating that aging oocytes may be more important than aged sperm in causing fetal waste.

6. Mechanisms of Nondisjunction

6.1. Nucleolar Organization

Two of the chromosomes (numbers 13 and 21) that have been identified in maternal-age-related autosomal trisomies are also involved in nucleolar organization. It has been suggested that with maternal aging, persistence of nucleoli during meiosis could result in nondisjunction of these nucleolar organizing chromosomes (Evans, 1967). Evidence for nucleolar persistence includes the observation of frequent acrocentric chromosome association in human meiotic and mitotic cells (Bennett, 1966; Cooke, 1972; de Capoa *et al.,* 1973).

The involvement of nucleolar organization in the production of chromosomal nondisjunction also provides a mechanism for a viral effect: a virus attached to the nucleolar organizing regions of a chromosome might inhibit nucleolar disruption and lead to nondisjunction of nucleolar organizing chromosomes. Only two of the four common chromosome trisomies, however, involve nucleolar organizers. In addition, the most common trisomy (trisomy-16) found in human fetuses does not involve a nucleolar organizing chromosome (Boué and Boué, 1973). Therefore, although nucleolar persistence might contribute to chromosomal nondisjunction, it cannot account for all the observed maternal-age-related disorders.

6.2. Univalent Formation

A second mechanism that has been suggested to be responsible for the increased frequencies of aneuploid offspring observed in aging mothers is the formation of univalents in oocytes. Univalents result when a pair of homologous chromosomes fail to pair and form chiasmata during the first meiotic division. Random segregation of these univalents can result in monosomic and trisomic oocytes. Henderson and Edwards (1968) examined frequencies and positions of chiasmata in mouse oocytes as a function of maternal age. In the CBA strain, which features premature reproductive decline, a statistically significant decrease in the number of chiasmata per metaphase was observed in animals between 2 and 12 months of age. In the C57BL6 strain, however, the average number of chiasmata per metaphase was not significantly decreased with maternal aging. Studies of spermatocytes revealed no decrease in chiasmata number in CBA males aged 2–9 months. This observation is in contrast to a previous observation by Crew and Koller (1926), who noted a small decline in chiasma frequency with age in male mice.

Increased incidence of univalents correlated well with decreased chiasmata. The number of univalents per oocyte in the CBA strain increased approximately tenfold between 2 and 12 months, while no increase was observed in C57BL6 mice. No correlation was found between chromosome size and susceptibility to univalent formation. On the basis of these observations, the authors proposed a "production-line" model with oocytes formed early in development having larger numbers of chiasmata than those formed late in development. If oocytes were ovulated in the same sequence as they were formed, oocytes with more univalents would occur in older animals.

Although direct proof of the "production-line" model does not exist, many other examples of reduced chiasmata and increased univalents have been reported to occur with increasing maternal age. Luthardt et al. (1973) compared chiasmata and univalent frequencies in C57BL/6J and ICR females between 1.5 and 15 months of age. Although the decline in chiasmata number was similar for the two strains, ICR females had a higher incidence of true univalents (homologues widely separated). The authors concluded that efficiency in pairing of homologous chromosomes was greater in the inbred C57BL/6J strain. R. G. Edwards (1970) found a similar relationship between maternal age and chiasma frequency in human oocytes.

Because chiasmata formation and recombination appear to be functionally related, several studies have measured recombination frequencies as a function of age. Bodmer (1961) noted a significant decline in recombination with maternal age for the genetic markers "pallid" and "fidget" in mice. Similarly, Reid and Parsons (1963) noted a decline in recombination between the loci "leaden" and "fuzzy" with maternal age, while a slight increase was noted with paternal age.

6.3. Premature Centromere Division

The majority of trisomic offspring thus far analyzed have been found to result from nondisjunction at the first maternal meiotic division. Cases of nondisjunction at the second meiotic division have also been documented, however, and may result from premature centromere division. Examination of the chromosomal complements of normal women has revealed that more than 2% of all mitotic metaphases contain fragments the size of large C-group chromosomes. Autoradiography and chromosome-banding techniques have revealed that these fragments are X chromosomes in which the centromere has divided prematurely (Fitzgerald *et al.*, 1975). Perhaps the most interesting observation was an increasing frequency of premature centromere division with increasing age in women. Women 60 years and older had four times as many such "fragments" as women under 40. This centomeric dysfunction may be responsible for the somatic-cell aneuploidy that has been observed as a function of human aging, since the most frequently lost chromosome appears to be the X (Fitzgerald *et al.*, 1976). If premature centromeric division also occurs in germ cells, it may be responsible for the high frequency of sex-chromosome aneuploidy observed with maternal aging.

7. Approaches to Studying Parental-Age Effects

Because of the practical and ethical limitations on human experimentation, the majority of the studies of the maternal-age effect in man have been epidemiological. A search has therefore been made for appropriate animal models to examine the mechanisms of the maternal-age effect. Examination of the chromosome complement of newborn mice derived from aged females (15+ months) revealed no aneuploidy (Goodlin, 1965). Subsequent studies were directed at analyzing the chromosome complement of fetuses obtained from young and old mouse mothers (Fabricant and Schneider,

1978; Gosden, 1973; Yamamoto *et al.*, 1973). Results from these three different laboratories revealed a significant increase in chromosomally abnormal fetuses as a function of mouse maternal aging. These studies indicate that in the mouse, prenatal selection against aneuploid fetuses may be more severe than in man. Aneuploidy also appeared to correlate well with fetal morphological alterations (Fabricant and Schneider, 1978). The mouse may therefore be a good experimental model for examining many of the etiological factors proposed for the maternal-age effect.

In contrast to the situation with the maternal-age effect, there have been few experimental studies of paternal-age-related disorders. This paucity of studies is probably related to the low frequency of their occurrence as well as to the absence of a unifying feature, such as chromosomal alteration, that can be readily identified.

8. Prevention by Genetic Counseling and Prenatal Diagnosis

The advent of prenatal diagnosis by amniocentesis now allows us to take positive steps toward preventing parental-age-related disorders. Amniocentesis involves the insertion of a needle into the amniotic cavity of a pregnant woman and the removal of approximately 5–15 ml of amniotic fluid. This fluid contains cells derived from the fetus. When placed in the appropriate culture medium, these cells will proliferate, and after 3–4 weeks, sufficient cells will be available for chromosomal analysis. In this way, the chromosomal complement of the fetus can be accurately determined.

It is vital that genetic counseling accompany prenatal diagnosis. The parents should be informed of the risks of having an affected child at their age as well as the risks of the procedure. Extensive studies of prenatal diagnosis at many centers throughout the United States have indicated that these risks are minimal. The incidence of abortions occurring after amniocentesis does not appear to be significantly higher than would be expected at similar stages of pregnancy. There does exist, however, the rare possibility of fetal injury.

To date, more than 10,000 procedures have been conducted (Golbus, 1977). The major indication for prenatal diagnosis has been maternal age. Many prenatal diagnostic centers recommend that all mothers over 35 should have prenatal diagnosis, while others feel that 37 is a more reasonable age level. Deciding whether 35 or 37 is the right age is less important than providing mothers over 35 with the risk figures and allowing them to make the decision.

Since recent studies indicate that the mean maternal age for Down syndrome births may be declining (Lowry *et al.*, 1976), the recommended age for prenatal diagnosis may need to be revised. Other indications for prenatal diagnosis by amniocentesis include carriers of chromosomal translocations, previous Down syndrome offspring, and parents at risk for inherited biochemical disorders and neural tube defects. Of the 4855 pregnancies that were monitored by amniocentesis for advanced maternal age, 131 chromosomally abnormal fetuses were detected (Golbus, 1977). Thus, over 100 families were provided the opportunity to avoid the tragedy of having a genetically abnormal child.

Unfortunately, the techniques for prenatal diagnosis of paternal-age-related disorders are quite limited. The major difficulty is the lack of a unifying abnormality such as the aneuploidy observed as a function of maternal aging. In the future, it may be possible to diagnose specific paternal-age-related disorders such as achondroplasia by such techniques as fetoscopy (examination of the fetus directly by a fiber optic system) or X-ray examination of the fetus. Many of the disorders related to advanced paternal age, however, may not be as amenable as maternal-age-related disorders to prenatal diagnosis.

9. Summary

With parental aging, there is a significantly increased risk of having genetically abnormal offspring. Advanced paternal age is associated with an increased frequency of offspring with autosomal-dominant (or single-gene) disorders, while advanced maternal age is related to an increased incidence of chromosomally abnormal infants. Because of their higher frequencies, more attention has been paid to the maternal-age-related disorders. The risk of having a child with the Down syndrome may be as high as 1 in 20 births in mothers over age 45. The difference in frequency between maternal- and paternal-age-related disorders as well as their diverse presentation may be related to their contrasting germ-cell physiology. The long period that the oocyte remains in the first meiotic prophase (up to 50 years) may predispose the older oocyte to chromosomal nondisjunction. In contrast, spermatogonia are continually producing spermatocytes after age 13 and may be more susceptible to propagation of single-gene mutations.

Despite considerable speculation concerning the etiology of these parental-age effects, the exact mechanisms remain to be elucidated. Proposed etiological agents that may be responsible for the maternal-age effect include radiation, chemicals, and infectious agents. Altered immunity, genetic predisposition, and delayed fertilization have also been offered as contributing factors. Among the proposed mechanisms for the maternal-age effect are nucleolar organization, univalent formation, and premature centromeric division. It is anticipated that the availability of a mouse model for the maternal-age effect may allow for thorough evaluation of some of these proposed agents, factors, and mechanisms. The goal of these studies is to prevent the enormous fetal waste that occurs with maternal aging. Until this goal is achieved, however, prenatal diagnosis will remain the best alternative for the older pregnant mother.

Although little effort has been expended on paternal-age-related disorders, future research should be focused on this important area. Such an effort would be particularly timely, since paternal-age-related disorders cannot now be diagnosed by amniocentesis or other prenatal procedures.

The older parent should also be advised to avoid radiation exposure, as well as any nonessential drug ingestion, since both X-irradiation and chemicals have been demonstrated in laboratory animals to be capable of causing an increased frequency of abnormal offspring.

References

Alberman, E., Polani, P. E., Roberts, J. A. F., Spicer, C. C., Elliot, M., and Armstrong, E., 1972, Parental exposure to X-irradiation and Down's syndrome, *Ann. Hum. Genet.* **36**:195–208.

Austin, C. R., 1967, Chromosome deterioration in ageing eggs of the rabbit, *Nature (London)* **213**:1018–1019.

Barrai, I., Cann, H. M., Cavalli-Sforza, L. L., and Nicola, P., 1968, The effect of parental age on rates of mutation for hemophilia and evidence for differing mutation rates for hemophilia A and B, *Am. J. Human Genet.* **20**:175–196.

Bell, A. G., and Cripps, M. H., 1974, Familial aneuploidy: What risk to sibs?, *Can. J. Genet. Cytol.* **16**:113–119.

Bennett, D., 1966, Non-random association of chromosomes during mitotic metaphase in tissue cells of the mouse, *Cytologia* **31**:411–415.

Berry, W. T. C., 1958, A study on the incidence of mongolism in relation to the fluoride content of water, *Am. J. Ment. Defic.* **62**:634–636.

Blank, C. E., 1960, Apert's syndrome (a type of acrocephalosyndactyly)—Observations on a British series of thirty-nine cases, *Ann. Hum. Genet.* **24**:151–164.

Bodmer, W. F., 1961, Viability effects and recombination differences in a linkage test with pallid and fidget in the house mouse, *Heredity* **16**:485–495.

Bott, C. E., Sckhon, S. E. and Lubs, H. A., 1975, Unexpected high frequency of paternal origin of trisomy 21, *Am. J. Hum. Genet.* **27**:20.

Boué, J. and Boué, A., 1973, Anomalies chromosomiques dans les avortements spontanes, in: *INSERM Symposium: Les Accidents Chromosomiques de la Reproduction* (A. Boué and C. Thibault, eds.), pp. 29–56, Institut National de la Sante et da la Recherche Medicale, Paris.

Boyer, S. H., Ferguson-Smith, M. A., and Grumbach, M. M., 1961, The lack of influence on parental age and birth order in the aetiology of nuclear sex chromatin-negative Turner's syndrome, *Ann. Hum. Genet.* **25**:215–225.

Branden, A. W. H., and Austin, C. R., 1954, Fertilization of the mouse egg and the effect of delayed coitus and hot-shock treatment, *Aust. J. Biol. Sci.* **7**:552–565.

Broustet, A., Serville, F., Roger, P., and Gachet, M., 1975, X monosomy and 21 trisomy in a sibship, *Humangenetik* **27**:333–337.

Burger, P. C., and Vogel, S. F., 1973, The development of the pathologic changes of Alzheimer's disease and senile dementia in patients with Down's syndrome, *Am. J. Pathol.* **73**:457–476.

Burgio, G. B., Severi, F., Rossoni, R., and Vaccaro, R., 1966, Auto-antibodies in Down's syndrome, *Lancet* **1**:497–498.

Butcher, R. L., Blue, J. D., and Fugo, N. W., 1969, Overripeness and the mammalian ova. III. Fetal development at midgestation and at term, *Fertil. Steril.* **20**:223–231.

Butcher, R. L., and Fugo, N. W., 1967, Overripeness and the mammalian ova. II. Delayed ovulation and chromosome anomalies, *Fertil. Steril.* **18**:297–304.

Carter, C. O., and Evans, K. A., 1961, Risk of parents who have had one child with Down's syndrome (mongolism) having another child similarly affected, *Lancet* **2**:785–787.

Carter, C. O., Evans, K. A., and Stewart, A. M., 1961, Maternal radiation and Down's syndrome (mongolism), *Lancet* **2**:1042.

Chamberlain, J. G., and Kasahara, M., 1971, Influence of maternal age and parity on fetal mortality and congenital abnormalities induced in rats, *Growth* **35**:213–220.

Chrisman, C. L., 1974, Aneuploidy in mouse embryos induced by diethylstilbestrol diphosphate, *Teratology* **9**:229–232.

Cohen, B. L., and Lilienfeld, A. M., 1970, The epidemiological study of mongolism in Baltimore, *Ann. N. Y. Acad. Sci.* **171**:320–327.

Cohen, M. M., 1970, Drugs and chromosomes, *Ann. N. Y. Acad. Sci.* **171**:467–477.

Collman, R. D., and Stoller, A., 1962, A survey of mongoloid births in Victoria, Australia, 1942–1957, *Am. J. Public Health* **52**:813–829.

Cooke, P., 1972, Age-related variation in the number of secondary associations between acrocentric chromosomes in normal females and patients with Turner's syndrome, *Humangenetik* **17**:29–35.

Craig-Holmes, A. P., Moore, F. B., and Shaw, M. W., 1975, Polymorphism of human C-band heterochromatin. II. Family studies with suggestive evidence for somatic crossing over, *Am. J. Hum. Genet.* **27**:178–189.

Crew, F., and Koller, P., 1926, The sex incidence of chiasma frequency and genetical crossing over in the mouse, *J. Genet.* **26**:359–383.

Dallaire, L., and Fraser, F. C., 1964, Two unusual cases of familial mongolism, *Can. J. Genet. Cytol.* **6**:540–547.

Dallaire, L., and Leboeuf, G., 1973, Maternal autoimmunity and its relationship to reproductive failure, in: *INSERM Symposium: Les Accidents Chromosomiques de la Reproduction* (A. Boué and C. Thibault, eds.), pp. 333–339, Institut National de la Sante et de la Recherche Medicale, Paris.

Day, R. W., and Wright, S. W., 1964, Thyroid autoantibodies and sex-chromosome abnormalities, *Lancet* **2**:667.

de Capoa, A., Rocchi, A., and Gigliani, F., 1973, Frequency of satellite association in individuals with structural abnormalities of nucleolus organizer region, *Humangenetik* **18**:111–115.

Down, J. L. H., 1866, Observations on an ethnic classification of idiots, *Clin. Lect. Rep. London Hosp.* **3**:259–262.

Dunning, J. M., 1965, Current status of fluoridation, *N. Engl. J. Med.* **272**:30–34.

Edwards, J. H., Harnden, D. G., Cameron, A. H., Grosse, V. M., and Wolff, O. H., 1960, A new trisomic syndrome, *Lancet* **1**:787–789.

Edwards, R. G., 1970, Meiosis in males and females, in: *Human Population Cytogenetics* (P. A. Jacobs, W. H. Price, and P. Law, eds.), pp. 20–21, Williams and Wilkins Co., Baltimore.

Engel, E., 1967, Autoantibodies and chromosomal aberrations, *Lancet* **1**:1271–1272.

Erickson, D., and Cohen, M. M., 1974, A study of parental effects on the occurrence of fresh mutations for the Apert syndrome, *Ann. Hum. Genet.* **38**:89–96.

Evans, H. J., 1967, The nucleolus, virus infection, and trisomy in man, *Nature (London)* **214**:361–363.

Fabricant, J. D., and Schneider, E. L., 1978, Studies of the genetic and immunologic components of the maternal age effect (in prep.).

Fialkow, P. J., 1966, Autoimmunity and chromosomal aberrations, *Am. J. Hum. Genet.* **18**:93–108.

Fialkow, P. J., Thuline, H. C., Hecht, F., and Bryant, J., 1971, Familial predisposition to thyroid disease in Down's syndrome: Controlled immunoclinical studies, *Am. J. Hum. Genet.* **23**:67–86.

Fitzgerald, P. H., Pickering, A. F., Mercer, J. M., and Miethke, P. M., 1975, Premature centromere division: A mechanism of nondisjunction causing X chromosome aneuploidy in somatic cells of man, *Ann. Hum. Genet.* **38**:417–428.

Freeman, M. E., Butcher, R. L., and Fugo, N. W., 1970, Alteration of oocytes and follicles by delayed ovulation, *Biol. Reprod.* **2**:209–215.

Furguson-Smith, M. A., Anderson, J. R., Froland, A., and Gray, K. G., 1966, Frequency of autoantibodies in patients with chromatin-positive Klinefelter's syndrome and their parents, *Lancet* **2**:566–568.

Gates, A. H., and Beatty, R. A., 1954, Independence of delayed fertilization and spontaneous triploidy in mouse embryos, *Nature (London)* **174**:356.

German, J., 1968, Mongolism, delayed fertilization and human sexual behavior, *Nature (London)* **217**:516–518.

Giraud, F., Mattei, J. F. and Matei, M. G., 1975, Étude chromosomique chez les parents d'enfants trisomiques 21: Chromosomes marquers, remaniements, cassures et aneuploidies, *Lyon Med.* **233**:241–251.

Glass, H. R., and Ritterhoff, R. K., 1961, Mutagenic effect of a 5-r dose of X-rays in *Drosophila melanogaster, Science* **133**:1366.

Golbus, M. S., 1977, The prenatal diagnosis of genetic defects, in: *Advances in Obstetrics and Gynecology,* Williams and Wilkins Co., Baltimore.

Goodlin, R. C., 1965, Nondisjunction and maternal age in the mouse, *J. Reprod. Fertil.* **9**:355–356.

Gosden, R. G., 1973, Chromosomal anomalies of preimplantation mouse embryos in relation to maternal age, *J. Reprod. Fertil.* **35**:351–354.

Guerrero, R., and Rojas, O. I., 1975, Spontaneous abortion and aging of human ova and spermatozoa, *N. Engl. J. Med.* **293**:573–574.

Hamerton, J. L., Briggs, S. M., Giannelli, F., and Carter, C. O., 1961, Chromosome studies in detection of parents with high risk of second child with Down's syndrome, *Lancet* **2**:788–791.

Hara, Y. and Sasaki, M., 1975, A note on the origin of extra chromosomes in trisomies 13 and 21, *Proc. Jpn. Acad.* **51**:295–299.

Harlap, S., 1974, A time-series analysis of the incidence of Down's syndrome in West Jerusalem, *Am. J. Epidemiol.* **99**:210–217.

Hauschka, T. S., Hasson, J. E., Goldstein, M. N., Koepe, G. E., and Sandberg, A. A., 1962, an XYY man with progeny indicating familial tendency to nondisjunction, *Am. J. Hum. Genet.* **14**:22–30.

Heindrichs, E. H., Allen, S. W., and Nelson, P. S., 1963, Simultaneous 18-trisomy and 21-trisomy cluster, *Lancet* **2**:468.

Henderson, S. A., and Edwards, R. G., 1968, Chiasma frequency and maternal age in mammals, *Nature (London)* **218**:22–28.

Herrmann, J., 1966, Der Einfluss des Zeugungsalters auf die Mutationen zu Haemophile A, *Humangenetik* **3**:1–16.

Hertig, A. T., 1967, The overall problem in man, in: *Comparative Aspects of Reproductive Failure* (K. Benirschke, ed.), pp. 11–41, Springer-Verlag, Berlin.

Hsia, D. Y. Y., Justice, P., Smith, G. F., and Dowben, R. M., 1971, Down's syndrome: A critical review of the biochemical and immunological data, *Am. J. Dis. Child.* **121**:153–161.

Hutton, E. M., and Thompson, M. W., 1970, Parental age and mutation rate in Duchene muscular dystrophy, *Am. J. Hum. Genet.* **22**:26a.

Israsena, T., Quatrale, A. C., and Becker, K. L., 1967, Autoimmune disease and chromosomal instability, *Lancet* **2**:1226–1227.

Jagiello, G., and Lin, J. S., 1973, An assessment of the effects of mercury on the meiosis of mouse ova, *Mutat. Res.* **17**:93–99.

James, W. H., 1968, Mongolism, delayed fertilization and sexual behavior, *Nature (London)* **219**:279–280.

Jones, J. L., Smith, D. W., Harvey, M. A. S., Hall, B. D., and Quan, L., 1975, Older paternal age and fresh gene mutation: Data on additional disorders, *J. Pediatr.* **86**:84–88.

Jongbloet, P. H., 1975, The effects of preovulatory overripeness of human eggs on development, in: *Aging Gametes* (R. J. Blandau, ed.), pp. 300–329, S. Karger, Basel.

Juberg, R. C., and Davis, L. M., 1970, Etiology of nondisjunction: Lack of evidence for genetic control, *Cytogenetics* **9**:284–293.

Klinefelter, H. F., Reifenstein, E. C., and Albright, F., 1942, Syndrome characterized by gynecomastia, aspermatogenesis without α-Leydigism, and increased excretion of follicle-stimulating hormone, *J. Clin. Endocrinol.* **2**:615–627.

Kochupillai, N., Verma, I. C., Grewal, M. S., and Ramalingaswami, V., 1976, Down's syndrome and related abnormalities in an area of high background radiation in coastal Kerala, *Nature (London)* **262**:60–61.

Kogan, A., Kronmal, R., and Peterson, D. R., 1967, Viral hepatitis and Down's syndrome, *Lancet* **1**:615.

Langenbeck, U., Hansmann, I., Hinney, B. and Honig, V., 1976, On the origin of the supernumerary chromosome in autosomal trisomies—with special reference to Down's syndrome, *Hum. Genet.* **33**:89–102.

Leck, I., 1966, Incidence and epidemicity of Down's syndrome, *Lancet* **2**:457–460.

Lejeune, J., Gautier, M., and Turpin, R., 1959, Étude des chromosomes somatiques de neuf enfants mongoliens, *C. R. Acad. Sci.* **248**:1721–1722.

Lieznerski, R. L., and Lindsten, J., 1972, Trisomy 21 in man due to maternal nondisjunction during the first meiotic division, *Hereditas* **70**:153–154.

Lilienfeld, A. M., 1969, *Epidemiology of Mongolism,* Johns Hopkins University Press, Baltimore.

Lowry, R. B., Jones, D. C., Renwick, D. G. H., and Trimble, B. K., 1976, *Teratology* **14**:29–34.

Lunn, J. E., 1959, A survey of mongol children in Glasgow, *Scott. Med. J.* **4**:368–372.

Luthardt, F. W., Palmer, C. G., and Yu, P. -L., 1973, Chiasma and univalent frequencies in aging female mice, *Cytogenet. Cell Genet.* **12**:68–79.

Lynas, M. A., 1958, Marfan's syndrome in Northern Ireland: An account of thirteen families, *Ann. Hum. Genet.* **22**:289–301.

Lyon, M. R., 1961, Gene action in the X-chromosome of the mouse, *Nature (London)* **190**:372–373.

Magenis, R. E., Hecht, F., and Milham, S., 1968, Trisomy 13 (Dl) syndrome: Studies on parental age, sex ratio, and survival, *J. Pediatr.* **73**:222–228.

Mariona, F. G., 1975, Is pregnancy a risk in the elderly woman?, in: *Aging and Reproductive Physiology* (E. S. E. Hafez, ed.), pp. 167–192, Ann Arbor Press, Ann Arbor, Michigan.

Marmol, J. G., Scriggins, A. L., and Vollman, R. F., 1969, Mothers of mongoloid infants in the collaborative project, *Am. J. Obstet. Gynecol.* **104**:533–543.

Matsunaga, E., and Maruyama, T., 1969, Human sexual behavior, delayed fertilization and Down's syndrome, *Nature (London)* **221**:642–644.

Mikamo, K., and Hamaguchi, H., 1975, Chromosomal disorder caused by preovulatory overripeness of oocytes, in: *Aging Gametes* (R. J. Blandau, ed.), pp. 72–97, S. Karger, Basel.

Mikkelsen, M., Hallberg, A., and Poulsen, H., 1976, Maternal and paternal origin of extra chromosome in trisomy 21, *Hum. Genet.* **32**:17–21.

Miller, R. W., 1970, Neoplasia and Down's syndrome, *Ann. N. Y. Acad. Sci.* **171**:637–644.

Murdoch, J. L., Walker, A. A., Hall, J. G., Abbey, H., Smith, K. K., and McKusick, V. A., 1970, Achondroplasia: A genetic and statistical survey, *Ann. Hum. Genet.* **33**:227–244.

Murdoch, J. L., Walker, B. A., and McKusick, V. A., 1972, Parental age effects on the occurrence of new mutations of the Marfan syndrome, *Ann. Hum. Genet.* **35**:331–336.

Needleman, H. L., Pueschel, S. M., and Rothman, K. J., 1974, Fluoridation and the occurrence of Down's syndrome, *N. Engl. J. Med.* **291**:821–823.

Nichols, W. W., 1970, Virus induced chromosome abnormalities, *Annu. Rev. Microbiol.* **24**:479–500.

Nielsen, J., 1972, Immunological aberrations in patients with aneuploid chromosome abnormalities and their parents, *Humangenetik* **16**:171–176.

Nielsen, J., Brunn Petersen, G., and Therkelsen, A. J., 1973, Seasonal variation in the birth of children with aneuploid chromosome abnormalities, *Humangenetik* **19**:67–74.

Ohno, S., Kaplan, W. D., and Kinosita, R., 1959, Do XY and O sperm occur in *Mus musculus?*, *Exp. Cell Res.* **18**:382–384.

Patau, K., Smith, D. W., Therman, E., Inhorn, S. L., and Wagner, H. P., 1960, Multiple congenital anomaly caused by an extra autosome, *Lancet* **1**:790–793.

Pellie, C., Feingold, J., and Demos, J., 1973, Age parental et mutation à propos d'une enquéte sur la myopathie de Duchene deBoulogne, *J. Genet. Hum.* **21**:33–41.

Penrose, L. S., 1933, The relative effects of paternal and maternal age in mongolism, *J. Genet.* **27**:219–224.

Penrose, L. S., 1955, Parental age and mutation, *Lancet* **2**:312–313.

Race, R. R., and Sanger, R., 1969, Xg and sex chromosome abnormalities, *Br. Med. Bull.* **25**:99–103.

Rapaport, I., 1956, Contribution a l'étude due mongolisme: Rôle pathogenique du fluor, *Bull. Acad. Natl. Med.* **140**:529–531.

Reid, D. H., and Parsons, P. A., 1963, Sex of parent and variation of recombination with age in the mouse, *Heredity* **18**:107–108.

Robinson, A., and Puck, T. T., 1967, Studies on chromosomal nondisjunction in man. II. *Am. J. Hum. Genet.* **19**:112–129.

Robinson, J. A., 1973, Origin of the extra chromosome in trisomy 21, *Lancet* **1**:131–133.

Rodman, T. C., 1971, Chromatid disjunction of unfertilized ageing oocytes, *Nature (London)* **233**:191–193.

Rohrborn, G., and Hansmann, I., 1971, Induced chromosome aberrations in unfertilized oocytes of mice, *Humangenetik* **18**:184–198.

Rowe, R. D., and Uchida, I. A., 1961, Cardiac malformation in mongolism: A prospective study of 184 mongoloid children, *Am. J. Med.* **31**:726–735.

Sandler, L., Lindsley, D. L., Nicoletti, B., and Trippa, G., 1968, Mutants affecting meiosis in natural populations of *Drosophila melanogaster, Genetics* **60**:525–558.

Schedl, W., 1971, Unterschiedliche Fluoreszenz der beiden homologen Chromosomen Nr. 3 beim Menschen, *Humangenetik* **12**:59–63.

Schneider, E. L., Stanbridge, E. J., Epstein, C. J., Golbus, M., Abbo-Halbasch, G., and Rodgers, G., 1974, Mycoplasma contamination of cultured amniotic fluid cells: Potential hazard to prenatal diagnosis, *Science* **184**:477–479.

Searle, A. G., and Beechey, C. V., 1974, Cytogenetic effects of X-rays and fission neutrons in female mice, *Mutat. Res.* **24**:171–186.

Shaver, E. L., and Carr, D. H., 1967, Chromosome abnormalities in rabbit blastocysts following delayed fertilization, *J. Reprod. Fertil.* **14**:415–420.

Shaver, E. L., and Carr, D. H., 1969, The chromosome complement of rabbit blastocyte in relation to the time of mating and ovulation, *Can. J. Genet. Cytol.* **11**:287–293.

Smith, C. A. B., 1972, Note on the estimation of parental age effects, *Ann. Hum. Genet.* **35**:337–342.

Smith, D. J., and Joffe, J. M., 1975, Increased neonatal mortality in offspring of male rats treated with methadone or morphine before mating, *Nature (London)* **253**:202–203.

Smith, D. W., 1970, in: *Recognizable patterns of human malformation,* p. 129, W. B. Saunders and Co., Philadelphia.

Smith, S. W., and Wilson, A. A., 1973, What is a child with Down's syndrome like? in: *The Child with Down's Syndrome* (D. W. Smith and A. A. Wilson, eds.), p. 24, W. B. Saunders and Co., Philadelphia.

Smith, G. F., and Sachdeva, S., 1973, Paternal origin of the extra chromosome in trisomy 21, *Lancet* **1**:487.

Stevenson, A. C., Mason, R., and Edwards, K., 1970, Maternal diagnostic X-irradiation before conception and the frequency of mongolism in children subsequently born, *Lancet* **2**:1335–1337.

Stoller, A., and Collman, R. D., 1965, Virus aetiology of Down's syndrome (mongolism), *Nature (London)* **208**:903–904.

Swanson, T. E., 1970, Economics of mongolism, *Ann. N. Y. Acad. Sci.* **171**:679–682.

Szemere, G., and Chandley, A. C., 1975, Trisomy and triploidy induced by X-irradiation of mouse spermatocytes, *Mutat. Res.* **33**:229–238.

Tijo, J. H., and Levan, A., 1956, The chromosome number of man, *Hereditas* **42**:1–6.

Tunte, W., 1972, Human mutations and paternal age, *Humangenetik* **16**:77–82.

Tunte, W., Becker, P. E., and Von Knorre, G., 1967, Zur Genetik der Myositis ossificans progressiva, *Humangenetik* **4**:320–351.

Uchida, I. A., 1962, The effect of maternal age and radiation on the rate of nondisjunction in *Drosophila melanogaster, Can. J. Genet. Cytol.* **4**:402–408.

Uchida, I. A., and Curtis, E. J., 1961, A possible association between maternal radiation and mongolism, *Lancet* **2**:848–850.

Uchida, I. A., Ray, M., McRae, K. N., and Besant, D. F., 1968, Familial occurrence of trisomy 21, *J. Hum. Genet.* **20**:107–118.

Vanhaelst, L., Hayez, F., Bonnyns, M., and Bastenie, P. A., 1970, Thyroid autoimmune disease and thyroid function in families of subjects with Down's syndrome, *J. Clin. Endocrinol.* **30**:792–797.

Vickers, A. D., 1969, Delayed fertilization and chromosomal anomalies in mouse embryos, *J. Reprod. Fertil.* **20**:69–76.

Wagenbichler, P., Killian, W., Rett, A., and Schnedl, W., 1976, Origin of the extra chromosome No. 21 in Down's syndrome, *Hum. Genet.* **32**:13–16.

Witschi, E., 1952, Overripeness of the egg as a cause of twinning and teratogenesis: A review, *Cancer Res.* **12**:763–786.

Witschi, E., and Laguens, R., 1963, Chromosomal aberrations in embryos from overripe eggs, *Dev. Biol.* **7**:605–616.

Wren, P. J., Evans, D. A. P., Vetters, J. M., and Chew, A., 1967, Autoimmune antibodies in mongol families, *Lancet* **2:**186–188.

Yamamoto, M., Endo, A., and Watanabe, G., 1973, Maternal age dependence of chromosome anomalies, *Nature (London) New Biol.* **241:**141–142.

Zellweger, H., and Simpson, J., 1973, Is routine prenatal karyotyping indicated in pregnancies of very young women?, *J. Pediatr.* **82:**675–677.

Zuppinger, E., Engel, E., Forbes, A. P., Mantooth, L., and Claffey, J., 1967, Klinefelter's syndrome: A clinical and cytogenetic study in twenty-four cases, *Acta Endocrinol. (Copenhagen) Suppl.* **113:**5–48.

Chapter 9

Genetics of Longevity in Man

Edmond A. Murphy

As soon as we are born we begin to die and the end depends on the beginning.

Manilius *Astronomica IV* 16

1. Introduction

In this chapter, we shall consider three major topics: the evolutionary implications of the length of life, the light that genetics may throw on the nature of longevity, and the empirical evidence that there is a heritable component. It is wise to perceive at the start not only that these topics are elusive but also that they are posed inside an arbitrary conceptual framework. There is *a priori* no reason to believe that the terms of the question, or even the question itself, have any meaning; it may be that we think the questions are sound simply because, as reflecting animals, we are interested in prolonging life. Superficially, it appears a simple problem to explore, but the more we try to crystallize it with scientific investigation in mind, the more it becomes eroded by elimination of aspects that prove to be irrelevant.

2. Evolutionary Implications

There is a modest literature on the evolutionary aspects of life span, which Wilson (1974) reviewed compactly and with lucidity. It is heuristic in

Edmond A. Murphy • Division of Medical Genetics, Department of Medicine, Johns Hopkins School of Medicine, Baltimore, Maryland 21205

character and somewhat lacking in testable detail. Moreover, in the light of recent insights, it is in large part superficial, even naïve. An adequately formed theory would also take account of a few facts that I shall mention, but call for a much better insight into the immensely complex nature of evolutionary dynamics in the real world.

The mechanisms of reproduction are perforce conservative. A long and provocative discussion has raged in the last half century as to what load of mutations a population can tolerate and at what point this load may imperil the species (for a review of recent developments, see Lewontin, 1973). Whatever this load may be, it presumably has some limit, and transmission over thousands of years to each subsequent generation of all the genetic changes inherited by, or acquired in, the preceding one might transcend that limit. At each generation, then, the slate is wiped clean, or almost so: a small, and presumably tolerable, number of mutations occur in the germinal cells themselves, and form the basis of the comparatively slow changes of natural evolution. It is by no means clear that evolution occurs at a uniform rate over time (Stanley, 1975), but the genetic similarity of father and son when both were newborn is probably considerably greater than that between the newborn son and his father when the father is dying of cancer. The need for conservatism in maintaining the coherence of the personality may explain why the parenchymatous cells of the nervous system do not undergo mitosis in adult life, not even when it would be demanded by the normal process of repair.

Nevertheless, this conservatism operates in a strangely liberal way. It is a common belief from the era of Fabré that the behavior of insects is heavily, perhaps exclusively, programmed, though there are reasons for believing that these limitations are transcended by the anthill or the hive operating as a whole. The further up the evolutionary scale, the less rigidly activity is programmed. McDougal (1924) suggested many years ago that the helplessness of so many higher animals at birth is a necessary state if learning is to be reflective, and if intelligence is to be not stereotyped but flexibly developed by cultivating ingenuity when grappling with the unknown and the unexpected. Thus, in each generation, an apparently very inefficient process of learning occurs anew, but the dividend is that each creature has distinctive characteristics, which may properly be called unique. If the evolutionary watchword of the lower species is excellence-of-the-mean, that of the most sophisticated is excellence-in-diversification. A mass-produced genetic endowment would be as much wide of the mark of higher evolution as mass-produced instruction would be wide of the aims of education.

Thus, we see genetic components conservative at three levels: (1) physical structure, which, indeed, admits of little modification from without after birth; (2) programmed behavior of the type that, rather emptily perhaps (Bateson, 1972), we call reflex and instinctive, such as breathing, sucking, coughing, and blinking; and (3) capacity for diversifying in the face of a mutable environment (which may indeed be changing more rapidly than adaptive selection could cope with). Of course, these conserving mechanisms may at times be in open conflict. In principle (whether we can determine it or not), there is presumably one optimal phenotype for the present immediate situation; those that vary from this optimum must be, temporarily at least, at some disadvantage. Equally, however, when the environment changes, the optimum also changes, and the best adapted will no longer comprise the same genetic lines as now. Hence, the "best" is a continually moving target. Individual wisdom built up over a lifetime of practical experiences may be inapplicable in the next generation; on these terms, a petrification of this wisdom would be dysgenic. Thus, we may argue that the conservation of those, as it were, strategic structures and habits that have proved of value over a long time and (presumably) over a wide range of environmental challenges is eugenic, and for the rest, what is conserved is a *capacity* for tactical adaptation to the idiosyncrasies of the present, and of a vast and complex instinctive machinery for nurturing the young while learning is taking place.

Such an interpretation of the eugenic values of a short life span is seductively simple. Like so many evolutionary arguments, it has two major defects.

First, it is not an adequately quantitated statement. Where there is conflict in objectives (for instance, as clearly seems to be the case here, between excellence and diversity), we must suppose that there is some point that would be an optimal compromise between them. If long life is dysgenic, why does not life as a result of Darwinian selection get shorter and shorter? Presumably, it is because up to a certain point, long life is eugenic. There is, then, we must suppose, an optimal length of life, and the whole point of Darwinian evolution is the claim that selection makes or, at least tends to make, the phenotype conform to this optimum. But where is this optimum? We might estimate it empirically, but the difficulty arises that the indispensable logical basis for this empirical estimate must be precisely the assumption that it is indeed being pursued by selection. We cannot validly prove the argument by first assuming that which we set out to prove. This is an old broad criticism of Darwinian evolution as a scientific theory that has been raised by epistemologists and never adequately confronted. But its relevance is brought clearly in focus here. Mean survival in a species with a finite life span must assume *some* value, but if in trying to find the optimum we can do no better than estimate this actual value, we have no means of deciding whether age at death is influenced by evolution in any way at all. Hence, we may gain no empirical insight into the desirable. [I am aware that it is commonly said that we can make no useful inferences about values from empirical data; indeed, Moore (1903) argues that the good cannot be inferred: it is an irreducible postulate. But at least we might gain some insight into what constitutes a robust structure of a population, unless, as has been suggested, Darwinism is tautologous.]

The second criticism, which is more subtle but in the long run may prove much more devastating, is that the argument presupposes that we know what the point of the point is. Granted that there is Darwinian evolution in the broad sense—that is, that evolution is not simply a "random walk" with no polarization whatsoever—what is the level at which it operates? There has been a heavy emphasis, particularly in recent discussions on the neutralist–selectionist controversy, on the behavior of the isolated products of individual genes in populations. Convincing arguments have been put forward suggesting that the main factor in change is drift; other convincing arguments have been put forward suggesting that it is Darwinian selection. The disputants have been very ingenious, and the scholar might be at something of a loss to reconcile their arguments and find where the truth lies. It is not impossible, however, that the whole debate is irrelevant to the main issue. It is not difficult to devise simple systems involving interaction of two loci that lead to predictions—paradoxical selection of lethal genes, for example—that are very different from what one might expect considering either locus in isolation. Galtonian, or multivariate, control seems more often than not to be the pattern for genetic control of traits in higher organisms, and where many loci are involved, I know of no way of predicting what the global effect would be from study of individual loci, unless several not very appealing assumptions are made. Again, it is well known that a predator, if it is too efficient in its hunting and too fastidious in its choice of prey, may perish, while a less efficient predator would survive. Thus, Darwinian excellence in the short term would, in the long term, be dysgenic.

We hear the argument that since genetic fitness is expressed almost entirely before the age of 45, there can be no evolutionary value in the life span's being 70 rather than 60. This argument, however, is a hopeless confusion between genetic fitness and evolutionary fitness. Mere fertility guarantees nothing. Moreover, what is true for the individual may not at all be true of the group. An illuminating example is given in recent papers on the genetics in the *Hymenoptera* (Trivers and Hare, 1976), in which it is shown that the sterile workers that assume an "altruistic" role in the economy can by their behavior make a larger bequest than the highly fertile queen bee to the genetic endowment of the hive. This paradoxical result reflects the peculiarity of the mating system, but it should be a warning of the perils of "common sense" and superficial argument.

Postmenopausal mothers may still have to rear their youngest children to maturity. Grandmothers may care for the children while the mothers go to work. Sterile men may still be valuable hunters. The peak of useful experience and wisdom may be attained well into old age. Elderly people may harbor infectious diseases less and hence make better nurses. Listing such possibilities is a mere exercise in imaginativeness. The supposition that the target of selection is the gene merits, at the least, some questioning. The chromosome, cell, organ, body, family, tribe, ecology may in fact be selected on as a whole, and since effects are not necessarily, perhaps not even usually, additive, the whole may bear at best a remote relationship to the sum of the parts. In the face of these formidable difficulties, a purely theoretical approach to the evolutionary aspects of aging is unlikely to furnish an authoritative answer in the near future.

Sacher (1959) showed that in mammals for which data are available, the logarithm of the "characteristic oldest age" (i.e., the age at which the second oldest member of a cohort dies) can be expressed with considerable accuracy as a linear function of the logarithm of body weight and the logarithm of brain weight. Life span increases directly with brain weight and decreases with increasing body weight. These factors may reflect the subtlety of control mechanisms, on the one hand, and metabolic rate, on the other. The findings are interesting and persuasive. Sacher was clearly aware of the sensitivity of extreme values to sample size, but his claim that this effect could be adjusted for rests heavily on the supposed mathematical form of the survivorship curve. The argument seems somewhat questionable, but in the absence of precise data could hardly be improved on. There seems to be no good reason for ascribing the remarkable relationship to bias.

Cutler (1975) explored the evolutionary record as a means of assessing the dimensions of the genetic contribution to length of life. His argument rests principally on the rate of change of "maximum life span" in hominids and the maximum rate at which gene substitution has occurred in the last ten million years. The latter is based on Haldane's gene substitution arguments and on paleogenetic analysis. The doubling of maximum life span in that time appears to have been achieved with changes at not more than 250 loci. The argument is ingenious and plausible, although one might quarrel with details of both the data and the logic. It is not at all sure, for instance, that the genetic contribution is adequately assessed by changes in genes individually; indeed (as Cutler concedes), the important change may be at a higher level of organization—for instance, regulation, cytoplasmic factors, or redundancy—that would not show up on simple analyses of genes. Using different arguments involving regression analysis, Sacher (1975) also concludes that comparatively few genes are involved in the change.

3. Genetics and Length of Life

At first blush, it seems clear what is meant by aging. We think of old paintings cracking, buildings weathering, bridges falling down, and the like. We also look at the changes in the skin of old people, the brittleness of their bones, their eroding hairlines, and we equate the two types of processes, scarcely recognizing that we are perpetrating a specious metaphor. Whether the metaphor is of value or not remains to be seen. But it may not reflect any true equivalence whatsoever, and an analysis at a superficial level suggests that the two are indeed very different. It is a commonplace that life is essentially (I use the word in the strict sense) a dynamic process—that bone, for instance, is not a living fossil, but a vital structure with a rapid turnover of even its most "nonvital" mineral components. Thus, while metal fatigue, for instance, may operate on a physical structure, the changes in bone with age must impinge on a process. Again, the notion of "wear and tear" as a cause of the senile changes is another inadequate metaphor from the behavior of clothing; some stresses at least are essential to the sound structure and functioning of bone, and inactivation may do immense harm, as the orthopedic surgeon well knows. Morey *et al.* (1977) reported that in space flight, bone formation is completely arrested in rats.

We must beware of reifying senescence, of attempting to isolate as a process what we believe we have observed as an entity of experience. One could make a long list of such figments in the past, from the idea of witches and alchemy, to phlogiston, gravitation, and ether. Reflection points up the perils of trying to solve arbitrarily constructed, and perhaps meaningless, questions.

If with these caveats, we consider what the genetic insight into aging might be, three major classes of conjectures emerge.

3.1. Aging May Be Ineluctable

It may be that there is simply no way of devising a system as complex as the living organism that will prevent it from breaking down with certainty, sooner or later, even in a perfect environment, or that if such a system exists, it has not yet been unearthed by evolution. It is not easy to imagine where this Achilles' heel may be, but in a complex emergent (i.e., roughly, a "nonadditive") system, limitations of the imagination furnish puny arguments. Certainly one might appeal to the evidence of the Hayflick phenomenon, discussed elsewhere in this volume. But tissue culture is, after all, highly artificial, and it may be that some vital but unidentified component is not adequately provided. The phenomenon may thus be factitious.

An appeal to comparative biology does nothing to allay our misgivings. If there were something close to a uniform trend in the life span of animals, it would be reassuring. Bacteria, grains of corn, and other simple forms of life can remain alive over thousands of years, and one might suppose that a shortened life span is the penalty for complexity. But a detailed analysis of the higher vertebrates seems to be in conflict (Wolstenholme and O'Connor, 1959, *passim*). The turtle and the parrot can apparently live hundreds of years, the elephant and man perhaps 70 years or so, but interspersed there are animals of all sizes and complexities that show no uniform trend in survivorship, the analysis of Sacher (1959) notwithstanding. Of course, the very terms of the question are vague and ambiguous. The animals on which it is easy to keep records are often pampered, and might be expected to live longer than others. Even so, the facts are not reassuring that survival is inversely related to complexity. If death inevitably "cometh soon or late," it is difficult to devise a cogent test of the proposition at this stage.

Indirect arguments may have some value, and previously (Murphy, 1973), I explored the following question, which may be relevant: Granted that high blood pressure is deleterious, we would expect that selection has tended to produce a progressively lower blood pressure in the past, and will continue to do so in the future. On this argument we are driven to suppose (considering the massive scale on which high blood pressure occurs and the toll of morbidity and mortality it exacts, which could hardly be maintained by recurrent mutation alone) that we are very far from an equilibrium state. But we have no external evidence to support this idea of disequilibrium, and it is tempting to invoke stabilizing selection. This view is readily supported by appealing to extreme cases, since manifestly a zero blood pressure is incompatible with life. From available data, however, notably the published results of the Framingham Study (1968), I was unable to produce convincing evidence that the long-term mortality rate is a U-shaped function of age (that is, high at both extremes of blood pressure), which is broadly what one would expect with stabilizing selection. It seems reasonable, then, to infer that the present system of blood pressure regulation is being selected for as-a-whole, the deleterious effects on so many people in middle life being perhaps the price paid for the physiological advantages in earlier life.* This interpretation could scarcely be called more than a broad conjecture, which, to be tested, would call for much better directed collection and formal analysis of data. For a great many examples of these metrical traits, I am impressed by two general points that have proved to be recurrent stumbling blocks in genetic analysis. First, for non-

---

*Williams (1957) suggested that this kind of delayed pleiotropy may have wide importance in the evolutionary aspects of aging.

Mendelian common disease (e.g., hypertension, hyperlipidemia, gout, diabetes), the disease states seem most often to be associated with excesses rather than deficiencies; second, frequently, even usually, the distribution is positively skewed. (The latter characteristic invariably generates an antithesis between those who seek to resolve the distribution into components and those who propose to normalize it by the use of logarithmic transformations.) This pattern has been encountered so often as to make one wonder whether it is indeed some ineluctable consequence of vital processes.

3.2. Aging May Be a Programmed Self-Destruction

Such an argument is teleological, though perhaps in Ayala's sense of adaptive (Ayala, 1970, 1972). It may be programmed because it is eugenic, and here we may revert to the arguments at the beginning of this chapter. Certain body cells—in the epidermis, the intestinal mucosa, the holocrine glands, the blood cells—provide precedents, though perhaps for varying reasons. The blood platelet, for instance, dies in large part because its means of performing its functions, as in hemostasis or phagocytosis of foreign particles, involve self-injury, which may be lethal. The holocrine glands die because their function is to deliver their contents. In epidermal cells, it may be that the elaborate repair mechanisms they possess— mechanisms that are compromised in xeroderma pigmentosum and other genetic disorders (Cleaver and Bootsma, 1975)—are simply not elaborate enough, and since destruction cannot be staved off indefinitely, some means of replacement must be provided. Also, of course, cells on the skin, as on any surface structure (the intestine, the intima, the bladder), are removed by abrasion. In fact, there is a complex fail-safe system, elaborated in varying degree in various tissues and organisms, that we may now expound.

In Fig. 1 is represented a heuristic, and doubtless much over simplified, version of the chain of mechanisms that tend to keep the economy of the body functioning and to fend off the process that we have identified as senescence. We may start with the progeny. Some primitive organisms— viruses, for instance—consist simply of an elementary structure, with capacity to reproduce and the means to enter a host cell on which they are totally dependent for subsistence. I know of no cell in the human body that is quite so primitive. Most tissues have some endowment of consumable supplies, even when, as in erythrocytes, there are no more elaborate systems of reserve in the cell. Thus, the maintenance of an adequate concentration of red cells calls for continual replenishment from parent cells in the bone marrow. Without this continual bolstering from outside, death would result as the individual red cells gradually die, as seems to be

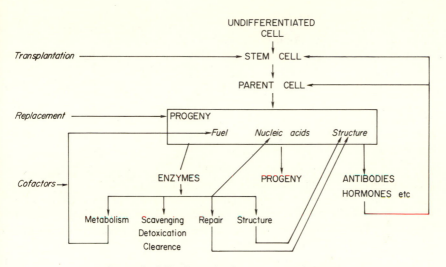

Fig. 1. The fail-safe mechanisms to meet vital needs.

the case in the aplastic anemias. The red cell has a relatively simple function, and the cause of its demise—structural or functional—is not altogether clear. The hemolytic anemia due to poorly fitting prosthetic valves suggests that purely structural change may be a limiting factor.

Cells with more complicated structures may be perpetuated in various ways. They may reproduce as the lymphocytes do, which allows a genealogical survival. They may preserve their individual existences because they are well-provided for, well-protected physically, and allowed the luxury of a protected function, as in the cells of the brain. They may be individually vulnerable, but the function of the type conserved by considerable redundancy, as in kidney cells. But, more generally, cells may survive by having elaborate housekeeping mechanisms, largely enzymic in nature, that preserve the status quo by metabolic processes that assimilate and process foods, that can repair structural damage or injuries to the nucleic acids, and that prevent the accumulation of harmful chemical substances. We recognize, also, that certain highly specialized mutual-security duties are assumed, such as scavenging (leukocytes and platelets), detoxication (liver), excretion (lungs and kidneys), and physical protection (osteoblasts).

With such a system, it is easy to see a great many points at which genetic factors could impinge, and indeed where they are known to impinge. It would be unwise to emphasize the exciting but exotic disorders such as xeroderma pigmentosum at the expense of these many other factors, since these genetic disorders are summarized in other chapters. There emerge, however, two points that seem important to my purpose.

First, it is likely that genetic factors in length of life operate in the Galtonian, or multifactorial, fashion. This conclusion will provide a strong incentive not to prune the data extensively. The very nature of our task is the analysis of an aggregation of factors which is, at present, unlikely to be resolvable into its component parts by any amount of refinement in analysis.

Second, the true pattern of inheritance is likely to be complex, and not necessarily amenable to the attractive limit theorems in which mathematical statistics abounds. In particular, we note that such complications as cybernesis, weakest-link failures, nonadditivity, and emergence must be reckoned with, but are commonly ignored by the probabilist.

Many of the more fundamental and elaborate cells, such as those of the blood, seem in principle capable of being sustained indefinitely in the absence of catastrophic changes in the stem lines. Many tissues multiply very efficiently in the face of damage and destruction. It is not obvious, however, why some, such as the kidney, cannot do so well as the liver and the lymph glands. The brain is, of course, unique in that its major function involves storage of information from the exterior, a function presumably not readily transmitted to a replacing cell; even so, there is reason to suspect that the predominant effect of age on brain is not a loss of cells, but a decrease in volume, perhaps of cytoplasm (Konigsmark and Murphy, 1972). The repair of the kidney by kidney tissue may involve problems of organization that are simply too great for postuterine life, though it is not easy to see why what is feasible *in utero* should be irrecoverably lost. The possibility nonetheless exists that as the body matures, it abdicates the means of surviving by repair.

3.3. Aging May Be an Exogenous Process

Alternatively, we may suppose that aging is due to the accumulation of insults or "hits" from the exterior. I shall deal first with the idea that it may be purely exogenous, that is, that there is no interior component, no heightened vulnerability, that contributes to the process. We might imagine this process of gradual attrition by wear and tear as having a literally continuous impact, or as consisting of discrete injuries delivered probabilistically from the exterior. If these results are cosmic, i.e., have no purely local component, it would be reasonable to suppose that they occur at constant hazard. Under such circumstances, whatever internal changes there may be, heightened or lowered susceptibility as a result of previous hits, the waiting time for each hit would follow an exponential distribution. If death is to result whenever a certain number of hits have arrived, the so-called "multiple-hit" model, the total waiting time until death would follow the sum of exponential distributions, the Erlangian distribution. If all injuries occur sequentially at constant risk, the waiting time will follow the gamma distribution. The gamma model fits the survival patterns of certain individual cells (notably erythrocytes and blood platelets) reasonably well, though the data are not such as to allow any stringent tests.

We are confronted at the start with three substantial facts. First, every exponential distribution is positively skewed; that is, the third moment about its mean is positive. Second, the sum (or convolution) of random variables, each of which is positively skewed, will itself be positively skewed (in fact, the skewness of the sum of independent random variables is the sum of the constituent skewnesses). Third, survivorship data, in man at least, are, with considerable consistency, negatively skewed. This discordance, which will be explored more fully later, calls for some revision of the simple multiple-hit model. It may be noted that even if the vulnerability of cells increases or decreases according to the amount of damage already sustained, the waiting time for each individual hit will still be exponential and the skewness of the whole positive. The risks might, of course, change systematically with time—for example, as a result of pollution—and under certain circumstances, this change would lead to negative skewness in the total waiting time. But it is not at all clear that such systematic cosmic changes occur with any great regularity. Certainly if data were available for constructing survivorships over a period of a thousand years or so, a distribution with persistently negative skewness would not be readily explained in this fashion. These ideas will be more fully developed in Section 5.

4. Analysis of Empirical Data

This topic is at once the most gratifying and the most exasperating of the three. It is gratifying in that the instincts of the scientist are to solve problems by appeal to the actual, rather than to the possible. It is exasperating because it brings clearly into focus the imprecision of the whole endeavor.

It is obvious that environmental factors bear on survival. A man in the prime of health may be killed by a meteor, which is as close to a purely random factor as one can imagine. The tendency in an analysis of the genetics of survivorship is to argue that such an occurrence is pure "noise"; that it cannot possibly tell us anything nontrivial about the process of senescence; that the analysis should be adjusted accordingly, as it would be were a subject lost to follow-up. But then, once this precedent is established, it is difficult to see, on principle and not merely by arbitration, where to stop. Cosmic rays seem to be every bit as much a purely random accident, and while they occur so much more frequently than meteors that over a matter of years their behavior may, in accordance with the laws of large numbers, be treated as though it were deterministic, there is no coherent ontological difference between the two. To introduce the qualification "we are not interested in bizarre and rare accidents" is an uncomfortably arbitrary constraint. How rare is a "rare" accident? It leads to difficult decisions as to whether death by being struck by lighting or drowned in a tidal wave should be eliminated. It is not clear whether accidental deaths should be excluded, or death from assaults, or in military service, or involvement in an overwhelming epidemic. To take the matter of adjustments to the extreme, we would compensate for all causes of death, the random causes because they are random and the nonrandom causes because they are nonrandom. Such adjusted data would show that everybody is immortal, and since the essence of genetic analysis is variation, we would have reached an impasse. There are genuine difficulties over infections, for example. A man might die of exposure to an infectious disease introduced from a distant planet. It might be argued that an ideal man would have resisted this infection. Equally, it might be said that since the human race has never been exposed to this infection, it is irrelevant to the genetics of survival, at least in an evolutionary context. But what if another man, also exposed to it, survives? Are we to adjust him "out of the data" also? What if we suspected, but could not prove, that he survived for random reasons that had nothing to do with resistance? But also, and less fancifully, on the basis of the argument of no previous exposure, what are we to do about the historical studies on the impact on the Eskimos of the introduction of measles?

All these are real issues, and I do not see any way of solving them in principle. We may use arbitrary decisions (as indeed we ourselves have done in dealing with our own data), but that they are arbitrary compels the belief either that the issue of genetic factors in survival is inadequately defined or that the question is fundamentally meaningless and hence has no solution at all. The problem is indeed much deeper and has much more widespread implications. The causal dichotomy—the question whether the cause of something is genetic or environmental—is a false one, as geneticists have long since recognized. The answer of quantitative genetics (Kempthorne, 1957; Falconer, 1960) has been to partition the variation of phenotypes according to its real, or apparent, origins. The method seems to have some utility, to judge by the advances in selective breeding, though whether they could have developed as quickly by the "black box" methods of the last century is not clear. But it is not always clear what the results of an analysis may mean scientifically. *Heritability,* a term used in various senses to mean the heritable component of the variance, is distressingly brittle, sensitive not only to the environment and (rather more disturbingly) to the genetic structure of the population, but also to the mathematical model that is assumed in the analysis. The latter fact is indeed obvious enough: the first and second moments are sufficient (in the technical sense) for the parameters of a multivariate normal distribution, but not, in general, for other distributions. For instance, in the mixed models of quantitative inheritance (Morton, 1967; Murphy and Bolling, 1967), they are not sufficient. Genetic components may reside in something other than the means, variances, and covariances of sample data.

These arguments demand two conclusions. First, whatever results we may obtain from the analysis are tentative and should always be handled provisionally and with the utmost circumspection. Second, we should give some serious consideration to the mathematical models that we intend to employ. The latter topic will now be the subject of further discussion.

5. Models of Aging

We may suppose three broad classes of models: a purely external process, a purely internal one, and a mixture of the two. Let us consider them separately.

5.1. External Models

We may suppose that the whole process is simply a matter of an insult or an accumulation of insults from the exterior. Some of these insults can be identified; for instance, we have reason to believe that cosmic rays cause aging. Because of their origin, we have excellent grounds for supposing their intensity to be on the whole fairly constant over time and, because of their hardness, their effect to be little influenced by some of the more common secular changes in the environment such as atmospheric pollution. In these circumstances, a single-hit process should have an exponential waiting time (which is positively skewed). If death results from the accumulation of such injuries, the net result is a multiple-hit or Erlangian function which, for any number of hits, is always positively skewed, though in the limit, the surviving time would be normal and therefore symmetrical. A familiar example of such a process is that in which the risk for each hit remains constant throughout, the so-called "gamma function," which we have applied extensively to analyze survival of blood platelets (Murphy and Francis, 1971), and which has been adopted as an analytical procedure by the International Committee for Standardization in Haematology (Belcher *et al.,* 1977). In fact, with suitable adjustment of parameters, the general Erlangian function can be approximated by the more stereotyped but also more tractable gamma function (Murphy, 1971). Taking this model as our starting point, we may modify it in various ways (Fig. 2).

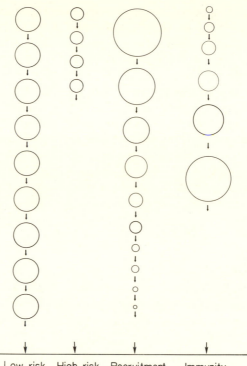

Fig. 2. Four variations on the multiple-hit model. Each column of circles represents a series of containers through which fluid is passing with complete mixing at every stage. Survivorship corresponds to the transit time through the entire system. Transitions from one container to another represent accumulation of further injuries. A big container represents a long mean transition time, and conversely. Where risk is low and damage small (first column) or both are high (second column) but all steps are similar, we have the gamma process. Recurrent insults may be progressively more easily produced and more damaging; i.e., recruitment occurs (third column). Such would be the case with recurrent acute glomerulonephritis or processes involving sensitization. Conversely, recurrent exposure may enhance resistance, and aging occurs more slowly (fourth column). Such systems could be elaborated and generalized in various ways.

Death may result from failure of any one of a number of vital organs. The heart, brain, kidneys, liver, adrenal glands may any one fail when destroyed by sufficient environmental insult. If one insult suffices to destroy each (not all are necessarily susceptible to the same size of insult or at uniform risk), survivorship should have an exponential distribution at a hazard equal to the sum of the hazards, or in more familiar terms, if there are k vulnerable targets and the average waiting time for the type of hit that will destroy the ith organ is m_i, then the average survival for the entire organism M is given by the familiar reciprocal formula from optics:

$$\frac{1}{M} = \frac{1}{m_1} + \frac{1}{m_2} + \cdots + \frac{1}{m_k}$$

This model may be made more elaborate and more realistic by supposing that these organs all have some reserve and that failure results only when a number of insults have been received. The results may be called (for obvious reasons) a *bingo model*. If the probability of bingo for the ith organ (i.e., it has received enough insults to destroy it) by time t is denoted by $F_i(t)$, and if it may be supposed that the events are all independent, the probability that the i is not destroyed is the complement, and hence the probability that all organs have survived, $S(t)$, is given by

$$S(t) = \prod_{i=i}^{k} [1 - F_i(t)]$$

The probability density may be found by taking the absolute value of the derivative.

The bingo model is one that has not received much attention,* even though it is an obvious means of representing failure in a multicomponent system. Let us consider some simple examples. Suppose that there are k vulnerable parts, each at the same risk (which, for simplicity and without loss of generality, we shall suppose to be of unit intensity) of destruction by a single insult. Then, as is well known, the probability of *not* being destroyed by any particular one of them in time x is given by e^{-x}. Hence, supposing independence, the probability of all k systems being intact at the end of that time is

$$(e^{-x})^k = e^{-kx}$$

which is simply an exponential process with risk intensity of k and therefore, like the constituent processes, positively skewed.

This system can be generalized so that it takes n hits to destroy a system. Then, it is well known (Murphy and Francis, 1971), the probability of survival of any particular system to time x is

$$e^{-x} \left[1 + x + \frac{x^2}{2!} + \cdots + \frac{x^{n-1}}{(n-1)!} \right]$$

*There is a hint of this idea in Wilson (1974): "To the extent that natural selection leads to a postponement of the effects of deleterious genes, there will tend to be a piling-up of such harmful, programmed effects toward the end of, or after a normal life span." He does not explicitly discuss, however, the mechanism of postponement or the impact on skewness (see below).

The joint probability of all k systems surviving to x is this quantity raised to the power k. This function may be differentiated and its sign changed to give the probability density function $f(x)$:

$$f(x) = ke^{-kx}\left(1 + x + \cdots + \frac{x^{n-1}}{(n-1)!}\right)^{k-1}\left(1 + x + \cdots + \frac{x^{n-2}}{(n-2)!}\right)$$

This distribution has interesting properties. Depending on the values of n and k, it may exhibit various degrees of skewness, including, for large values of n, negative skewness. Some results are shown in Fig. 3. To keep the scales manageable, each distribution is linearly transformed so that the time scale is reduced by a factor of n and the probability density increased by a factor of n (these rescalings do not change the shape or symmetry of the curves). In each diagram, the position of the mode is represented by a vertical line. Two values of k are selected, 10 because of interest in a small bingo process and 250, which was chosen because it is the number of loci Cutler (1975) believes germane. I have not endowed the latter number with any critical significance, but it is of interest that the degree of negative skewness encountered is comparable to that in human survivorship data. It will be evident that for small values of n, the distribution is positively skewed, and conversely for large values of n.

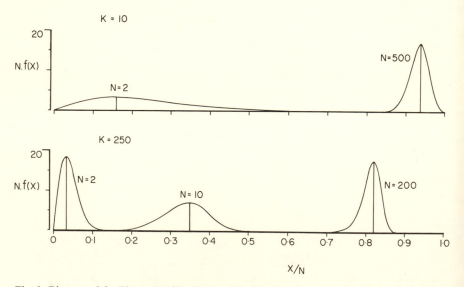

Fig. 3. Bingo models. The probability density functions are shown for 10 identical competing gamma systems (top) and 250 identical competing gamma systems (bottom). Where the order of the gamma process (N) is small, the distribution is positively skewed; i.e., its highest point is asymmetrically displaced to the left. Where (N) is large, the distribution is negatively skewed.

Table I.   Symmetry of the Bingo Model with 250 Competing Gamma
Processes of Order n

F_{max}/n ╲ n	Mode	Ascending limb			Descending limb		
		0.1	0.25	0.5	0.1	0.25	0.5
1	0.0000	—	—	—	0.0092	0.0055	0.0028
2	0.0316	−0.0307	−0.0293	−0.0218	0.0695	0.0566	0.0307
3	0.0875	−0.0691	−0.0576	−0.0430	0.0863	0.0668	0.0470
4	0.1416	−0.0954	−0.0767	−0.0553	0.0983	0.0769	0.0549
5	0.1891	−0.1116	−0.0879	−0.0623	0.1037	0.0817	0.0587
10	0.3480	−0.1353	−0.1027	−0.0705	0.1040	0.0829	0.0603
20	0.4984	−0.1291	−0.0962	−0.0651	0.0903	0.0724	0.0531
50	0.6597	−0.1022	−0.0753	−0.0504	0.0671	0.0540	0.0398
200	0.8200	−0.0606	−0.0443	−0.0295	0.0379	0.0305	0.0220
∞	1.0000	−0.0000	−0.0000	−0.0000	0.0000	0.0000	0.0000

NOTE: Each line is scaled by dividing through by n. The values shown are the distances from the mode at which the indicated fraction of the modal density is attained.

Table II.   Ratio of the Mode to the Median for a Bingo
Model with 250 Competing Gamma Processes of
Order n

n	Mode	Median	$\dfrac{Mode}{Median}$
1	0.00000	0.00277	0.000
2	0.06325	0.07633	0.829
3	0.26256	0.27306	0.962
4	0.56658	0.56819	0.997
5	0.94552	0.93593	1.010
10	3.47962	3.41065	1.020
20	9.9683	9.7989	1.017
50	32.986	32.603	1.012
100	75.111	74.484	1.008
∞	—	—	1.000

Unfortunately, the conventional measures of skewness are very tedious to compute for this model. Table I, however, shows some typical results for $k = 250$. The mode and the times for the mode at which ½, ¼, and ¹/₁₀ of the modal value are attained are shown for various values of n. For a symmetrical distribution, corresponding times should be symmetrically placed about the mode. Manifestly, they are not. For $n = 1$, there is no ascending limb at all. For $n = 50$, the values are all closer to the mode on the descending than on the ascending limb, indicating negative skewness. Another, more conventional, criterion is given in Table II. With $k = 250$, for low values of n, the mode is smaller than the median; for $n > 5$, the median is smaller than the mode. For $n = \infty$, the probability density curve is an infinite spike at n, and the median and the mode coincide.

5.2. Internal Models

It may be supposed that the environment has little to do with survival, which depends on some purely endogenous process. There is ample evidence from the study of both entire organisms and individual cells that survival varies appreciably. It is difficult to account for a describable random component without appealing to quantum mechanics, which seems an implausible explanation. Indeed, much of what has been written about the survivorship of individual cells (mostly blood cells) is based on the assumption of a deterministic process and a fixed life span. The methods of exhaustion of the reserves of a cell or a tissue were discussed in Section 3.2. It may be, then, that variation among individuals is ascribable to variation in their natural endowment, and there is no reason the survival curve should assume any particular form; at present, the biological mechanisms are too complex to attempt any real interpretation. The weakness of the model, however, lies much deeper. It seems scarcely believable that the process of aging is totally unrelated to the environment.

5.3. Composite Models

These models derive conceptually from the model of red-cell survival proposed by Mills (1947). It basically supposes that there is a finite fixed endogenous survival that may be cut short by a random exogenous process, the latter being, in Mills's instance, at constant hazard and thus tending in itself to produce an exponential survival. (His scheme could in fact be viewed mathematically, though not biologically, as a bingo model in which one process is exponential and the other is an infinite-hit process, which behaves deterministically since it has a coefficient of variation of zero.) The form of Mills's model is thus

$$S(t) = e^{-at} \qquad 0 < t < L$$
$$= 0 \qquad \text{elsewhere}$$

L being the length of the finite endogenous span. It is analytically easy to show (what intuition would suggest) that if $1/L$ is large relative to a, the random component becomes negligible and the whole behaves deterministically, and if it is small, the curve is indistinguishable from a simple exponential. Generalizations of the fixed component are not available (since whatever gives the earliest deterministic death will always define this component of the process), but there is no reason the exponential component should not be replaced by a gamma, Erlangian, or bingo process, or, for that matter, by any other process. There seems to have been curiously little interest in exploiting such models, although they are analytically much easier to handle than the bingo models.

We can understand the idea of a "mixed" model in another sense: that the aging depends on the external insult, but that the reaction depends on the native endowment of the organism. Thus, the "number of hits" to destruction may vary genetically; indeed, in the instance of xeroderma pigmentosum, such seems clearly to be the case, and other disorders are analyzed elsewhere in this volume. Alternatively, the threshold that an insult must attain to do damage may vary. For example, those with much skin pigment can tolerate strong sunlight much better than those without.

Recently, Woodbury and Manton (1977) proposed a random-walk model of aging. This model has certain nice properties, but the statistical details have not been worked out, nor is there any attempt to apply it to actual data. I confess to some disappointment at the total lack of concern with physiological details. The operation, one feels, is successful, but the patient has died.

5.4. Constructive Models

I shall use this term to designate what are at best feeble models in the biological sense, and which are in fact descriptive devices that the statistician has used because they happen to fit the data and could be used to "reconstruct" it fairly accurately. Sometimes there is a half-hearted attempt to attach biological meaning to the components of the models afterward, but often even this effort is not made. In consequence, while these models provide an excellent basis for interpolation or in multiple adjustments for covariables, their use in extrapolation is fraught with peril. Here I am indebted to Dr. Ann Zauber (1976), who reviewed the literature very fully and herself made extensive use of these methods in analyzing our data.

The cardinal idea in these models is the hazard function or the ratio of the density function to the complement of the distribution function. We may roughly state it in the following terms: Consider a member of the class (in this context a person) who at some particular time t is still alive. We will suppose that the probability of dying in some very small interval of time of length h immediately following t is $h \cdot a$; that is, the probability of death between t and $(t + h)$ is ha. Then a is referred to as the hazard. Now a may be a constant (as it is in the exponential process), or it may be a function of one or more variables—e.g., of time or the age or sex of the patient. For the general Perks (1932) function, if we let the variable of interest be time t, the hazard function $H(t)$ is

$$H(t) = \frac{A + e^{B+Ct}}{1 + e^{D+Ct} + Ke^{-x}}$$

where A, B, C, D, and K are all constants. If we let $K = 0$ and D becomes infinitely negative, the hazard function assumes the form

$$H(t) = A + e^{B+Ct}$$

which is the Makeham model. If we further let $A = 0$, we have

$$H(t) = e^{B+Ct}$$

which is the Gompertz model. If, finally, we let $C = 0$, we have

$$H(t) = e^{B}$$

which is a constant and constitutes an exponential process. Thus, by specialization of a general function, we may generate all the major functions that have been of interest in this context.

These models have been shown to have a considerable utility in that they fit observed data well. They have the advantage that with a suitable choice of constants (tending to make B small relative to C), the resulting model has a negative skewness. The problem from the standpoint of the biologist is the interpretation of these processes in physiological terms. I know of no interpretations of the logistic model that have any relevance to the present problem. Greenwood (1928) gave the following interpretation of the Makeham model: A is the environmental component and e^{B+Ct} is the "physiological constitution," which I would take to mean a purely endogenous process. Greenwood comments that the separation is an unrealistic one, but my criticism would lie deeper. Why would the hazard change with the age of the patient? The formulation smacks of a *deus ex machina* to deal with the problem of fitting the data, without having any interpretation to which meaning can readily be given. We are driven back on the old problems. We may suppose that there is some intrinsic process that makes the subjects more vulnerable to external injury, and not only is there no hint as to what this process is, but also there is no suggestion as to why it should operate. Anything we have learned in the last fifty years about human physiology suggests no such process. If, on the other hand, we suppose (as Greenwood hints) that there is some external process that alters the susceptibility of the subjects to insults, it is very far from clear why this should have anything to do with the *age* of the patient and not with the passage of *time*. To be sure, the two are highly related, but one would make three distinctions showing that the ideas are not interchangeable: First, the hazards from the exterior may change over time, and thus (if this is the source of the change in susceptibility) ''aging'' may occur at different rates from time to time. Second, if the subject is protected from the external injury, ''aging'' should be capable of being slowed down or possibly prevented altogether. Third, and most important, these distinctions, which might be trivial in a deterministic process, assume major force in a stochastic process.

There is another point about the foregoing hazard–function approaches that must not be obscured by the complexities of the models. They are all one-hit processes, which implies that the first encounter is lethal. It is not difficult to imagine situations (earthquakes, for instance) in which this assumption may be compelling. There are plenty of instances, however, in which an encounter may or may not be fatal, but a nonfatal outcome does not mean that the episode disappears without trace; susceptibility to, or the course of, subsequent results may be modified. Examples include recurrent acute glomerulonephritis or pneumonia before the era of sulfanilamide. A one-hit process would necessarily imply that provided the subject survived the attack, it would make survival in any subsequent attack exactly the same as though the first attack had not occurred: risk of death would depend only on the age of the patient. These claims for all types of possible lethal diseases would not appeal to many physicians or biologists.

6. Studies of the Inheritance of Longevity

6.1. Previous Studies

The belief that there is a heritable component in longevity is widespread, ancient but so far lacking substantiation. It is not necessary to point out that the existence of familial components is not unequivocal evidence of genetic factors, since much more is shared among members of a family than genes alone—culture, psychological atmosphere, climate, diet, and so forth. But it seems a reasonable argument that the converse applies—that if there is no familial component, there is probably no genetic component.

While one must regret the lack of good evidence, a realistic appraisal will make it clear wherein the difficulties lie and why so many writers have had recourse to flawed data. Human genetic studies are never easy, especially where, as the arguments of Sacher (1959, 1975) and Cutler (1975) suggest, the pattern of inheritance is unlikely to be simple. Age-dependent manifestation of inherited traits, such as Wilson's disease or polyposis coli, adds further complications, and manifestly longevity is the age-dependent trait *par excellence*. The difficulties of maintaining such studies over the long period of time necessary to obtain interpretable results are formidable, especially from a logistic and fiscal standpoint, as the investigators of coronary diseases and other chronic diseases know to their cost. Finally, there are so many known or suspected environmental factors that influence length of life and that have been changing rapidly over the last two hundred years or so that even striking correlations within families are liable to be ascribed to some source of bias. I do not imply that these difficulties should be glossed over. The exigencies of logic can make no concessions to the elusiveness of evidence. Empirical proof of heritability of longevity is difficult to obtain, and it is easy to understand why the topic has not been popular and investigators have resorted to easier and more immediately rewarding, if less direct, sources of evidence. I am indebted to an excellent review by Cohen (1964) for a fair-minded but critical perspective on the literature, a source that those interested in details are advised to consult.

In the face of the constraints outlined above, investigators have had recourse to three types of studies.

First are studies of genealogies, such as those of Bell (1918), Yuan (1931), Pearl and Pearl (1934), and many others. If the issue were a Mendelizing trait, this approach would be entirely appropriate, since the members of the family would segregate into groups, the genetic evidence residing in the contrast between the groups, and the segregation ratios would be testable against the predictions of the Mendelian model. But so often, families were selected because of remarkable longevity among some of the members. If they are selected because of remarkable longevity, what can one expect but that they should be remarkably longevous? It is difficult to think what they are to be compared with or what findings would have been expected if there were no genetic component in longevity. For the more far-flung genealogies, one may wonder about the quality of data in early centuries, and so forth.

Second are studies on total populations, such as that of Preas (1945). Here, in principle at least, one is on firmer ground, since there is a population of reference of which the families are representative, and the subjects are thus not being selected because they are extraordinary (as a result, perhaps, of chance aggregation alone). But there remain major problems of attrition and differential weighting by fertility, itself a function of age. There is a large group of studies, which Cohen (1964) reviewed in some detail, in which the subjects are relatives of holders of life insurance policies. The problems are that those accepted for insurance are selected, in part, because of family history, and the information on the ages and causes of death in relatives is hearsay evidence and usually not authenticated by other means. One must wonder not only how accurate the information is, but also what sources of bias may be operating.

Third, studies have been done on longevity of twins, notably by Kallmann (1957) and his associates and by Hauge *et al.* (1963). They show considerable similiarity, more marked in monozygous than in dizygous twins, although the study by the former group shows that the mean difference decreases with age (the latter finding is doubtless an artifact arising from the constraint imposed on the variance by progressive increase in the age of the proband). In many ways, data of this kind are the most satisfactory from a genetic standpoint. Nevertheless, one must acknowledge a general feeling of disillusionment among geneticists about the utility of twin studies. Results from them for a wide variety of different traits and diseases show the foregoing kind of pattern with considerable regularity; one would perhaps have expected some major exceptions and, lacking them, may wonder about the power of this method. Would it still give the same pattern of result if the characteristic studied had no genetic component whatsoever? Moreover, contrary to what is commonly supposed, dizygotic twins are more closely related than sibs because, among other matters, they share a common uterine environment, and monozygotic twins probably share it more intimately than dizygotic. Again, postnatal management will in most cases be influenced by what zygosity is, or is believed to be. I have pointed out elsewhere (Murphy, 1972) that it would be of interest to compare phenotypes in twins of each type of zygote according to whether or not the parents believed them identical. To my knowledge, the point has not been exploited. Some of the newer techniques, notably the comparison of half-sibs with the progeny of identical twins (Nance, 1973; Christian *et al.,* 1976), may be fruitful in this regard.

It is of interest that Cohen (1965) and her associates are engaged in a study of familial factors in the cause and age of death. So far, only limited preliminary results have been published, and the later findings will be awaited with great interest.

Philippe (1976) recently gave a brief presentation on the results of a population-based study of longevity. No details of this study are available at the time of writing, but the heritable component is small.

6.2. The Baltimore Longevity Study

Between 1920 and 1934, Pearl and Pearl (1934) conducted a study on longevity in man. The data on some 2300 persons who had attained the age of 90 were individually ascertained. For each, the sum of the ages at death of the parents and the grandparents was divided by 6 to give a "total index of ancestral longevity" (TIAL). The mean TIAL was compared with that computed for patients attending the Pearls' clinic for "constitutional" diseases, which was a kind of precursor of a clinic for medical genetics. Not unexpectedly, perhaps, the investigators found a much higher average value in the parents of the nonagenarians.

The results are difficult to interpret. A superficial criticism would condemn the study as totally unacceptable by modern standards, and we ourselves have stated some of the more obvious defects (Hawkins *et al.,*

1965). Yet it would be difficult to defend these criticisms in detail or to justify the alternate procedures that a modern epidemiologist would propose, and this difficulty stems precisely from the ambiguities in the fundamental issue that have been discussed previously. This subject is one in which the sterotypes of epidemiology are inadequate. For instance, consider the choice of controls. We have objected that the ancestors of a patient attending the Pearls' clinic because of tuberculosis are likely themselves to have tuberculosis and a shortened life on that account; thus, the Pearls have biased controls. But is this a legitimate criticism? Is not the clustering or the absence of clustering of tuberculosis within families precisely one of the familial contributors to longevity or the lack of it? It will be argued, of course, that such a factor may be familial, but, tuberculosis being infectious, not genetic. The conclusion, however, is scarcely warranted. The environmental and the genetic components are completely confounded in such a study in exactly the same way that they are in familial studies of coronary disease (Murphy, 1967, 1975). That there are undoubted genetic factors in resistance to tuberculosis is shown by the total resistance of certain species to the infecting organism. Is it unreasonable to suppose that one of the genetic factors operating in the nonagenarians was a genetic resistance to tuberculosis in them and their stock? This is not a mere quibble. Nobody would argue either that falciparal malaria is not infectious or that sickle hemoglobin is not a clear hereditary trait. Least of all would anyone argue that they are totally unrelated. Yet what method would the conventional investigator propose for getting unrelated controls to study longevity in carriers of sickle trait living in a malarious district?

Or, again, we have criticized the Pearls for their ascertainment of cases, which depends on a haphazard collection of sources: newspaper cuttings and the like. There is, by the modern canons, a deplorable lack of any population of reference. The conclusions from the Pearl study, however, were not *logically* dependent on the probands: they were not about the probands seen as a representative sample of nonagenarians, but inferences about their ancestors, conditioned on the probands. To be sure, even the latter may be unrepresentative, but while biases may exist in principle, they can be given substance by only the most contrived surmises—for example, that the ascertainment of the probands *depends* on the age of death of their ancestors. Indeed, whatever criticisms may be leveled on this score of bias apply equally well to our own studies on descendants of the probands, which are conditioned on ascertainment in the same way.

6.3. Our Extension of the Baltimore Study

In 1960, the Pearls' data, long sequestered in dark places, came to light, and the opportunity was seized to explore the pattern of survival in the progeny of the probands. The tracing of the records (Hawkins *et al.,* 1965) and the compiling of the data have been under the direction of Abbott. The study was terminated in 1970, and the results, already partially published (Abbott *et al.,* 1974), are still being analyzed. The tracing, though tedious, is surprisingly efficient, some 90% of the families explored having been completely traced (see Section 6.3.2).

6.3.1. Principles of Preliminary Analysis

Preliminary analysis was conducted in accordance with the principles stated below, some of which are admittedly more or less arbitrary and open to dispute. It is to be remembered, however, both that these decisions were made *a priori* and not *a posteriori* and that they are uniformly applied throughout the data.

1. Deaths by violence and by accident are so unlike death from other causes that they should be analyzed separately.

2. Deaths in infancy, childhood, and adolescence are highly atypical and, since they preclude reproduction, are unlikely to bear on genetic components of extreme longevity. Accordingly, all progeny who did not attain the age of 20 were eliminated from the analyses.

3. Since expected life span is greater in women than in men, survival to age 90 is more remarkable in a man than a woman and, insofar as it is heredity, reflects a more remarkable genetic endowment. Accordingly, the analysis of the data should take account of sex both in the parent and in the progeny—for instance, by a 2 × 2 grouping. (A similar argument would be applicable to studies on body height.)

4. The most reasonable surmise would be any genetic component in survival should reflect contributions from both parents. Analysis must take account of the age at death of the nonproband parent as well. (Because this datum is missing in a few cases, we have been obliged to group data when using distribution-free methods.)

5. The most efficient means of analysis is likely to be one that uses measures of nonindependence (especially convariation or conditional expectations). The probands have, by definition, attained the age of 90, and few will live to be more than 100; thus, the variation due to the probands is small, especially in relation to the errors in the recorded ages in such a group. Moreover, there are some logical difficulties in treating this variation as if it applied to a random variable. In contrast, the age attained by the nonproband parent exhibits considerable variation, and there are no difficulties in seeing it as a random variable, in large part at least. Accordingly, considerable emphasis is given in the analysis to this factor. Logically, the survival of the nonproband parent may be viewed either as a source of variation that allows genetic factors in *length of life* to be explored or as a

covariable (nuisance variable) obscuring the inheritance of *longevity* (arbitrarily defined, for example, as survival to age 90) and one calling for appropriate adjustment.

6. It is more than likely that survival will reflect other factors, e.g., occupation and place of birth and death. These factors may be of considerable interest in both epidemiology and gerontology, but in the narrower context of genetics, they are covariables which it is desirable to eliminate. For nonparametric analyses this elimination is accomplished simply (if perhaps nonefficiently) by analyzing individually the results within groups.

7. In the first place, in the interest of simplicity, and for lack of any well-authenticated mathematical model, we have used the nonparametric or actuarial method. The entire survivorship curve is of interest and may be informative. We shall be content to present the sample means and standard deviations. These primitive methods have been used without prejudice to more refined methods, which will be applied to the data subsequently.

6.3.2. Completeness of Tracing

The methods of tracing the progeny of the Pearls' probands, though surprisingly effective despite the lapse of time, are nevertheless tedious to apply. I have been fortunate in both my collaborators and the devoted labor of our technical staff; we also must acknowledge the support of the National Institutes of Health, which funded this work for ten years.

Even so, it has not proved possible to trace all the families, and it was recognized at the start that this incompleteness would lead to risks of bias. Simply to study families easy to trace would undermine the representativeness of the sample. For instance, it is easier to trace families in which there are many offspring still alive; thus, a sample so compiled would be weighted in favor of more longevous offspring and hence perhaps exaggerate the apparent genetic component. To offset this defect, we argue as follows: With incompletely traced data, the opportunities for bias are least where almost all or almost none of the data are available. If 98% are traced and 15% are dead, the true sample proportion dead cannot be less than 15% or more than 17%. Likewise, if only 3% are traced, however unrepresentative this 3% may be, it will involve little distortion because it makes a very small contribution to the whole. But 50% tracing neither makes a small contribution nor allows setting of narrow limits on the proportion dead. Accordingly, the probands were grouped into consecutive batches of 100 following the original numbering system of the Pearls, and each technical assistant confined attention to one such group until tracing was complete or very close to it.

The completeness of tracing is indicated in Fig. 4, in which traced families are shown in white, untraced in black. Most groups are almost all

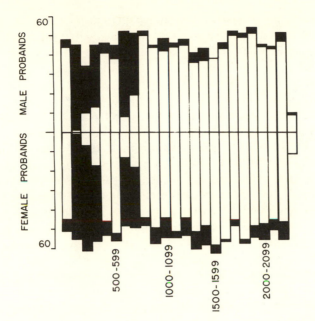

Fig. 4. Completeness of tracing. Each column represents a group of 100 consecutively numbered probands of the Pearls' series. Total families traced are represented in white, untraced in black. There are few groups in which the proportion traced is neither very low nor very high. Figures 4–8 reproduced from the *Johns Hopkins Medical Journal* by kind permission of the editor.

white or all black. The overall completeness of tracing was 78% for male probands and 74% for female, but in about half the groups, tracing was 90% or over (details are given in Abbott *et al.,* 1974). The incomplete families include those in which the proband was born outside the United States, so that (subject to this condition) the representativeness of those traced is even better assured than is apparent from Fig. 4, since the true rate of completion is higher. The "completeness" of the data does not mean, of course, that all the progeny are dead. A tracing is complete if at some stage in the study the age at death, or age when last heard of, was obtained for each progeny.

6.3.3. Analysis of Survivorship Curves

From the data are constructed standard survivorship curves. The mean survival is then easily estimated by finding the area under the survivorship curve (using the trapezoidal rule), and the variance may be found by differencing and computation by the usual method. (It should be pointed out that since the "effective sample size" is steadily decreasing, the standard error of the mean cannot be estimated in the usual fashion by dividing the estimate of the standard deviation by the square root of the sample size.)

To explore the genesis of longevity, it is clear that as in all genetic studies, a source of variance must be available. As pointed out above, the probands have by definition attained the age of 90 and, even under the best of circumstances, cannot be expected to live many years longer. There is thus little "opportunity" for variance from this source. Of course, if extreme longevity is a Mendelian trait, variation in the phenotype of the proband is unnecessary. Age at death of the progeny should be bimodal (in accordance with the inheritance or noninheritance of the gene). Bimodality should show up as a double sigmoid survivorship curve that should be, as it were, ξ-shaped rather than S-shaped. On the other hand, if we believe that what genetic component there is relates not to a category "longevity" but to a quantitative variate "length of life," the other parent should be a substantial contributor to the outcome, with the added advantage that in the absence of constraints, there is a large component of variance with which variance in the progeny may be compared. Arguments are given in Section 6.3.1 for grouping both the probands and the progeny separately by sex, in view of well-established differences in mean survival.

The ordinary system for studying the impact of length of parental life on that of the progeny would be by bivariate regression analysis. The main obstacle to this simple approach is that often the ages at death of the progeny (and occasionally of the parents) are unknown, because they are lost to follow-up, or are still alive. Thus, we do not always know the outcome value, merely a lower limit on it. In such circumstances, the obvious remedy is to construct a parametric model and estimate the final length of life in those cases in which it is not known.

6.3.4. Analysis of Longevity Studies

The analysis is proceeding in two steps, nonparametric and parametric. Nonparametric analysis by the so-called "Greenwood life-table" or actuarial method (Greenwood, 1926) has the virtues of simplicity, familiarity, and freedom from controversy. Its main defects are its relatively low statistical efficiency, its inelasticity, and its failure to throw any light on fundamental mechanisms. The method furnishes a survivorship curve that in any real situation is doubtless accurate, and a standard error can be derived from which at least approximate confidence limits can be constructed. These limits are relatively wide, but are sound. We might reasonably require that any parametric model, to be acceptable, should give a fitted cohort curve that for most of its length falls within these confidence limits.

Of course, it would be hoped that the parametric model would generate its own test of goodness of fit, but it must in any case meet this criterion.

The defects of the life-table method, however, must also be weighed. Given a homogeneous set of data, the curve can be fitted, although we cannot expect it to be smooth, especially for small samples. In this study, however, the surmise of heritability implies that the data are *not* homogeneous, but that survivorship should depend on age at death of the parents. The actuarial method is not designed to cope with such a continuous variation. Accordingly, we have had to be content to divide the data by sex of proband, sex of progeny, and into three classes by age at death of the nonproband parent—12 classes in all. The results are displayed graphically in Figs. 5–8, and a few simple statistics are given in Table III. Note that this solution is marred by two defects: (1) First, the grouping by survival of the nonproband parent is coarse, one group (< 60) comprising a very broad subpopulation. But finer grouping creates the familiar problem of small sample size and exacerbation of the consequences of sampling variation. Even the broad grouping, however, gives us some indication of the existence and size of trends. The other problem is misclassification. A parent aged 84 and still alive when last heard from creates no problems, but one of 65 will be classed in the middle group (Age at death . . . 61–80), although the actual age at death may be 90. Only a few of the parents yield such ambiguous results, however, and I have no doubt that the distortion is small and that the results, for what they are, are sound. Note, however, that there are many other items of information (see below) that may bear on survival.

Table III. Estimated Mean and Standard Deviation of Life Span by Sex of Proband, Sex of Progeny, and Age of Nonproband Parent at Death[a]

Sex of proband	Sex of progeny	Age of nonproband parent at death (years)	Number of progeny	Estimated mean	Estimated S.D.
Male	Male	$\leqslant 60$	295	67.6	18.8
		61–80	676	71.4	18.8
		> 80	596	73.2	18.6
	Female	$\leqslant 60$	334	73.8	19.4
		61–80	764	74.1	18.0
		> 80	570	77.2	18.7
Female	Male	$\leqslant 60$	442	67.0	20.0
		61–80	928	69.3	18.8
		> 80	461	70.9	18.7
	Female	$\leqslant 60$	394	73.0	19.7
		61–80	955	73.5	19.2
		> 80	455	73.3	20.5

[a]From Abbott *et al.* (1974).

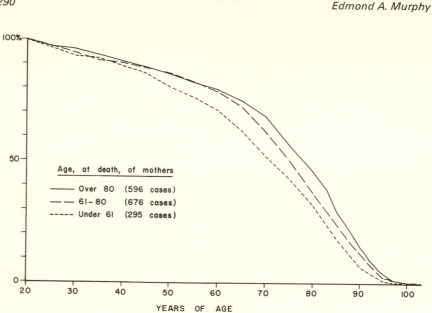

Fig. 5. Actuarial survivorship curves in sons of male probands, grouped by life span of their mothers. Here and in Figs. 6–8, there is no evidence of more than one inflection point such as would accord with a unilocal trait.

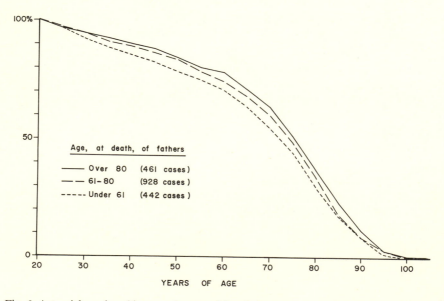

Fig. 6. Actuarial survivorship curve in sons of female probands, grouped by life span of their fathers.

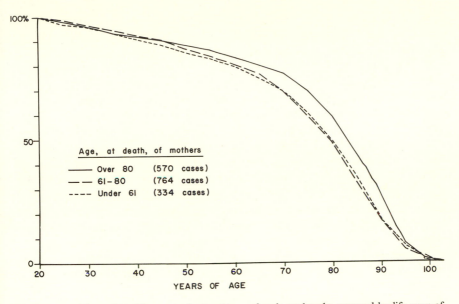

Fig. 7. Actuarial survivorship curves in daughters of male probands, grouped by life span of their mothers.

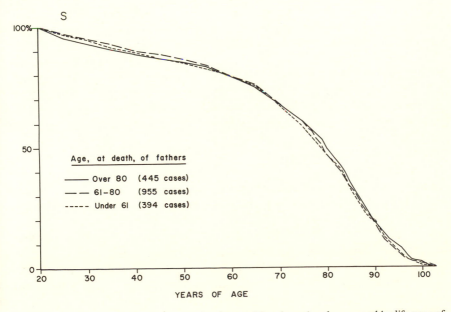

Fig. 8. Actuarial survivorship curves in daughters of female probands, grouped by life span of their fathers.

To analyze these results adequately calls for extensive subclassification and analysis, which involves much calculation based on progressively smaller samples.

The details are not altogether consistent, but the broad trends are clear enough. Parental age does have some impact on length of life. The results are most striking for sons, less so for daughters, especially where the proband is female (i.e., where we are looking at the impact of paternal age). Detailed tables (Abbott *et al.,* 1974) suggest that the familial component bears no clear relationship to year of birth, and that the maternal contribution is perhaps twice that of the paternal. Even in the latter case, the difference in the mean values for the offspring in the most, and the least, longevous mothers is only about 5 years, although the difference in the mean survival of the nonproband mothers is (by definition) well over 20 years. The familial component is therefore comparatively small, especially where the fathers are concerned. The question must arise as to what these results may mean.

1. The familial component may be genetic. Here we think of four broad groups of mechanisms. Mendelian traits in which life is shortened are numerous, and the normal alleles would be associated with long life. It was recently claimed (Glueck *et al.,* 1977) that the condition hypobetalipoproteinemia apparently protects against coronary disease and conduces to long life. The findings are promising. But in general, we have an embarrassing lack of well-established "supergenes" that would promote health and lead to unusual longevity; whether this lack is an artifact due to the mode of ascertainment of most Mendelian traits in man (more often than not from genetic clinics) remains to be seen. This explanation, however, does not help us explain why in our study the maternal influence on survival is greater than the paternal. In some small degree, it can be accounted for by nonpaternity, but this can scarcely account for a 50% reduction.

Other genetic mechanisms are somewhat more helpful. Galtonian (multifactorial or polygenic) inheritance seems, in the light of common sense and the studies of Sacher and Cutler quoted earlier, a much more plausible route. To be sure, ordinary mechanisms would not account for the sex difference, but it is well known (Murphy and Chase, 1975) that sex differences occur where there is reason to suppose a threshold of expression, for instance, in congenital pyloric stenosis. The possibility exists that such a mechanism may lead to a quasi-qualitative change that bears on some as yet unidentified critical phenomenon of, say, middle life.

The third possibility is that length of life may be related to minor chromosomal changes. Again, one may appeal to many instances of such changes that lead to a shortening of life, or even neonatal death, but I know of no precedent of a chromosomal change leading to enhanced fitness, although there are some examples of neutral chromosomal polymorphisms known. The data do not quite square with some known effects of parental sex on transmission of chromosomal anomalies. For translocations, for instance, it appears that carrier mothers are something like ten times as likely to transmit the trait to their progeny as carrier fathers are, this effect operating regardless of the sex of the offspring. In our longevity data, however, it is the progeny, not the parents, who exhibit the sex difference.

The same criticisms apply to the fourth possibility, that the mode of transmission is cytoplasmic.

2. Environmental factors may lie at the bottom of the familial effects. We must then find a mechanism to account for the sex differences. Certain of them have been explored in detail (Abbott *et al.,* 1970, 1974, 1977).

For example, we might argue that sons, especially the oldest sons, are most likely to inherit the family business or farm and that they are therefore exposed to the parental environment longer than the daughters, who are likely to marry and move elsewhere. We have several ways of testing this hypothesis. The trend is much the same whether the son had the same occupation as the father or not. For sons (but not for daughters), the trend is greater if the father and progeny both lived in similar domiciles in either a rural or an urban area. There is a similar but less clear difference in the sexes where the issue is concordance or nonconcordance with the usual residence of the mother. It might be argued that unmarried daughters (who would probably live at home) would show the same pattern as the sons, and this proves to be so. But curiously enough, the trend is much the same whether the daughter habitually lived in the same state as the parent or in a different state. Firstborn sons are more like their fathers than later sons, but this difference is abolished if we compare fathers and sons who died in different states.

We might expect that where the cause of death of the parent and of the child of the same sex (father and son or mother and daughter) is the same, there would be a marked trend, and there is indeed approximately 14 years difference in the mean for the highest and lowest parental age groups, which is remarkably consistent over all groups. This age trend is the steepest in any factor we have explored. It is largely an artifact, however, since age of onset and death vary from one disease to another, and also since (in the diagnostician's mind) the plausibility of a diagnosis is influenced, at least partially, by the age of the patient at presentation. It is noteworthy that where the causes of death in parent and child differ, there seem to be no trends at all.

We are thus led to surmise that the familial component in survivorship may be in large part mediated through the cause of death. This conclusion seems to have two implications. First, the familial component is perhaps negative—not a tendency to long life, but an absence of a tendency to short life. The blood β-lipoprotein level, quoted above, would be one such example. I make this point with some diffidence, not merely because of the crudity of the present analyses, but also because of the possibility of artifacts arising from the rather artificial constraints of death certification (there seems little doubt that in many cases the "cause of death" is far from clear, but the requirements of death certification call forth a spurious clarity). The second implication is that the uncertainty as to whether the familial component is genetic or not remains clearly unresolved. Despite widespread complacency among clinicians on the point, it is still far from clear whether the familial aggregation of such common disorders as coronary diseases, hypertension, and diabetes is to be ascribed to genetic factors or to diet, trace metals, infectious processes (such as slow viruses), or other environmental factors. Furthermore, our skepticism should not be blunted because one can produce several rare types of each of these disorders that are undoubtedly Mendelian (Murphy, 1973, 1975; Rimoin and Schimke, 1971).

a. Parametric Approaches. Zauber (1975) explored extensively the applicability of multiple-hit models to the foregoing data. The cardinal problem is that, as has been previously mentioned, the distribution of survival in these data, as in most other published material, is negatively skewed, whereas all Erlangian models without competing pathways give positively skewed distributions. It is of course well known that certain transformations, such as the use of logarithms, will make skewness less or even negative. If we were prepared to suppose that the hazard is increasing such that on a logarithmic scale the process would become time-homogeneous, we would perhaps be able to develop a negatively skewed survival function from a multiple-hit process. This solution to the problem is rather contrived, however, and does not lead to any biologically illuminating insight. On the other hand, the bingo model described above is both plausible and promising, but the development of the bingo model described above is too new to have been applied to our data.

b. Constructive Models. In the course of a doctoral thesis, Zauber (1976) made extensive use of the Makeham model (see above) as a descriptive device for our data. The goodness of fit is excellent. A representative curve is shown in Fig. 9. The method of maximum likelihood was used to estimate the parameters, which allows all data, whether completed life span is known or not, to be utilized. Estimated mean survival and the appropriate parameters are given in Table IV.

This way of representing the results points up the weaknesses and the strengths of constructive models. Goodness of fit of the curve to the actuarial (Greenwood) results is excellent (Fig. 9), with the added advantages of smoothness and the assurance that the analysis is statistically efficient. The main problem is in interpreting the parameters themselves.

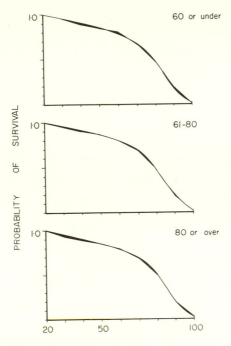

Fig. 9. Goodness of fit of the total survivorship curve to the best-fitting Makeham curve determined by maximum likelihood estimation. Discrepancies are indicated in solid black, so that the degree of congruity can be easily assessed. Considering that the actuarial curve is rounded to 10-year intervals, the fit is excellent. Drawn from the data of Zauber (1976).

Zauber shows that in fact the estimates are not independent, and one might surmise as much from Table IV, for although the estimated *mean survivals* show reassuring trends (which only in the last line fail to show the expected increase), the trends in the estimates of the *parameters* are anything but orderly, as can be seen by inspection. Of course, it is clear that an aberration in one parameter can, because of correlatedness, be compensated for by a contrary aberration of the others. If, however, we were to take Greenwood's interpretation of the parameters of the Makeham model literally—that *A* is an environmental component, whereas the other term in the hazard function is a physiological component representing aging—then we are further than ever from a coherent understanding of what is going on. Of course, it is neither fair nor useful to criticize this otherwise excellent method for failing at what it is not designed to do; I merely wish to make the point that to the geneticist's mind, there is more to analyzing data than precision, power, and the other virtues extolled in statistical textbooks.

Table IV. Point Estimates for the Parameters of the Makeham Model[a]

Proband	Progeny	Age of nonproband parents at death (years)	Maximum likelihood estimates			Mean survival (years)
			$A\ (\times 10^5)$	B	$C\ (\times 10^2)$	
Male	Male	60 or less	53.2	−9.96	9.31	67.67
		61–80	40.6	−10.58	9.88	71.41
		81 or more	44.5	−11.95	11.37	73.15
	Female	60 or less	45.1	−11.81	11.05	73.65
		61–80	37.5	−11.43	10.70	73.99
		81 or more	40.0	−14.03	13.45	77.20
Female	Male	60 or less	69.6	−10.96	10.48	67.11
		61–80	52.6	−10.65	10.11	69.02
		81 or more	43.6	−10.70	10.03	71.01
	Female	60 or less	48.9	−12.08	11.39	73.19
		61–80	45.2	−11.97	11.28	73.62
		81 or more	51.3	−12.30	11.54	73.56

[a]Data of Zauber (1976). This model is most succinctly represented by its hazard function: $\mu = A + e^{B+CT}$.

7. Summary and Conclusion

It will be evident that this field of investigation has been impeded by a general failure to confront the fundamental issues. In some degree, solving the problem of the genetic control of length of life is a trivial one that will answer itself from common experience alone. We cannot accept the notion that harmful alleles relatively shorten life without accepting the tautologous conclusion that the nonharmful alleles relatively lengthen life. Differences in length of life from one species to another, which not only are a matter of common sense but also have been extensively documented, clearly imply a genetic factor if we are prepared to accept that from a biological standpoint, the "executive" mechanism that accounts for the differences among species is genetic programming. Those who believe that behavior is ascribable ultimately to the unfolding of the individual genetic constitution would argue, with reason, that habits of life that impinge on survival and are commonly considered environmental are in fact simply indirect, rather than direct, manifestations of genetic factors. None of these ideas would be repugnant to common sense, but on these terms, it is difficult to imagine how studying them could fall within the domain of science. What manner of experiment or collection of data could refute them? If proving that the familial component of life span is not due to some direct and regrettably elusive impact on life-force but, more prosaically, to an immunity to infectious disease or to a gut that absorbs cholesterol more slowly, we have done nothing to our assessment of genetic factors, merely to their explication.

In this inquiry the real dichotomy—if we must make one—is not the old and rather meaningless distinction between "genetic" and "environmental" components, but rather between systematic and random components. Here we are obliged to take a little care in our terminology, for segregation of genes is ordinarily thought of as a random process, whereas the main emphasis I would like to make is on the random *accidental* component. Inasmuch as the scientist in general and the actuary in particular are interested in prediction, they must regard the cutting short of life by being struck by a meteor as totally accidental. I find it very difficult to imagine how such a process could have any relevance to genetics, although perchance it might have a profound effect on evolution. On the other hand, a predilection for climbing mountains may lead to accidental death and yet have a large component of the systematic, and therefore have important genetic implications.

A second major issue arises from the confusion surrounding the word *longevity*. *Webster's* (1970) gives (among others) two meanings: "a long duration of individual life" and "length of life." From the geneticist's standpoint, the difference would be analogous to that between "hypertension" and "blood pressure." In approaching it, we might either set up a category "longevity" and look perhaps for a segregation of the life spans of the progeny into a small number of groups; or treating length of life as a continuous variable, we might look at partitions of variance, correlation coefficients, and the like. The two approaches would follow the familiar analyses furnished by Mendelian and Galtonian genetics, respectively. The design of the Baltimore study has in fact allowed us to test both approaches. If longevity were a dominant trait, we might look for bimodality, or even segregation into clear groups, in the distribution of the length of life in the progeny. There has been no evidence of this pattern in any of the populations studied, as is evident from Figs. 5–8, in which none of the curves has more than one inflection point. But we can also capitalize on the variation in the age at death of the nonlongevous parent to test for a Galtonian component. As we have discussed at length, there seems undoubted evidence of the existence of such a relationship between parent and child, although the regression coefficient seems to be considerably less than 10%. On the other hand, detailed analysis of the results shows no readily recognizable pattern, and while we may speculate about cytoplasmic inheritance or purely cultural factors, cogent means of testing for them or arriving at clear interpretations have eluded us so far.

There are those who may wonder how worthwhile it is to explore characteristics so intricate and so broad as length of life, rather than to focus sharply on precisely defined biochemical mechanisms such as are discussed elsewhere in this volume. I have three arguments to put forward. First, there is little to be said for looking for explanations of familial longevity until there is evidence that it indeed exists. The prospector always precedes the chemical engineer in the rational society. Second, nature abhors a vacuum, and while the fastidious may disdain the use of black-box analysis of empirical data, the physician and the actuary are often content to make use of conclusions based on vague experience that does not meet even the minimal canons of sound empirical sampling. A Galtonian analysis can, at the very least, improve on that. But most of all, a long accumulation of evidence and experience has cast doubt on the facile assumption that the characteristics of the organism are nothing but the aggregate of isolated effects from individual genes. There are now several lines of inquiry suggesting that evolution and the operation of fitness are not vested in the locus but in the complex emergent phenotype, which may have properties that are in no way to be inferred from the parts. In the same way (to quote a familiar illustration), one could not readily infer the wetness of water from the gaseousness of hydrogen and oxygen. The whole topic of emergence is too large and too complex to discuss here, but the conflicting and paradoxical nature of the data unearthed in the course of the drift–

selection controversy of the last five years may find its resolution in the idea of a pattern that transcends the Mendelian trait. Certainly, despite small early triumphs, we seem to have made little progress in our understanding of the genetics of coronary disease in the last quarter century.

The following broad conclusions seem to be warranted by the data adduced herein:

1. In those who have survived to the age of 20, there is a clear and almost uniform familial component in the length of life. Expressed as a regression, this does not seem to amount to more than a 1-year increase in survivorship in the progeny for every 10 years in the parent.

2. There is no clear evidence to suggest whether this aggregation is due to genetic factors (including genetic factors influencing behavior) or to purely cultural or environmental factors that would be transmitted equally well to adopted children. Preliminary analyses suggest that part, at least, of the mechanism is of the latter type.

3. On the supposition of genetic inheritance of one type or another, the details of the pattern of transmission do not conform to any well-recognized mechanisms, and the possibility of some unusual mechanisms such as cytoplasmic inheritance must be borne in mind. On the other hand, the complex patterns observed may be the resultant of several different mechanisms.

4. A detailed resolution of the components of inheritance must await the practical development of some promising analytical developments that have recently become available.

References

Abbott, M. H., Murphy, E. A., Bolling, D. R., and Abbey, H., 1970, The hereditary component in longevity, Proceedings of the annual meeting of the American Society of Human Genetics, Indianapolis, *Am. J. Hum. Genet.* **22**:19a (abstract).

Abbott, M. H., Murphy, E. A., Bolling, D. R., and Abbey, H., 1974, The familial component in longevity. A study of offspring of nonagenarians. II. Preliminary analysis of the completed study, *Johns Hopkins Med. J.* **134**:1–16.

Abbott, M. H., Murphy, E. A., Bolling, D. R., and Abbey, H., 1977, The familial component in longevity. A study of offspring of nonagenarians III. Intrafamilial studies (in prep.).

Ayala, F. J., 1970, Teleological explanation in evolutionary science, *Philos. Sci.* **37**:1–15.

Ayala, F. J., 1972, The autonomy of biology as a natural science, in: *Biology, History and Natural Philosophy* (A. D. Breck and W. Yourgrau, eds.) pp. 1–16, Plenum Press, New York.

Bateson, G., 1972, *Steps to an Ecology of Mind,* Chandler, Toronto.

Belcher, E. H., Berlin, N. I., Ernisse, J. G., Garby, L., Glass, H. I., Heimpel, H., Lee, M., Lewis, S. M., McIntyre, P. A., Mollison, P. L., Murphy, E. A., Najean, Y., Pettit, J. E., and Szur, L., 1977, Recommended methods for radioiostope platelet survival studies: A report by the panel on diagnostic application of radioisotopes in haematology by the International Committee for Standardization in Haematology, *Blood* (in press).

Bell, A. G., 1918, *The Duration of Life and Conditions Associated with Longevity: A Study of the Hyde Genealogy,* Genealogical Record Office, Washington, D.C.

Benjamin, B., 1959, Actuarial aspects of human lifespan, in: *Ciba Found. Colloq. Ageing* (G. E. W. Wolstenholme and M. O'Connor, eds.), Vol. 5, *The Lifespan of Animals,* pp. 2–15, Little, Brown and Co., Boston.

Christian, J. C., Cheung, S. W., Kang, K., Harmath, F. P., Huntzinger, D. J., and Powell, R. C., 1976, Variance of plasma free and esterified cholesterol in adult twins, *Am. J. Hum. Genet.* **28:**174–178.

Cleaver, J. E., and Bootsma, D., 1975, Xeroderma pigmentosum: Biochemical and genetic characteristics, *Annu. Rev. Genet.* **9:**19–38.

Cohen, B. H., 1964, Familial patterns of mortality and life span, *Q. Rev. Biol.* **39:**130–181.

Cohen, B. H., 1965, Family patterns of longevity and mortality, in: *Genetics and the Epidemiology of Chronic Diseases* (J. V. Neel, M. W. Shaw, and W. J. Schull, eds.), pp. 237–263, U.S. Department of Health, Education and Welfare, Washington, D.C.

Cutler, R. G., 1975, Evolution of human longevity and the genetic complexity governing aging rate, *Proc. Natl. Acad. Sci. U.S.A.* **72:**4664–4668.

Falconer, D. S., 1960, *Introduction to Quantitative Genetics,* Ronald Press, New York.

Framingham Study, 1968, *An Epidemological Investigation of Cardiovascular Disease,* Section 19, U.S. Government Printing Office, Washington, D.C.

Glueck, C. J., Gartside, P. S., Mellies, M. J., and Steiner, P. M., 1977, Familial hypobetalipoproteinemia: Studies in 13 kindreds, *Clin. Res.* **25:**517 (abstract).

Greenwood, M., 1926, A report on the natural duration of cancer, *Rep. Public Health Med. Subjects* **33:**1–26.

Greenwood, M., 1928, "Laws" of mortality from the biological point of view, *J. Hyg.* **28:**267–94.

Hauge, M., Harvald, B., and Degnbol, B., 1963, Hereditary factors in longevity, in: *Genetics Today* (S. J. Geerts, ed.), Proceedings of the 11th International Congress of Genetics, Pergamon, New York.

Hawkins, M. R., Murphy, E. A., and Abbey, H., 1965, The familial component in longevity. A study of offspring of nonagenarians. I. Methods and preliminary report, *Bull. Johns Hopkins Hosp.* **117:**24–36.

Kallmann, F. J., 1957, Twin data on the genetics of ageing, in: *Ciba Found. Colloq. Ageing* (G. E. W. Wolstenholme and M. O'Connor, eds.), Vol. 3, *Methodology of the Study of Ageing,* pp. 131–143, Little, Brown and Co., Boston.

Kempthorne, O., 1957, *An Introduction to Genetics Statistics,* John Wiley & Sons, New York.

Konigsmark, B. W., and Murphy, E. A., 1972, Volume of the ventral cochlear nucleus in man: Its relationship to neuronal population and age, *J. Neuropathol. Exp. Neurol.* **31:**304–316.

Lewontin, R. C., 1973, Population genetics, *Annu. Rev. Genet.* **7:**1–17.

McDougal, W., 1924, *Outline of Psychology,* pp. 130ff, Scribner, New York.

Mills, J. N., 1947, The life-span of the erythrocyte, *J. Physiol.* **105:**16p–17p.

Moore, G. E., 1903, *Principia Ethica,* Cambridge University Press, London.

Morey, E., Haller, R., and Baylink, D., 1977, Cessation of bone formation during space flight, *Clin. Res.* **25:**498A (abstract).

Morton, N. E., 1967, The detection of major genes under additive continuous variation, *Am. J. Hum. Genet.* **19:**23–34.

Murphy, E. A., 1967, Some difficulties in the investigation of genetic factors in coronary disease, *Can. Med. Assoc. J.* **97:**1181–1192.

Murphy, E. A., 1971, The estimation of blood platelet survival. III. The robustness of the basic models, *Thromb. Diath. Haemorrh.* **26:**431–449.

Murphy, E. A., 1972, Application of genetics to epidemiology, in: *Trends in Epidemiology* (G. T. Stewart, ed.), pp. 102–138, Charles C. Thomas, Springfield, Illinois.

Murphy, E. A., 1973, Genetics in hypertension: A perspective, *Circ. Res.* 21 (Suppl. 1):129–137.

Murphy, E. A., 1975, Genetic factors in coronary heart disease, in: *Sandorama,* November, Vol. II, pp. 4–6, Sandoz, Barcelona.

Murphy, E. A., and Bolling, D. R., 1967, Testing of single locus hypotheses where there is incomplete separation of the phenotypes, *Am. J. Hum. Genet.* 19:322–334.

Murphy, E. A., and Chase, G. A., 1975, *Principles of Genetic Counseling,* Yearbook, Chicago.

Murphy, E. A., and Francis, M. E., 1971, The estimation of blood platelet survival. II. The multiple hit model, *Thromb. Diath. Haemorrh.* 25:53–80.

Nance, W. E., 1973, Monozygotic twin kinships: A new model for the analysis of quantitative inheritance in man, *J. Clin. Invest.* 52:60a (abstract).

Pearl, R., and Pearl, R. D., 1934, *The Ancestry of the Long-Lived,* Johns Hopkins University Press, Baltimore.

Perks, W., 1932, On some experiments in the graduation of mortality statistics, *J. Inst. Actu,* 63:12–40, cited in Benjamin (1959).

Philippe, P., 1976, Genetics of longevity, *Excerpta Med. Int. Congr. Ser.* 397:192 (abstract).

Preas, S., 1945, Length of life of parents and offspring in a rural community, *Milbank Mem. Fund Q.* 23:180–196.

Rimoin, D. L., and Schimke, R. N., 1971, *Genetic Disorders of the Endocrine Glands,* C. V. Mosby, St. Louis.

Sacher, G. A., 1959, Relation of lifespan to brain weight and body weight in mammals, in: *Ciba Found. Colloq. Ageing* (G. E. W. Wolstenholme and M. O'Conner, eds.) Vol. 5, *The Lifespan of Animals,* pp. 115–133, Little, Brown and Co., Boston.

Sacher, G. A., 1975, *Antecedents of Man and After,* Vol. 1, *Primates: Functional Morphology and Evolution* (R. Tuttle, ed.), pp. 417–441, Mouton, The Hague, cited in Cutler (1975).

Stanley, S. M., 1975, A theory of evolution above the species level, *Proc. Natl. Acad. Sci. U.S.A.* 72:646–650.

Trivers, R. L., and Hare, H., 1976, Haplodiploidy and the evolution of social insects, *Science* 191:249–263.

Webster's Seventh New Collegiate Dictionary, 1970, G. & C. Merriam Co., Springfield, Massachusetts.

Williams, G. C., 1957, Pleiotropy, natural selection and the evolution of senescence, *Evolution* 11:398.

Wilson, D. L., 1974, The programmed theory of aging, in: *Theoretical Aspects of Aging* (M. Rockstein, ed.), pp. 11–22, Academic Press, New York.

Wolstenholme, G. E. W., and O'Connor, M. (eds.), 1959, *Ciba Found. Coloq. Ageing,* Vol. 5, *The Lifespan of Animals,* Little, Brown and Co., Boston.

Woodbury, M. A., and Manton, K. G., 1977, A random-walk model of human mortality and aging, *Theor. Popul. Biol.* 11:37–48.

Yuan, I. C., 1931, Life tables for a southern Chinese family from 1365 to 1849, *Hum. Biol.* 3:157–179.

Zauber, A. G., 1975 (unpublished).

Zauber, A. G., 1976, Multiple regressions with censored survivals in a Makeham model with application to longevity, Ph.D. thesis, Johns Hopkins University, Baltimore.

Chapter 10

A Longitudinal Study of Aging Human Twins

Lew Bank and Lissy F. Jarvik

1. Introduction: History, Methodology, and Purpose

Just about a century ago, Galton (1876) initiated the use of twins in human research, thus taking advantage of the regular natural occurrence of both monozygotic (one-egg or identical) and dizygotic (two-egg or fraternal) twins. Inasmuch as monozygotic (MZ) twins are genetically identical— whereas dizygotic (DZ) twins are no more alike in terms of their genes than any pair of nontwin siblings—and since twin partners generally share a similar environment from conception on, comparisons of differences between the two members of a twin pair provide cues to genetic and environmental influences on various traits. To say it another way, if within-pair differences are significantly smaller for one-egg than for two-egg pairs (i.e., if the one-egg pairs have the significantly higher concordance rates), then we have presumptive evidence for a significant influence of genetic factors on that trait.

Another method of gaining helpful information from the lives of twins is to observe a group of MZ twins with their cotwins in different life conditions or under different planned regimes. This method, called the "co-twin control method," is also useful when natural discordance takes place (e.g., one psychotic and one nonpsychotic twin, or one married and one

Lew Bank • Department of Psychology, University of California at Los Angeles; Veterans Administration Hospital, Brentwood, Los Angeles, California   *Lissy F. Jarvik* • Department of Psychiatry, University of California at Los Angeles; Veterans Administration Hospital, Brentwood, Los Angeles, California

unmarried twin). In such cases, "longitudinal comparisons of aging patterns, biochemical tests, or psychometric scores may prove illuminating as to etiology, diagnostic classification, treatment procedures or personality assessment, provided the given twins are monozygotic" (Kallmann and Jarvik, 1959).

Literally hundreds of twin studies investigating human attributes and behaviors have been performed since Galton's time. The majority of these twin studies, however, concentrate on children and younger adults, and obviously these studies cannot provide information on the later stages of life. The study of elderly twins allows comparisons over virtually the entire human life span. Thus, childhood and adulthood factors may relate to particular adult and senescent traits and behaviors; in addition, relationships between these life-history variables and survival may be studied.

The particular study on which this chapter will focus is the New York State Psychiatric Institute Study of Aging Twins, begun in 1946 by Franz Kallmann and Gerhard Sander, in the course of which data from over 2000 twins were collected for a long-term investigation of hereditary aspects of aging and longevity (Kallmann and Sander, 1948, 1949). Data analyses were limited to 1603 twin "index cases" who had reached the age of 60 and were residents of New York State or neighboring areas. A subset of intact pairs in this sample was selected for psychological testing based on further restrictions, including fluency in English—so that language difficulties would not obscure interpretation of psychological test results—and availability of both twins at the time of field visits (a period of several months). In addition, among the DZ twins, only same-sex partners were used so as not to confound zygosity differences with sex differences. Initially, 120 pairs fit all constraints (Feingold, 1950). In 1949, 14 more pairs were added, giving a total sample of 268 subjects. These 268 subjects have either been followed to the completion of their lives or are still alive; they were originally tested in 1947–1949 (Kallmann and Sander, 1949; Feingold, 1950), and survivors were retested in 1955, 1957, 1967, and 1973. As of 1973, there were 61 survivors, and 21 of them were still alive at last contact.

A great deal of information has emerged from this longitudinal study of senescent twins, the only such study reported to date, and some of this information will be reviewed in this chapter.

2. Genetic Factors and Survival

In one of their initial reports on the senescent twins, Kallmann and Sander (1949) tested the hypothesis that heredity is a significant factor in determining the human life span. Though only 58 twin pairs had completed their life histories at that time, the results were clear: intrapair differences in life span were significantly smaller for MZ than for DZ twins.* Mean intrapair differences ranged from 36.9 months for MZ twins to 126.6 months for opposite-sex DZ twins, with same-sex DZ partners averaging 78.3 months between their deaths.

Successive biennial analyses on deceased MZ and same-sex DZ twins showed increasing intrapair differences in longevity for the one-egg twins; in contrast, those for two-egg pairs decreased for males and increased for females (Jarvik *et al.,* 1960). The average intrapair differences were, however, greater at all times for the DZ than for the MZ group, even when the sexes were examined individually. This observation is in accord with expectation, since, as the study continued, the passage of time allowed more extreme intrapair differences in survival to manifest themselves; hence, the increasing life-span differences for one-egg pairs (Kallmann and Jarvik, 1959). Further, as more and more twins approached the asymptotic portion of the survival curve, similarity in length of life was bound to increase as the result of the limited human life span. This tendency is clearly illustrated by the converging of life spans of *both* male and female twin partners in *both* zygosity groups (Jarvik, 1971). Even at the oldest ages (over 80 years of age), however, intrapair differences in life span were still less for MZ than for DZ partners, although not significantly so.

The data permitted examination of intrapair differences not only in survival, but also in certain diseases. Thus, Jarvik and Falek (1961, 1962) reported malignant neoplastic disease (cancer) in 68 of the 1603 twin index cases.† Interestingly, cancer was a cause of death in 9.2% of both MZ and same-sex DZ twins, a finding that does not support the higher rate expected in MZ twins according to the hypothesis of Macklin (1940) that twinning represents a tendency toward tumor formation (Jarvik and Falek, 1961). It is also noteworthy that the rate of 9.0% cancer deaths among the aging twins (including opposite-sex DZ and "unclassified" twins) was lower and not higher than the rate of cancer deaths in the New York State population for the same age group (16.5%). The lowered cancer death rate existed for twins of both sexes, both zygosity groups, and all three age groups (60's, 70's, and 80's), and could reflect the diagnostic rigor of the twin study, which undoubtedly resulted in failure to identify some unknown number of deaths due to cancer. The discrepancy may also be due in part to artifacts, as, for example, a reluctance among physicians to make the diagnosis of cancer for a deceased twin when there is a known surviving cotwin (Jarvik and Falek, 1961). There are other explanations; to name just one more, twins selected for survival beyond age 60 could thereby also have been selected for resistance to malignant neoplasia (Jarvik and Falek, 1961).

---

*All relationships in this chapter reported to be statistically significant are significant at or beyond the 0.05 level (i.e., $p \leq 0.05$).

†Jarvik and Falek (1961, 1962) also discuss 26 nonindex twin cases with cancer. Although those additional cases will not be considered here, including them would not alter the results.

Concordance rates for cancer among MZ and DZ twins were compared; the assumption was that similar percentages would indicate a lack of significant genetic factors in the etiology of the disease. Concordance rates were 25% for MZ and 4.3% for DZ pairs (Jarvik and Falek, 1962), in general agreement with four earlier studies of cancer in twins (Busk *et al.,* 1948; Harvald and Hauge, 1956, 1958; von Verschuer and Kober, 1956; Nielsen A., and Clemmesen, 1957); the average concordance rates for these five studies were 9.8% for 255 MZ and 5.1% for 704 DZ pairs. This difference between the two zygosity groups was statistically significant, leading Jarvik and Falek to conclude that some form of genetic control for cancer (resistance or susceptibility) exists, even though exogenous factors undoubtedly play a major role in the etiology of various forms of cancer. Because cancer does not appear to be a single disease entity, it is quite possible that genetic factors specific to particular forms of cancer are obscured in comparisons of the type noted here. Twin studies large enough to enable comparisons of each of the many forms of neoplastic disease are therefore necessary.

The importance of genetic predisposition even when the presence of a known infectious agent is a *sine qua non* in the etiology of a disease is illustrated by findings with regard to tuberculosis (derived from a twin study observing younger subjects) (Kallmann and Jarvik, 1957). Here, too, concordance rates were significantly—and dramatically—higher for MZ (61.5%) than for DZ (18.3%) twins or siblings (18.9%). The magnitude of the MZ–DZ difference for concordance rates on tuberculosis as compared with cancer may be due to the fact that tuberculosis is a single disease entity (tubercle bacillus). Genetic predisposition for the disease is not obscured by the confounding influence of a multitude of etiologies, as in cancer.

Illnesses linked to stressful life situations in our society (e.g., hypertension and ulcers) have become as threatening to human life as diseases such as cancer. A genetic propensity for marked physiological reactivity to situational stressors may exist. Bank and Jarvik (1976) examined the relationship between stress and survival in a group of 14 surviving intact twin pairs (12 MZ and 2 DZ) who had responded to items concerning childhood and adult stressors, including adult health stress variables (e.g., smoking, drinking coffee and alcohol). Initial analysis of the data revealed that no single stress factor or combination of factors could be used to discriminate between longer- and shorter-lived members of twin pairs. When the 28 twins were analyzed as individuals (i.e., without regard to the twin/cotwin relationship), however, a combination of factors I (stability of childhood home environment) and III (adult health) predicted survival with statistical significance.

These findings, though based on a small number of observations, suggest that differences in the life spans of genetically identical (and long-lived) twin partners cannot be predicted by the usual stressful events of daily life. In contrast, the same predictors worked quite well with genetically dissimilar subjects. Taken together, these results indicate a strong role for heredity in determining longevity, with normal external stressors contributing a significant, but less potent, effect.

3. Genetic Factors and Mental Functioning

3.1. Test-Battery Description and Initial Assessment

The data reviewed thus far have been concerned with associations between genetic factors and survival. Mental functioning can also be influenced by heredity, and particular psychological variables may be associated with survival. As mentioned above, 268 twins constituting 134 intact pairs, who were English-speaking, white, residing in or near New York State, and 60 years of age or older, participated in the psychological testing program. This test population closely resembled the population of New York State with regard both to sex ratio (male/female ratio 1:1.26 in twins, 1:1.2 in New York whites 60 years and older) and education (29% with high school degree or better among twins, in comparison with 27% in New York State). There were, however, proportionately more farmers in the sample than in the population of New York State, and correspondingly fewer residents of metropolitan areas; this difference was due to the large number of twins drawn from rural areas with stable populations.

Practically none of the twins had ever taken a psychological test before, and a major consideration in selecting the tests was to make the experience as interesting and nonthreatening to a group of elderly persons as was possible (Feingold, 1950). Further, since testing was done in the subjects' homes, constraints of practicality dictated that the tests be easily transported and administered. The battery included five subtests from the Wechsler–Bellevue (Wechsler, 1944): Similarities, Digits Forward, Digits Backward, Digit Symbol Substitution, and Block Design; Vocabulary List 1 (Terman, 1916) of the Stanford–Binet; and a simple paper-and-pencil Tapping test to evaluate hand–eye coordination. The formats of all tests except the Tapping test are commonly known. The Tapping test consisted of a 10×10 matrix of boxes. Subjects were instructed to put a dot into as many of the 100 boxes as they could within a 30-sec interval; single- as well as multidotted boxes counted for 1 point, and stray dots were ignored (Feingold, 1950).

The initial test round (Kallmann and Sander, 1949; Feingold, 1950; Kallmann *et al.*, 1951) revealed no significant differences between scores achieved by the twins (ranging in age from 60 to 89 years) and by the oldest standardization groups (ages 50–54 and 55–59 years) of Wechsler (1944). Since Wechsler sums Digits Forward and Backward to obtain a single score (Digit Span), only four subtest scores could be compared (Table I). Since

Table I.   Mean Psychometric Test Scores for Aged Population Samples (with Standard Deviations)[a]

Sample (investigator)	Age (years) group	N	Test			
			Digit span	Similarities	Block design	Digit symbol
Single-born	50–54	45	7.7 ± 3.11	8.8 ± 2.94	8.0 ± 2.91	6.8 ± 3.22
(Wechsler)	55–59	36	7.5 ± 3.23	7.9 ± 3.38	6.7 ± 3.55	5.9 ± 2.85
Twin pairs,						
present study	60–89	190–238	7.1 ± 2.61	7.5 ± 3.37	6.8 ± 2.74	6.5 ± 2.48

[a]From Kallmann *et al.* (1951). Copyright 1951 by the University of Chicago Press. Reprinted with permission.

the twins were on the average 15 years older than Wechsler's subjects, and since they did not exceed the educational level achieved by the general population of New York State, their scores evidenced no significant decline in ability on these measures. In addition, their performance indicated that twins, at least twins over 60, appear to be every bit as good as singletons on these tests (Wechsler's standardization group consisted of single-born individuals). This finding stands in contrast to results reported for school-age twins, in which performance of twins averaged below that of singletons (e.g., Byrns and Healy, 1936; Mehrotra and Maxwell, 1949).

First-round psychometric test scores were also used to compare MZ and DZ twin pairs. It is particularly interesting that the mean *intrapair* differences in test scores measuring abstract intellectual functioning were smaller for MZ than for DZ twins. For women, these MZ–DZ comparisons attained statistical significance on the Vocabulary, Digits Backward, Digit Symbol, Block Design, and Similarities tests. There was a similar trend for the male zygosity groups, but differences were not statistically significant. The failure to find significantly larger mean within-pair differences in DZ than in MZ male pairs may indicate that changes in intellectual abilities (at least the ones reported here) occur at an earlier age in men than in women (Feingold, 1950; Kallmann *et al.*, 1951). Women have a longer life span than men. Thus, it may be that there is a difference between the developmental patterns of the two sexes, with intellectual change occurring later in women than in men. A longitudinal study of men and women from around age 50 or 55 (rather than 60 and over) is necessary for an accurate comparison of the sexes.

3.2. Longitudinal Changes in Psychological Test Performance

Half the original test pairs were retested about 1 year after the initial evaluation period (Feingold, 1950), while the remaining half the sample were retested over a 2- to 3-year period; in a third assessment, available surviving twins were tested again about 8 years after the initial test round (Jarvik *et al.,* 1957). A fourth round, approximately 9 years after the first assessment, succeeded in obtaining data from only 17 surviving twins; this dearth of subjects resulted from a lack of funding and experimenter hours, rather than from the demise of an extraordinarily large number of twins (Jarvik *et al.,* 1962*a,b*).

The first retest data revealed no significant changes in any of the tests, whether the entire retested sample was considered together or separately for the four zygosity × sex subgroups (i.e., MZ male, MZ female, DZ male, DZ female.) Test–retest intraclass correlations were above 0.9 for each subtest, with a high of 0.996 for Vocabulary. The magnitude of these correlations demonstrated adequate reliability of assessment and provided baseline data for subsequent retests.

Due to various health problems (e.g., visual and auditory impairments), not all subtests could be administered to the 79 twins tested at the second retest period (26 MZ and 10 DZ intact pairs plus 7 broken-pair survivors, mean age 74.5 years). In fact, for one subject, no usable scores could be obtained. The number of subjects taking each test ranged from a low of 66 (Block Design) to a high of 78 (Similarities). Although the average performance on each test declined over the 8-year interval, the decrements in *nonspeeded* tasks were small, ranging from 3.0 to 6.5% and statistically not significant (see Table II). In contrast, decreases in performance on the speeded tasks (Block Design, Digit Symbol, and Tapping) ranged from 12.1 to 21.6% and were statistically significant. In general, over the years, there was considerable variability among test score patterns, with some subjects consistently declining, others staying much the same, and still others improving in performance (Jarvik *et al.,* 1957).

Working with the data from 48 subjects who completed all subtests at all three testings, Jarvik *et al.,* (1962*a*) found consistently higher scores

Table II.   Longitudinal Data on Intellectual Decline in Senescence[a]

Test	Number of index cases		Mean test scores of total sample (1947)	Mean test scores of retested subsample		
	Total sample	Sub-sample		1947	1955	Decline (%)
Vocabulary	240	72	28.40	30.74	29.82	3.0
Digit Symbol	190	67	27.81	29.31	25.75	12.1
Block Design	206	66	13.39	15.09	12.65	16.2
Similarities	230	78	8.85	10.35	9.68	6.5
Tapping	240	75	66.10	72.61	56.92	21.6
Digit Span	239	74	9.98	10.28	9.88	3.9

[a]From Jarvik *et al.* (1957). Copyright 1957 by S. Karger AG, Basel, Switzerland. Reprinted with permission.

than were exhibited by Wechsler's standardization group on the five Wechsler–Bellevue subtests. The Digit Span (Digits Forward plus Digits Backward) and Similarities test scores remained stable, while performance on the two speeded tasks—Digits Symbol Substitution and Block Design— showed some decline. Analyses on all seven subtests revealed significant decline in score only on the Tapping and Digit Symbol tests; the decrease in Block Design scores was not significant. Since the subgroup of 48 healthy subjects should be representative of the elderly functioning well in the community, comparisons of this subgroup with the Wechsler standardization group appear to be justified.

After a 12-year testing hiatus, 81 surviving twins participated in the 1967 follow-up round. Of these twins, 46 had taken the psychological test battery three times (1947, 1955, and 1967); for statistical analysis, however, 11 cotwins were removed from the sample. Mean ages for the remaining 12 men and 23 women were 85.7 and 84.6, respectively. Analyses revealed that significant declines had occurred for both sexes on all subtests with the single exception of Vocabulary. On this test, women scored slightly lower, but not statistically significantly lower, than they had in 1947 (Blum *et al.,* 1970).

These data suggest that at least among subjects who are sufficiently healthy and cooperative to continue to participate in a study over a 20-year span, there is general stability of nonspeeded cognitive performance to age 75 and possibly even longer. During the ninth decade of life, however, many abilities will decline. The notable exception found indicates that women, with a longer life span than men, seem to retain beyond age 85 what is perhaps the most basic tool of cognitive functioning, vocabulary.

It should be pointed out that the first retest showed a general *increase* in scores, an unexpected finding that was attributed to test familiarity acquired during the first test round. After all, most of the twins had been out of school at least 40 years at the time of the first test round and had no prior experience with the kinds of tests used in the study. Nonetheless, as noted earlier, some decline in performance—especially on speeded tasks— was seen at the second testing. In general, given an elderly non-test-wise group of subjects, one would expect artificially low initial scores, and substantial practice effects on subsequent retests. Thus, to gain a clearer perspective on changing (or stable) scores in a longitudinal study, plans should be made to administer a test battery on at least three different occasions (Jarvik *et al.,* 1962*a*).

The importance of the stability of scores on nonspeeded tasks, (at least to age 75) as compared with a general decline on the speeded tasks, ought to be emphasized. These results indicate that aging processes affect diverse skills differently. In fact, a factor analysis showed almost every variable forming its own specific factor; only Vocabulary and Similarities shared a factor (*verbal* ability), and Digits Forward and Backward loaded on the same factor, but Digits Backward did not load nearly so high as Digits Forward (Jarvik *et al.*, 1962*b*). It may therefore be appropriate, as the authors pointed out, to revise our thinking so as not to concentrate on intelligence *per se* in the elderly, but rather on a number of readily distinguishable intellectual functions. Besides, the intelligence construct itself has proved valid only in predicting an individual's educational success; even if we possessed a reliable measure of intelligence for the aged, we would hardly be interested in predicting their success in school. Working with individual mental abilities would do away with such problems as dealing with the importance of speed in assessing the intelligence of an aging population. Currently, the assessment of *competence* in the aged has been recognized as vital, and work in progress (e.g., Krauss, 1976; Marquette, 1976; Ohta, 1976; Schaie, 1976; Scheidt, 1976) is concentrating on the measurement of individual abilities.

Another way of looking at longitudinal change in the psychological tests is, of course, to compare MZ and DZ intact twin pairs. The obvious hypothesis is that MZ twins are more similar than DZ twins. As already noted, initial mean intrapair difference scores were smaller for MZ twins than DZ twins on all seven subtests. These differences were statistically significant on four of the seven.

By 1955, although the same trend was evident, the differences were no longer statistically significant, and the mean intrapair difference on Digit Span was smaller for the DZ than for the MZ group (Jarvik *et al.*, 1957; Falek *et al.*, 1960). The lack of statistical significance might have been due to the small numbers of intact twin pairs tested in 1955 (26 MZ and 10 DZ pairs) in comparison with 1947 (75 MZ and 45 DZ pairs), and the increased intrapair variability observed among MZ twins.

Based on scores from the 1967 follow-up, Jarvik *et al.* (1972) compared mean intrapair differences of 13 MZ and 6 DZ twin pairs. By this time, the gradually increasing variability among the MZ twins and the now evident decrease in variability among the DZ twins had resulted in highly similar intrapair differences between the zygosity groups; only on Digit Symbol Substitution did the MZ pairs still demonstrate substantially smaller mean intrapair differences than the DZ pairs. What these data suggest is unclear at present, but it is likely that a meaningful part of the variance can be explained by the selective nature of all longitudinal studies. As the twins grew older, those DZ pairs not endowed with a similar genetic propensity for survival were eliminated from analyses through the death of one partner, while the more similar DZ pairs remained intact. While based on limited data, blood groups are consistent with this hypothesis, with 5 of the the 6 DZ pairs participating in the 1967 test round showing very few within-pair differences (Jarvik *et al.*, 1972). If one assumes that survival and cognitive functioning are related, then decreasing variability on test performance within DZ pairs seems reasonable.

For the genetically identical MZ pairs, the additional years (1947–1967) allowed environmental factors to play a larger role in determining intellectual change. Thus, as the surviving intact pairs grew closer and closer to completing their lives (in 1967, the mean age for the 19 intact pairs was over 83), there was a tendency for intrapair differences between MZ and DZ twins to become more and more similar. This process was noted earlier in discussing genetic factors and survival (Section 2), and it appears to operate in the realm of cognitive functioning as well.

3.3. Psychological Testing and Prediction of Survival

In 1955, 168 of the original 268 twins were alive and 100 were dead. The retested survivors were found to have scored higher at initial testing on *each* of the seven subtests than had the nonsurviving twins. It was reasoned that these differences might reflect a positive relationship between ability and survival (Jarvik *et al.*, 1957).

In an effort to investigate the relationship between psychometric test score and survival, each of the 78 subjects participating in the 1955 follow-up study was labeled as increased, decreased, or unchanged on each of the seven subtests (Jarvik and Falek, 1963). Operationally defined, an increased score indicated a higher score in 1955 (the second retest round) than at either of the earlier testing periods; conversely, a decreased score represented poorer performance at the third than at either of the first two test rounds. A subject with a score neither higher nor lower than either of the first two test round scores was said to be unchanged for that particular ability. Percentages of the third-round sample labeled as increased, decreased, or unchanged are shown for each subtest in Table III. Note that the mean ages for each category do not associate increasing age with decreasing score, as might be expected were intellectual decline to be a direct function of aging. Only Block Design shows subjects with decreased performance to have a higher mean age at the last testing than subjects with unchanged or increased scores. For the four nonspeeded tasks, from 67.1 to 86.9% of the twins either improved or remained unchanged. Even on the speeded tasks, 36.3, 59.1, and 20.3% of the sample either remained unchanged or improved on Digit Symbol, Block Design, and Tapping, respectively. A general lack of consistency on subtest change for individual profiles was found, with increased or unchanged scores on some tests and decreased scores on others seeming to be the rule.

At the time of the report by Jarvik and Falek (1963), 14 of the 78 subjects with three test points had died. The remaining subjects had survived their test session by 2½ to more than 6 years. Using 5-year posttest survival as a criterion, subjects were classified as: (1) survivors, i.e., survived more than 5 years since last testing (this group included 1

Table III. **Mean Ages at Last Testing for Subjects with Increased, Unchanged, or Decreased Retest Scores**[a]

		Mean age (years)		
	Number of subjects	Increased scores[b]	Unchanged scores[b]	Decreased scores[b]
Vocabulary	75	75.8 (22.7%)	75.7 (45.3%)	75.6 (32.0%)
Digit Symbol	66	74.1 (13.6%)	77.7 (22.7%)	74.6 (63.6%)
Similarities	76	76.2 (17.1%)	75.4 (50.0%)	75.4 (32.9%)
Block Design	66	72.2 (16.7%)	74.7 (42.4%)	76.5 (40.9%)
Digits Forward	76	75.4 (23.7%)	76.0 (63.2%)	74.8 (13.2%)
Digits Backward	75	75.4 (17.3%)	75.9 (56.0%)	75.5 (26.7%)
Tapping	64	76.4 (3.1%)	77.9 (17.2%)	75.0 (79.7%)

[a]Jarvik and Falek (1963). Copyright 1963 by the Gerontological Society. Reprinted with permission.
[b]Figures in parentheses are percentages of subjects in each group.

person who died 9 years after his last testing), 34 persons; (2) nonsurvivors, i.e., survived less than 5 years, 13 persons; or (3) alive, but fewer than 5 years elapsed since the last testing, 31 persons. Subjects in the third category could be classified neither as survivors nor as nonsurvivors, so analyses were performed on the first two groups only.

A statistically significant relationship obtained with Vocabulary such that survivors were more likely to have improved or remained stable and nonsurvivors to have declined in this ability. For no other subtest did a significant difference between the two groups result until an *annual rate of decline* (ARD) was computed:

$$\text{ARD} = \frac{T_H - T_L}{T_H \times Y} \times 100$$

where T_H is the highest score on either of the first two testings, T_L is the score on the last testing, and Y is the years intervening between T_H and T_L. This computation demonstrated a relationship between 5-year survival and an ARD greater than 10% on the Similarities test, and greater than 2% on the Digit Symbol Substitution test. In accord with these findings, the concept of *critical loss* was developed and used to describe a change in score consisting of at least two of the following: a yearly decrement of 10% or greater on Similarities and 2% or greater on Digit Symbol, as well as any decline on Vocabulary. Returning *(post hoc)* to the subsample of twins with complete data on each of the three critical tests for each of the three test rounds, 22 of the 26 twins without critical loss were survivors, while seven of the eight persons with critical loss were deceased. It is worth noting that the deceased twins with critical loss constituted the *youngest* subgroup. It is also interesting that two of the three predictor subtests are not speeded, and Digit Symbol, the predictor task with a time component, requires an associative process (Birren *et al.,* 1962). Siegler (1975), however, in her thorough review of the "terminal drop" literature, notes that among WAIS subtests, Digit Symbol Substitution (DSS) is the most highly correlated with reaction time, which presumably is a pure measure of speed. Siegler comments that a "confusing aspect of the NYS studies is the assertion that speeded measures are age-related (Tapping and Block Design) while DSS is a critical loss subtest." Siegler's point is well taken, but since the Tapping subtest—which is a pure test of speed (with hand–eye coordination)—did not predict survival, whereas DSS did, it is possible that the sensitivity of DSS is due mostly to the associative processes operating. Consistent with this hypothesis are the results of factor analysis showing high loading on one of the factors (VI) for both the DSS and the Similarities test. In addition, another factor (V)—apparently a "speed" factor—had fairly low DSS loading (Jarvik *et al.,* 1962*b*).

By 1967, all the twins could be classified as either having survived the test round by 5 years or more (60 persons) or having died within 5 years of the third testing (18 persons). A total of 14 survivors and 2 decedents had not taken the three critical tests on all three occasions, and consequently had to be omitted (Jarvik and Blum, 1971). Only 4 of the 46 remaining survivors, but 11 of the 16 decedents, had shown critical loss. Jarvik and Blum (1971) also examined the data from 26 intact twin-pairs, a subgroup of the 1955 sample of 78. In 16 of the pairs, both members were 5-year survivors, 1 twin was deceased in each of 9 pairs, and in one pair, neither twin had survived 5 years beyond the last testing. There was no evidence for greater concordance in survival for one-egg than for two-egg twins in this group; this result can be attributed, however, to the small number of DZ twin-pairs still intact (5) and to the likelihood of the members of the intact DZ twin-pairs being selected for survival. One-egg twins did show greater concordance for critical loss (actually, the absence of critical loss) than did two-egg twins (13 or 21 concordanct pairs for MZ twins as compared with 2 of 5 for DZ twins), but once again, the small number of intact DZ twin pairs makes this comparison unreliable. In 10 of 11 pairs discordant for critical loss, the deceased twin was the one with the critical loss; in the 11th pair, both twins survived, but the twin who had shown a critical loss was suffering from severe organic brain syndrome, whereas his cotwin was judged to be in good health. Although these predictions were in a sense *post hoc* (see above), that a total of 53 correct predictions of 62 were made tends to suggest the validity of the critical loss construct. These findings support the terminal drop hypothesis, which Kleemeier (1962) described: " . . . factors related to the death of the individual cause a decline in intellectual performance. . . . It therefore appears that we have strong evidence for the existence of a factor, which might be called terminal drop, or decline, which adversely affects intellectual performance and is related to impending death of the aged person."

A case history of two MZ twin sisters, "A" and "L," demonstrates the relationship between intellectual decline on the critical subtests and earlier death. These two women lived their entire lives together, with the exception of a 6-year period in their early 20's during which they were separated, with work duties requiring their living in different cities. The twins were extraordinarily similar at their first testing, but at the third testing, "A" showed a critical loss, whereas "L" had maintained her performance on Vocabulary and Similarities, and had, in fact, increased her score on DSS. Within 3 years of the third testing, "A" had died; many years after her sister's death, "L," when last seen at age 87, was still a vital, active person. Possibly the onset of myocarditis in "A's" late 50's was the crucial factor differentiating the life histories of the twins (Jarvik and Blum, 1971). Another possible sign of the sisters' diverging survival potential was that "L" outweighed "A" by 15–20 pounds for much of their adult lives.

The weight difference brings to mind reports of "twin transfusion syndrome," in which one twin gains a greater share of placental nourishment than the other (e.g., Babson *et al.*, 1964; Churchill, 1965); a 500-g or greater discrepancy in weight of MZ twins at birth has been used as a criterion for twin transfusion syndrome (Munsinger, 1977), but "A" and "L" reported themselves as having weighed the same at birth.

Although the explanation for critical loss and earlier mortality in one twin and not the other remains unclear, in MZ twins, the observed discordance can be attributed neither to genetic variability nor to an age difference.

"A" and "L" comprised one of the 8 MZ twin pairs discordant for critical loss; these 8 pairs failed to show statistically significant intrapair differences in mean scores at any time. At the time of the third test round, however, the twins with critical loss had declined significantly not only on the three tests of critical loss, but also on all four other subtests; their cotwins also showed general decline, but decrements reached statistical significance only on Tapping and Block Design, two *speeded* tasks. Once again, we see that declines in cognitive functioning portend impending death (and are probably pathognomonic of cerebral disease: Jarvik, 1967;

Birren, 1968), while decreases in performance on speeded psychomotor tasks are probably "normal" (though not necessarily inevitable) concomitants of aging.

Considering the 8 cotwins who did not exhibit critical loss, 3 were still alive at the time of the 1967 test round (approximately 11 years after their last testing), and the other 5 had died on the average 5.6 years after their third testing. Of the 8 critical-loss twins, 7 died an average of 3.1 years after test round three, while the lone survivor was a victim of severe organic brain syndrome (compared with a very healthy cotwin as indicated above). These data are sufficiently striking to suggest the use of the critical-loss subtests as periodic assessors of the elderly, perhaps at the time of health exams. Identification of at-risk cases, with possible intervention, could help many people to additional years of satisfying, more optimally functioning lives.

A case study that illustrates the potential of the at-risk diagnosis is that of the "W" twins. The MZ "W" twins were 70.5 years of age at the time of their third testing in 1955. Both were in good health and were vigorous and strong men; they refused to consult with a physician until 2 years later, when CW suffered a sudden diabetic coma that proved to be fatal. Had the meaning of CW's psychological scores been understood (critical loss was indicated) at the time, he might have been persuaded to see a physician and could possibly have survived an additional 8 years, as did his cotwin (Jarvik and Blum, 1971).

Additional analyses performed on the 1967 follow-up sample as well as continued observation of the lives of the surviving twins (as in the 1973 follow-up) have strongly supported the results already stated (Blum *et al.,* 1973). In particular, the healthy twins have shown relatively small decline in intellectual ability, and for the deceased and dying twins, critical loss has continued to predict the closeness of death, whereas no such relationship between death and decline on speeded tasks has been exhibited.

3.4. Test Performance, Ability, and Education as Factors in Aging

It is apparent from the preceding sections that a strong relationship exists between genetic similarity and similar psychological test performance. It is also well known, however, that late-life mental functioning is related to educational and life-history variables (Birren and Morrison, 1961). The twin data permit assessment of the effects of these variables.

The 1967 follow-up found 81 senescent twins still living; of these, 73 twins were tested, including 19 intact pairs. Blum and Jarvik (1974) investigated the relationships of ability and education to psychometric test performance. To avoid any possible effects of "twinning," the 19 cotwins of the intact pairs were eliminated from the analytical procedures (members of each of the intact pairs were randomly labeled as "twin" or "cotwin").

Initial ability was determined by each subject's first-round Vocabulary test score. The high correlation of vocabulary with general intelligence as well as the previously noted stability of vocabulary with advancing age (Thorndike and Gallup, 1944; Jones, 1959) justify its use as an indicator of ability. Remember, the subjects had attended school before the turn of the century, and therefore before the advent of intelligence testing. High and low ability were defined as scores one half of a standard deviation or more above or below the mean, respectively. Classified in this way were 17 high- and 18 low-ability twins; the remaining 19 cases fell within one half standard deviation of the mean and were omitted from analyses. Results indicated higher scores for the more able than the less able twins on all seven subtests, both at the first testing and at the 1967 follow-up testing. All differences were statistically significant except for Block Design (first test round) and Digit Symbol (1967 round). Regression to the mean, predicted by Baltes *et al.* (1972), failed to materialize. In fact, every one of the seven subtests evinced a greater percentage decline for the low- than for the high-ability group.

Entrance into high school operationally defined the high-education group (32 twins), whereas the low-education group (22 twins) did not attend school beyond the elementary grades. Subtest means for the high-education twins exceeded those of the low-education twins at both test periods for all tests. The first-round test differences were significant for four tests: Vocabulary, Similarities, DSS, and Tapping. By 1967, differences on all seven subtests were statistically significant. The percentage decline was greater for the less educated group on every test.

The difference between the more and less favored groups clearly emerged with both the ability and the education classifications. Presumably, a relationship between high ability and high education does exist, and therefore, not unexpectedly, the two high–low dichotomies were not independent of each other. The groups were *far* from identical, however, with 29% of the high-*ability* group classified as less *educated,* and 11% of the low-*ability* group classified as more *educated.* As Blum and Jarvik (1974) point out, the sample was most characteristic of the average: neither a lack of the formally educated nor a glut of Ph.D's (or even college graduates) marked the education groups; analogously, evidence of extremely high or low intellectual accomplishment was infrequent in the ability groups. "It is remarkable, therefore, that even under such limiting circumstances, the 'low' categories consistently showed larger declines than the 'high' categories" (Blum and Jarvik, 1974).

Apparently, then, age is less deleterious to the initially more able. This finding extends beyond intellectual functioning to survival itself. Survivors as of the 1955 third-round testing achieved higher mean scores initially than had the decedents (see above); this finding has now been supported by numerous other longitudinal studies (for reviews, see Jarvik and Blum, 1971; Jarvik *et al.*, 1973*a*).

It seems likely that a positive relationship between continued mental activity and successful aging exists; utilizing "activity" data (described by Jarvik *et al.*, 1973*b*) from this same longitudinal study, De Carlo (1971) found evidence supporting this hypothesis. Better-educated persons are likely to engage in more frequent intellectual activities throughout their lives, including senescence, and this mental exercise probably protects against cognitive declines. If it is true that the better educated are more likely to continue intellectual endeavors throughout their lifetimes, then their enjoyment of mental activity rather than their extended school years may be the valuable attribute.

The education–test performance relationship has also been evaluated in another way (Feingold, 1950; Jarvik and Erlenmeyer-Kimling, 1967). From the original group of 120 senescent twin pairs, 23 were discordant for formal education; the criterion for discordance was 1 year or more discrepancy in education. Of these twin pairs, 15 differed by 1–3 years (Group 1), and the remaining 8 (Group II) by 4 years or more. Figure 1 illustrates the intrapair differences for each of these 23 twin pairs on all seven subtests. One might expect the Group II DZ pairs to vary most on the psychometric subtests, with the better-educated (and most likely more capable) twin consistently scoring higher than the cotwin. Though borne out by 1 of the 4 Group II DZ pairs, Fig. 1 clearly does not affirm this hypothesis. Other individual cases contradict this commonsense prediction as well. For example, Lester, of the "L" twins, concluded his formal education in grade 7, whereas his cotwin graduated from law school. Lester performed better on Similarities, Block Design, and Tapping (Jarvik and Erlenmeyer-Kimling, 1967).

MZ pairs exhibit even less consistent trends. One pair, the "D" twins, had rather divergent educations and work careers, with the professionally educated twin enjoying a successful and apparently stimulating position and the less educated cotwin drifting from one job to the next, including numerous ill-fated business ventures. Despite these disparate educational and work histories, their psychometric test scores were quite similar, except for DSS, on which the less-educated twin outscored his cotwin, and Similarities, on which the better-educated twin excelled.

There is a statistically nonsignificant trend toward higher scores for the better-educated twin partner, but the most striking configurations of Fig. 1 are (1) the low variability on Digits Forward and Backward, Vocabulary, and Similarities (in that order), and the far greater variability on the three tasks with speed components (Block Design, Digit Symbol, and Tapping);

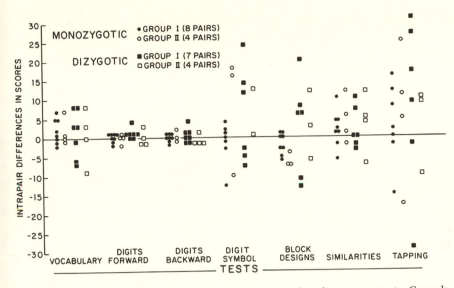

Fig. 1. Intrapair differences in raw scores of 23 senescent twin pairs on seven tests. Group I: education of one twin exceeded cotwin's by 1–3 years; Group II: education of one twin exceeded cotwin's by 4 or more years. Positive difference indicates higher score made by more educated partner; negative differences indicates higher score made by less educated partner. From Jarvik and Erlenmeyer-Kimling (1967). Copyright 1967 by Grune and Stratton, New York. Reprinted with permission.

and (2) the exhibition by the DZ groups of variability equal to or greater than that of the MZ groups on each subtest.

Intellectual decline in senescence could account for the inability to demonstrate the expected educational–psychological test performance relationship in these 23 twin pairs, but this rationale seems unlikely in light of the findings of cognitive stability with the larger ("parent") sample.

Combining these results with the analyses of Blum and Jarvik (1974), it appears that formal education does in some way exert an influence on intellectual functioning, but whatever differences can be accounted for in this way are frequently not sufficiently powerful to overcome genetic endowment, as is exemplified by the lack of consistent intrapair differences in the data of Jarvik and Erlenmeyer-Kimling (1967) just reviewed.

4. Chromosome Change and Survival

We have already discussed the relationships between genetic factors and survival and mental functioning and survival, and have concluded that genetic factors influence both cognitive abilities and life duration. It seems reasonable, therefore, to hypothesize the existence of an underlying biological mechanism that is responsible for the occurrence of these observed associations.

One such common cause could be the reproduction and accumulation of aberrant cells. Human cells characteristically have 46 chromosomes. If enough cells are inspected, however, cells with fewer or more than 46 chromosomes can be found. Such cells have been termed *aneuploid,* and were first reported to increase with age by Jacobs *et al.* (1961, 1963, 1964). It is possible that mitotic errors are propagated throughout the course of a lifetime, "with the eventual attainment of a level at which homeostatic mechanisms can no longer cope with primary and secondary metabolic dysfunctions" (Jarvik, 1965). At that level, the organism can no longer survive. Aneuploid changes in the brain (especially in the glial cells, which are known to reproduce) may then contribute to cognitive decline through the degeneration of neural support tissue.

The relationship between chromosomal change and aging is discussed in depth in Chapter 2 of this volume. In this section, the studies of chromosomal change in aging twins will be reviewed.

Jarvik and Kato (1969, 1970) examined the relationship between aneuploidy and age in 61 of the 81 surviving senescent twins whose peripheral leukocytes were cultured successfully. They ranged in age from 77 to 93 years, and for purposes of comparison, leukocyte cultures were also obtained from 15 male and 15 female volunteers between the ages of 17 and 34 years. The implicit assumption in the use of leukocytes is that the changes in aneuploidy with age are indicative of similar changes in glial cells; the relative ease of obtaining a blood sample as compared with a brain biopsy is obvious.

Aneuploid cells were classified either as hypodiploid (fewer than 46 chromosomes) or hyperdiploid (more than 46) for purposes of analysis. A significantly greater number of hypodiploid cells was found in the elderly female twins than in the younger women. No such difference obtained, however, when comparisons of the younger and older male groups were performed. Specific comparisons of the female group differences revealed that proportions of cells missing one, two, and three or more chromosomes were all significantly more prevalent in the aged than in the young women. Correlations of age with hypodiploidy for each sex *within* each of the two age groups, however, all proved to be low and nonsignificant. This finding combined with the significant mean differences in hypodiploid cells between young and old women indicates a gradual loss of chromosomes in women. This chromosome loss is present in some but not all old women.

Within-age-group comparisons resulted in oppositely directed significant differences: young males averaged more hypodiploid cells than young females, whereas aged males had fewer hypodiploid cells than aged females.

Additional analyses indicated no reliable differences in hyperdiploidy between age group or sex.

Calculating expected chromosome loss on the basis of size (instead of a random loss expectation) and comparing with actual loss, aged men were observed to have lost significantly more "G-group" chromosomes than was anticipated. No other chromosome group loss diverged significantly from its expected value.

Finally, comparison of chromosome counts for the 13 MZ and 4 DZ intact senescent twin pairs for whom leukocytes had been successfully cultured disclosed no greater similarity for the one-egg than for the two-egg twins. Further analyses, matching the MZ twins pairs as closely as possible with twins from broken pairs, resulted in larger intrapair differences in the intact MZ pairs than in the unrelated ones. The difference between the groups was not, however, statistically significant. Apparently, then, genotype is not a crucial factor in determining the development of aneuploid cells—at least not in this group of persons selected for prolonged survival. [Note that Jarvik *et al.* (1971*a*) reported evidence suggestive of greater heterogeneity between pairs than within pairs of aged MZ twins with regard to relative lengths of chromosomes.]

Since the Y chromosome belongs to the G-group, the pronounced loss of G-group chromosomes in aged males is provocative; unfortunately, banding techniques, which are helpful in determining the absence of a Y chromosome, were not yet available when these analyses were performed. A comparable C-group loss, corresponding to a possible loss of the X chromosome, was not found in the aged females. This result has been obtained, however, in numerous other studies (e.g., Hamerton *et al.*, 1965; Court Brown *et al.*, 1966; Nielsen, J., 1968; Goodman *et al.*, 1969), and was confirmed in the same laboratory in the course of a later follow-up of the same twin subjects (Jarvik *et al.*, 1973*c*).

The first longitudinal study with chromosome data from aged subjects (mean age 89.7 years) is consistent with the cross-sectional findings (Jarvik *et al.*, 1976). Over an interval of approximately 6 years, hypodiploidy, hyperdiploidy, and monosomy C increased significantly in the 11 female subjects; 8 of the women showed both greater hypodiploidy and hyperdiploidy than they had 6 years earlier, and 10 of the women had higher monosomy C. For the 6 male subjects, no statistically significant changes in chromosome aberration frequencies were found, though a mean loss in G-group chromosomes did occur. These results demonstrate by means of a longitudinal follow-up that women, but not men, undergo significant chromosome loss in the aging process.

5. Chromosome Change and Mental Functioning

Psychological tests administered to the 61 twins for whom chromosome data were available included the Memory-for-Designs test of Graham
and Kendall (1960) and the Stroop Color–Word test (Comalli et al., 1962),
as well as the seven-subtest battery of intellectual functioning used
throughout the longitudinal study. The subjects were also psychiatrically
evaluated for organic brain syndrome (OBS) according to the diagnostic
criteria of Goldfarb (1964), and were classified as OBS present or absent; if
present, OBS was further defined as mild, moderate, or severe. Complete
data were not obtained for all 61 twins, so the numbers of subjects vary
from one analysis to another. Detailed reports of the methodology and
findings can be found in previous publications (Jarvik et al., 1971b; Bettner
et al., 1971). Summaries of the results from work with these psychological
data as they relate to chromosome loss are included in papers by Jarvik
(1973a–c). Only the most salient findings will be discussed here.

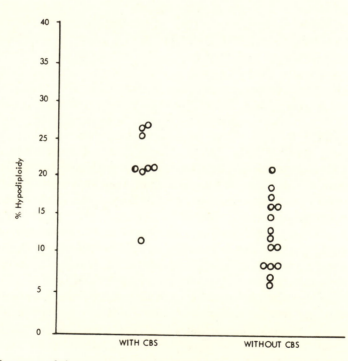

Fig. 2. Frequency of chromosome loss (% hypodiploidy) in 23 aged women with and without
organic brain syndrome. Nine subjects with suspected cerebral arteriosclerosis were excluded.
From Jarvik et at. (1971b). Copyright by the Physicians Postgraduate Press. Reprinted with
permission.

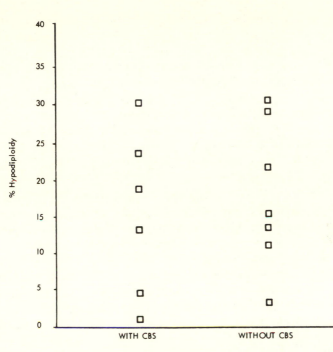

Fig. 3. Frequency of chromosome loss (% hypodiploidy) in 13 aged men with and without organic brain syndrome. Ten subjects with suspected cerebral arteriosclerosis excluded. From Jarvik *et al.* (1971*b*). Copyright by the Physicians Postgraduate Press. Reprinted with permission.

Because cerebral arteriosclerosis is itself known to cause OBS, a relationship between OBS and chromosome loss could be masked if subjects with arteriosclerosis were included. Hence, only persons judged to be free of cerebral arteriosclerosis were used for analysis; this restriction limited the sample to 13 men and 23 women. OBS was found to relate significantly to hypodiploidy in women; no similar relationship obtained for males. Figures 2 and 3 demonstrate the OBS–hypodiploidy relationship in women and its absence in men.

Analyses of the psychological test results indicated that for women, on all of the seven subtests of intellectual functioning, poorer scores were associated with greater hypodiploidy. The Graham–Kendall test as an indicator of memory loss and the Stroop test, which has been used as a measure of cognitive decline and may measure at least some aspects of OBS, were both significantly related to chromosome loss in female twins: the more hypodiploidy, the poorer the performance. The absence in males of any relationships between test performance and hypodiploidy is intriguing and remains unexplained. To date, only one other investigator has looked at the relationship between hypodiploidy and mental functioning, and his results are in agreement with our findings (Nielsen, J., 1970).

Greater mental impairment, as measured by psychiatric evaluation, correlated significantly with higher Graham–Kendall and Stroop scores among women; nonsignificant associations obtained for the men. The important Stroop factor for women was shown to be color difficulty, a task in which the name of a color (e.g., red) is printed in ink of a different color (e.g., green), and the subject must then report the color of the ink, rather than read the *name* of the color (e.g., green, not red); no particular Stroop factor emerged as salient for men.

That there is a relationship between hypodiploidy and general mental impairment seems likely, but this information still leaves us in a rather perplexed state regarding chromosome loss and intellectual decline, as well as the consistently emerging sex differences. Whether chromosome loss is actually related to long-term intellectual decline or is associated only with deficits in memory will remain unknown until the completion of longitudinal and prospective studies of chromosome loss covering at least the senescent years of the human life span (approximately 55 and on).

We know that both OBS and cognitive decline are predictive of mortality; it is also established that women live longer than men. Yet, hypodiploidy was associated with OBS and poor test performance only in women. It is possible that the human female, with two X chromosomes, is capable of sustaining a higher rate of chromosome loss than the male, since women are equipped with more chromosomal material than men. The X chromosome is approximately three times the size of the Y chromosome. It may also be that the excess genetic material on the X chromosome constitutes a survival mechanism in the presence of chromosome damage and loss, and such a mechanism could indeed account for the female's greater longevity (Jarvik, 1973c).

The actual consequences of chromosome loss, whether deleterious or beneficial, should "reflect the balance between loss of malfunctioning and optimally functioning DNA" (Jarvik *et al.*, 1974). It is possible that the mental impairment associated with hypodiploidy in women represents an undesirable accompaniment of what we have suggested (see above) may be a successful mechanism for survival (i.e., the loss of an X chromosome).

A recent report of chromosome examinations from our own laboratory (Yen *et al.*, 1976) was based on chromosome counts for the 38 female and 23 male twins for whom leukocytes were cultured in 1967, with a second chromosome examination obtained for 7 of the women with an approximate 2½-year lapse between the first and second gathering of blood samples. As of 1973, 6 years after the 1967 test round, only 28 (19 female and 9 male) of the 61 twins were still alive. Comparison of the 19 surviving women with the 19 female decedents showed greater hypodiploidy as well as greater C-group chromosome loss in the deceased group; these differences, however, were not significant. Similarly directed (though also nonsignificant) differences in hyperdiploidy, G-group loss, and chromosome breaks were also found.

In men, though differences were small and nonsignificant, the trend was reversed, with the 9 survivors exhibiting higher frequencies of the chromosome abnormalities than the 14 male decedents. No relationship between survival following the 1967 examination and any of the aberrant chromosome characteristics measured emerged for either sex. The 7 female twins with a second chromosome examination showed a statistically significant increase in the loss of C-group chromosomes; of the 6 women who actually showed a loss, however, 5 were among the decedents.

The 6-year longitudinal study of Jarvik *et al.* (1976) (noted in Section 4) sheds some additional light on this rather clouded area. No significant changes in aneuploidy were found in men, while women showed significant overall increases in hypodiploidy, hyperdiploidy, and monosomy C. Though only a small number of subjects (17) participated in this study, the sex difference in chromosome loss seems clearly established; at least among octogenerians, the loss of C-group chromosomes (as well as the total number of aneuploid cells) is a concomitant of aging in females, but not in males.

6. Sex Differences and Survival

Although sex differences have been noted at various places throughout this chapter, the topic is a sufficiently important one to be considered separately.

While no one would argue that differences between boys and girls at birth are determined largely by genetic factors, many of the differences observed between men and women have clearly been reinforced by environmental factors, and may in fact have little or no genetic basis.

It is commonly known that women outlive men. Metropolitan Life Insurance Company (1972) estimates for life expectancy in the United States are 75.1 years for females and 67.4 years for males. This sex difference in life span was observed by Kallmann and Sander (1948) when they noted that among 1602 twin index cases, 697 were men and 905 women; among those twins who resided outside of institutions, 464 were men and 584 were women. These figures were found to agree well with the New York State sex ratio of 478:570 for the over-65 population of males and females, respectively. Kallmann and Sander (1948) conclude provocatively that "the powerful trend toward a final excess of females over males, which reverses the original sex ratio existing at birth (100 females to 106 males), apparently reflects either the consequence or the illusiveness of the popular notion that this is still a man's world.''

Jarvik *et al.* (1960) compared both zygosity and sex in the survival trends of the longitudinal twin study population. Concordance rates for survival were 15.4 and 15.5% among male MZ and DZ twin pairs, respectively, and 33.6 and 27.5% among female MZ and DZ pairs, respectively. It appears, then, that zygosity exerts no effect on survival, but on the average, females of both zygosities outlive males of both zygosities.

It is still popular to attribute the greater longevity of women in comparison with men to the stressful and sometimes physically hazardous daily lives of men. Fiske Lowenthal (1975), however, recently observed that although middle-aged men have a higher incidence of hypertension and coronary thrombosis, it is middle-aged women who are in the psychologically most stressful position. Jarvik (1963) noted that the hypothesis attributing a shorter life span in men to occupational stressors failed to account for some basic phenomena. For example, females tend to outlive males throughout the animal kingdom (Wolstenholme and O'Conner, 1959). Observed differences in life span between the sexes all favor females, and include an advantage of 2 days in fruit flies (31 days for males, 33 for females), of 171 days in spiders (100 days for males, 271 for females), and of 150 days in laboratory rats (750 days for males, 900 for females). The difference in humans is about 8 years.

Also suggestive of biological responsibility for the sex differences in life span are the discrepant chromosome findings in the two sexes as previously described. Though the reasons for the discrepancies are not understood at present, it is believed that a sex-linked survival mechanism that accounts for greater longevity in women may be operating, but may also have deleterious effects on intellectual function.

7. Sex Differences and Mental Functioning

In the course of this 30-year longitudinal study of senescent twins, detailed descriptions of sex differences and mental functioning have been reported by Feingold (1950), Blum (1969), Blum *et al.* (1970, 1972), and Jarvik (1975). Only the most salient findings will be discussed here.

At the time of the first testing, mean scores for women exceeded those for men on five of the seven psychometric subtests; men achieved higher scores only on Digits Forward and Backward (Wechsler's Digit Span), and these differences were not significant. In contrast, sex differences on the Tapping, DSS, and Block Design were statistically significant in favor of women. Since women enjoy a longer life span than men, it is likely that the superior performance exhibited by the female twins is a reflection of differential rates of aging in the sexes, with earlier declines in men presaging earlier mortality. However, the facts that (1) women excel on verbal tasks in comparison with men (Maccoby, 1966; Maccoby and Jacklin, 1974; Jarvik, 1975), and (2) some of the Wechsler–Bellevue subtests used load high on verbal ability (Wechsler, 1958), when added to the finding of minimal decline in intellectual functioning through the third test round for both sexes, strongly suggest that the observed differences favoring women reflect, at least in part, the stability into senescence of the greater verbal facility of women compared to men.

The 1967 follow-up revealed that for the 54 subjects included for analyses (19 members of intact pairs were omitted), the *initial* mean score differences again showed women to be superior to men on all tests except Digit Span; significant differences were found only for Tapping and DSS for this small and select group of "20-year" survivors. (The intertest interval was approximately 20 years, 1947–1967; mean ages for the 20 males and the 34 females were 65.38 and 64.46 in 1947, and 84.67 and 84.06 in 1967, respectively. The prolonged first round of testing is responsible for within-sex mean differences in age being less than 20 years.) The 1967 test round again favored the women, but this time on all tests excepting only Digits Backward; moreover, the differences on Vocabulary and Similarities as well as Tapping and DSS now reached significance. In addition, computation of ARD showed more rapid losses for men than women on all but the Tapping and DSS tests (see Table IV). ARD for the last 12 of the 20 years (1955–1967), the interval during which the greatest declines took place, was greater for men than women on all tests, with the single exception of Digits Backward. Thus, although lifelong sex differences (especially on Vocabulary, Similarities, and DSS) are probably exerting some influence, it appears that senescent men *do* decline more rapidly than their female contemporaries on tests of intellectual functioning. It is interesting to note that the three tests found useful for the prediction of critical loss and

Table IV. Comparison of Mean Annual Rates of Change for Men and Women Between Mean Ages 64 and 84 years[a]

Type of test	Men			Women		
	N	M	S.D.	N	M	S.D.
Vocabulary	20	− 3.85	8.64	34	− 1.91	6.80
Similarities	19	− 12.53	26.87	32	− 7.25	16.71
Digits Forward	20	− 4.40	7.56	33	− 1.64	11.57
Digits Backward	20	− 7.05	12.42	31	− 1.61	15.97
Tapping	17	− 13.35	17.90	32	− 16.81	10.91
Block Design	14	− 20.43	30.52	29	− 16.10	17.58
Digit Symbol	16	− 19.50	12.80	32	− 21.28	16.71

[a]Blum *et al.* (1972). Copyright 1972 by the American Psychological Association. Reprinted with permission.

impending death are, in fact, Vocabulary, Similarities, and DSS, tests on which women of all ages tend to do better than their male counterparts.

Additional evidence bearing on this issue is that there are smaller mean intrapair differences for MZ than for DZ twin pairs. Among women, mean zygosity difference scores reached statistical significance on all but the Tapping and Digits Forward tests, but among men, no such differences appeared, though the trends were similar (Kallmann *et al.,* 1951). The absence of a clear MZ–DZ difference in men may be, as suggested in the discussion of initial assessment (Section 3.1), the result of the shorter male life span and concomitant earlier changes in the intellectual functioning of men as compared with women.

8. Summary and Conclusions

The longitudinal study of senescent twins has thus far extended over three decades. Among the many findings discussed in this chapter, some of the more salient ones include: (1) there is strong support of the hypothesis that heredity is a significant factor in determining the human life span. As is shown in Table V, data from several studies are consistent with this hypothesis; (2) maintenance of nonspeeded cognitive functioning, at least to age 75, was demonstrated by the healthy, surviving twins; (3) psychological test scores and survival were found to be positively associated; (4) for certain tests, heredity was found to relate to cognitive abilities; (5) women both outlived men and outscored men on most of the psychological tests administered; (6) data on chromosome change supported the hypothesis that hypodiploidy is a frequent concomitant of aging in women, but not in men; and (7) again only among women, hypodiploidy related significantly both to organic brain syndrome and to poorer psychological test performance.

Many questions have been raised in the course of this study. For instance, why is the relationship between chromosome loss and cognitive decline observed in women and not in men? What are the mechanisms underlying the observed association between chromosome loss and intellectual decline, and how can we intervene to prevent the latter?

Similarly, when we turn to cognitive decline and critical loss, in particular, the very same questions asked of chromosome loss and related variables are equally appropriate. Our knowledge of the critical loss phenomenon is sufficient at this point, however, to suggest that those persons found to be at risk on the basis of psychometric testing should be thoroughly examined. A standard list of medical tests to be performed on the at-risk aged should be compiled, made available to physicians, and brought to the attention of medical schools and their students.

Table V. Hypotheses Pertaining to the Role of Genetic Factors in Aging: Confirmation or Rejection from the Longitudinal Study of Aging Twins

Hypothesis	Data consistent?[a]	N	References
1. Heredity is a factor in determining life span. Intrapair differences in life span are smaller for MZ than for DZ pairs.	Yes	116	Kallmann and Sander (1949)
2. There is a genetic propensity for cancer.	Yes	68	Jarvik and Falek (1961, 1962)
3. Heredity is a factor in determining cognitive ability. Intrapair differences in psychological test performance are smaller for MZ than for DZ pairs.	Yes	240	Kallmann *et al.* (1951)
4. Heredity is a factor in determining chromosome loss. Intrapair differences in aberrant cells are smaller for MZ than for DZ twins.	No	34	Jarvik and Kato (1970)
5. Sex differences			
a. Chromosome loss			
i. Cross-sectional data	Yes	61	Jarvik and Kato (1970)
ii. Longitudinal data	Yes	17	Jarvik *et al.* (1976)
b. Survival	Yes	972	Jarvik *et al.* (1960)
c. Intellectual functioning	Yes	240	Feingold (1950)
	Yes	54	Blum *et al.* (1972)
Related observations			
1. Stress variables failed to predict the longer-lived cotwin (implying significant hereditary influence on longevity).	—	28	Bank and Jarvik (1976)
2. Discordance for education within twin pairs failed to predict psychological test performance (implying significant hereditary influence on cognitive functioning).	—	46	Jarvik and Erlenmeyer-Kimling (1967)

[a]A "Yes" in this column indicates that data for the particular study cited were consistent with the hypothesis, and the relationship exhibited was statistically significant at least at the 0.05 level.

The fact that so much new knowledge has been gained and so many more questions have been generated in the course of this single study will serve, it is hoped, as encouragement to other researchers to undertake new longitudinal as well as cross-sectional studies of the aging populace.

References

Babson, S. G., Kangas, J., Young, N., and Bramhall, J., 1964, Growth and development of twins of dissimilar sizes at birth, *Pediatrics* **33**:327–333.

Baltes, P. B., Nesselroade, J. R., Schaie, K. W., and Labouvie, E. W., 1972, On the dilemma of regression effects in examining ability level-related differentials in ontogenetic patterns of intelligence, *Dev. Psychol.* **6**:18–26.

Bank, L., and Jarvik, L. F., 1976, The effects of stress on longevity of twins, Paper presented at the 1976 annual meeting of the Gerontological Society, New York.

Bettner, L. G., Jarvik, L. F., and Blum, J. E., 1971, Stroop color-word test, non-psychotic organic brain syndrome and chromosome loss in aged twins, *J. Gerontol.* **26**:458–469.

Birren, J. E., 1968, Psychological aspects of aging, *Gerontologist* **1**:16–20.

Birren, J. E., and Morrison, D. F., 1961, Analysis of the WAIS subtests in relation to age and education, *J. Gerontol.* **16**:363–369.

Birren, J. E., Riegel, K. F., and Robbin, M. A., 1962, Age differences in continuous word associations measured by speech recordings, *J. Gerontol.* **17**:95–96.

Blum, J. E., 1969, Psychological changes between the seventh and ninth decades of life, Ph.D. dissertation (unpublished), St. John's University, Jamaica, New York.

Blum, J. E., and Jarvik, L. F., 1974, Intellectual performance of octogenarians as a function of education and initial ability, *Hum. Dev.* **17**(5):364–375.

Blum, J. E., Jarvik, L. F., and Clark, E. T., 1970, Rate of change on selective tests of intelligence: A twenty-year longitudinal study of aging, *J. Gerontol.* **25**:171–176.

Blum, J. E., Fosshage, J. L., and Jarvik, L. F., 1972, Intellectual changes and sex differences in octogenarians: A twenty-year longitudinal study of aging, *Dev. Psychol.* **7**(2):178–187.

Blum, J., Clark, E. T., and Jarvik, L. F., 1973, The New York State Psychiatric Institute Study of Aging Twins, in: *Intellectual Functioning in Adults* (L. F. Jarvik, C. Eisdorfer, and J. Blum, eds.), pp. 13–19, Springer Publishing Co., New York.

Busk, T., Clemmesen, H., and Nielsen, A., 1948, Twin studies and other investigations in the Danish Cancer Registry, *Br. J. Cancer* **2**:156–163.

Byrns, R., and Healy, J., 1936, The intelligence of twins, *J. Genet. Psychol.* **49**:474–478.

Churchill, J. A., 1965, The relationship between intelligence and birthweight in twins, *Neurology* **15**:341–347.

Comalli, P. E., Wapner, S., and Werner, H., 1962, Interference effects of Stroop color-word test in childhood, adulthood and aging, *J. Genet. Psychol.* **100**:47–53.

Court Brown, W. M., Buckton, K. E., Jacobs, P. A., Tough, I. M., Kuenssberg, E. V., and Knox, J. D. E., 1966, Chromosome studies in adults, Monograph XLII, Cambridge University Press, London.

De Carlo, T., 1971, Recreation patterns and successful aging: A twin study, Ph.D. dissertation, Columbia University, New York, New York.

Falek, A., Kallmann, F. J., Lorge, I., and Jarvik, L. F., 1960, Longevity and intellectual variation in a senescent twin population, *J. Gerontol.* **15**:305–309.

Feingold, L., 1950, A psychometric study of senescent twins, Ph.D. dissertation (unpublished), Columbia University, New York, New York.

Fiske Lowenthal, M., 1975, Psychosocial variations across the adult life course: Frontiers for research and policy, *Gerontologist* **15**:6–12.

Galton, F., 1876, The history of twins, as a criterion of the relative powers of nature and nurture, *J. R. Anthropol. Inst. Gr. Br. Irel.* **6**:391–406.

Goldfarb, A. I., 1964, The evaluation of geriatric patients following treatment, in: *The Evaluation of Psychiatric Treatment* (P. H. Hoch and J. Zubin, eds.), Grune and Stratton, New York.

Goodman, R. M., Fechheimer, N. S., Miller, F., Miller, R., and Zartman, D., 1969, Chromosomal alterations in three aged groups of human females, *Am. J. Med. Sci.* **258**:26–34.

Graham, F. K., and Kendall, B. S., 1960, Memory-for-designs test: Revised general manual, *Perceptual and Motor Skills, Monogr. Suppl.* **2-VII**:147–188.

Hamerton, J. L., Taylor, A. I., Angell, R., and McGuire, V. M., 1965, Chromosome investigations of a small isolated human population: Chromosome abnormalities and distribution of chromosome counts according to age and sex among the population of Tristan da Cunha, *Nature (London)* **206**:1232.

Harvald, B., and Hauge, M., 1956, Catamnestic investigation of Danish twins: Preliminary report, *Dan. Med. Bull.* **3**:150–158.

Harvald, B., and Hauge, M., 1958, Catamnestic investigation of Danish twins: Survey of 3100 pairs, *Acta Genet. Stat. Med.* **8**:287–294.

Jacobs, P. A., Court-Brown, W. M., and Doll, R., 1961, Distribution of human chromosome counts in relation to age, *Nature (London)* **191**:1178–1180.

Jacobs, P. A., Brunton, M., Court-Brown, W. M., Doll, R., and Goldstein, H., 1963, Change of human chromosome count distributions with age: Evidence for a sex difference, *Nature (London)* **197**:1080–1081.

Jacobs, P. A., Brunton, M., and Court-Brown, W. M., 1964, Cytogenetic studies in leukocytes on the general population: Subjects of ages 65 years and more, *Ann. Hum. Genet.* **27**:353–365.

Jarvik, L. F., 1963, Sex differences in longevity, in: *Advances in Sex Research* (H. G. Beigel, ed.), Harper and Row, New York.

Jarvik, L. F., 1965, Chromosomal changes and aging, in: *Contributions to the Psychology of Aging* (R. Kastenbaum, ed.), Springer Publishing Co., New York.

Jarvik, L. F., 1967. Survival and psychological aspects of aging in man, in: *Aspects of the Biology of Aging,* 21st Symposium of the Society for Experimental Biology, Sheffield, England, *Symp. Soc. Exp. Biol.* **21**:463–482.

Jarvik, L., 1971, Genetic aspects of aging, in: *Clinical Geriatrics* (I. Rossman, ed.), pp. 85–105, J. B. Lippincott, Philadelphia.

Jarvik, L. F., 1973*a,* Memory loss and its possible relationship to chromosome changes, in: *Psychopharmacology and Aging* (C. Eisdorfer and W. E. Fann, eds.), pp. 145–150, Plenum Press, New York—London.

Jarvik, L. F., 1973*b,* Genetic disorders late in life, *Medical World News, Geriatrics,* 13–16.

Jarvik, L. F., 1973*c,* Mental functioning related to chromosome findings in the aged, in: *Proceedings of the Vth World Congress of Psychiatry, 1971, Excerpta Med. Int. Congr. Ser.,* No. 274.

Jarvik, L. F., 1975, Human intelligence: Sex differences, *Acta Genet. Med. Gemellol.* **4**:189–211.

Jarvik, L. F., and Blum, J. E., 1971, Cognitive declines as predictors of mortality in twin pairs: A twenty-year longitudinal study of aging, in: *Prediction of Life Span* (E. Palmore and F. C. Jeffers, eds.), D. C. Heath and Co., Lexington.

Jarvik, L. F., and Erlenmeyer-Kimling, L., 1967, Survey of familial correlations in measured intellectual functions, in: *Psychopathology of Mental Development,* Grune and Stratton, New York.

Jarvik, L. F., and Falek, A., 1961, Cancer rates in aging twins, *Am. J. Hum. Genet.* **13**:413–422.

Jarvik, L. F., and Falek, A., 1962, Comparative data on cancer in aging twins, *Cancer* **15**:1009–1018.

Jarvik, L. F., and Falek, A., 1963, Intellectual stability and survival in the aged, *J. Gerontol.* **18**:173–176.

Jarvik, L. F., and Kato, T., 1969, Chromosomes and mental changes in octogenarians: Preliminary findings, *Br. J. Psychiatry* **115**:1193–1194.

Jarvik, L. F., and Kato, T., 1970, Chromosome examinations in aged twins, *Am. J. Hum. Genet.* **22**:562–573.

Jarvik, L. F., Kallmann, F. J., Falek, A., and Klaber, M. M., 1957, Changing intellectual functions in senescent twins, *Acta Genet. Stat. Med.* **7**:421–430.

Jarvik, L. F., Falek, A., Kallmann, F. J., and Lorge, I., 1960, Survival trends in a senescent twin population, *Am. J. Hum. Genet.* **12**:170–179.

Jarvik, L. F., Kallmann, F. J., and Falek, A., 1962a, Intellectual changes in aged twins, *J. Gerontol.* **17**:289–294.

Jarvik, L. F., Kallmann, F. J., Lorge, I., and Falek, A., 1962b, Longitudinal study of intellectual changes in senescent twins, in: *Social and Psychological Aspects of Aging* (C. Tibbits and W. Donahue, eds.), Columbia University Press, New York.

Jarvik, L. F., Yen, F. S., Fleiss, J., Kato, T., and Moralishvili, E., 1971a, Chromosome measurements in aged monozygotic twins, *Hum. Hered.* **21**:557–576.

Jarvik, L. F., Altshuler, K. Z., Kato, T., and Blumner, B., 1971b, Organic brain syndrome and chromosome loss in aged twins, *Dis. Nerv. Syst.* **32**:159–170.

Jarvik, L. F., Blum, J. E., and Varma, A. O., 1972, Genetic components and intellectual functioning during senescence: A 20-year study of aging twins, *Behav. Genet.* **2**:159–171.

Jarvik, L. F.. Eisdorfer, C., and Blum. J. (eds.), 1973a. *Intellectual Functioning in Adults,* Springer Publishing Co.. New York.

Jarvik, L. F., Bennett, R., and Blumner, B., 1973b, Design of comprehensive life history interview schedule, in: *Intellectual Functioning in Adults* (L. F. Jarvik, C. Eisdorder, and J. Blum, eds.), pp. 127–136, Springer Publishing Co., New York.

Jarvik, L. F., Klodin, V., and Matsuyama. S. S., 1973c, Human aggression and the extra Y chromosome—Fact or fantasy? *Am. Psychol.* **28**(8):674–682.

Jarvik, L. F., Yen. F. S., and Moralishvili, E., 1974, Chromosome examinations in aging institutionalized women. *J. Gerontol.* **29**(3):269–276.

Jarvik, L. F., Yen, F. S., Fu, T. K., and Matsuyama, S. S., 1976, Chromosomes in old age: A six year longitudinal study, *Hum. Genet.* **33**:17–22.

Jones, H. E., 1959, Intelligence and problem solving, in: *Handbook of Aging and the Individual* (J. Birren, ed.), University of Chicago Press.

Kallmann, F. J., and Jarvik, L. F., 1957, Twin data on genetic variations in resistance to tuberculosis, *Genetica della Tubercolosi e dei Tumori: Atti del Simposio Internazionale, Collana di Monografie 6, Analecta Genetica,* Torino, pp. 15–33.

Kallmann, F. J., and Jarvik, L. F., 1959, Individual differences in constitution and genetic background, in: *Aging and the Individual* (J. E. Birren, ed.), University of Chicago Press.

Kallmann, F. J., and Sander, G., 1948, Twin studies on aging and longevity, *J. Hered.* **39**:349–357.

Kallmann, F. J., and Sander, G., 1949, Twin studies on senescence, *Am. J. Psychiatry* **106**:29–36.

Kallmann, F. J., Feingold, L., and Bondy, E., 1951, Comparative adaptational, social, and psychometric data on the life histories of senescent twin pairs, *Am. J. Hum. Genet.* **3**:65–73.

Kleemeier, R. W., 1962, Intellectual changes in the senium, *Proc. Soc. Stat. Sect. Am. Stat. Assoc.* **1**:290–295.

Krauss, I., 1976, Predictors of adult competence, Paper presented at the 1976 annual meeting of the Western Psychological Association, Los Angeles.

Maccoby, E. E. (ed.), 1966, Sex differences in intellectual functioning, in: *The Development of Sex Differences,* Stanford University Press, Stanford, California.

Maccoby, E. E., and Jacklin, C. N., 1974, *The Psychology of Sex Differences,* Stanford University Press, Stanford, California.

Macklin, M. T., 1940, An analysis of tumors in monozygous and dizygous twins, *J. Hered.* **31**:277–290.

Marquette, V. W., 1976, The trans-situational generalizability of adult competence, Paper presented at the 1976 annual meeting of the Western Psychological Association, Los Angeles.

Mehrotra, S. N., and Maxwell, J., 1949, The intelligence of twins: A comparative study of eleven-year-old twins, *Popul. Stud. (London)* **3**:295–302.

Metropolitan Life Insurance Company, 1972, Table of life expectancies in the United States, by sex, age and ethnicity.

Munsinger, H., 1977, The identical twin transfusion syndrome: A source of error in estimating IQ resemblance and heritability, unpublished manuscript.

Nielsen, A., and Clemmesen, J., 1957, Twin studies in the Danish Cancer Registry 1942–1955, *Br. J. Cancer* **11**:327–336.

Nielsen, J., 1968, Chromosomes in senile dementia, *Br. J. Psychiatry* **114**:303–309.

Nielsen, J., 1970, Chromosomes in senile, presenile, and arteriosclerotic dementia, *J. Gerontol.* **25**:312–315.

Ohta, R. J., 1976, The role of cautiousness in research on adult competence, Paper presented at the 1976 annual meeting of the Western Psychological Association, Los Angeles.

Schaie, K. W., 1976, The assessment of competence in adulthood and old age, Paper presented at the 1976 annual meeting of the Western Psychological Association, Los Angeles.

Scheidt, R. J., 1976, Situational factors in the assessment of adult competence, Paper presented at the 1976 annual meeting of the Western Psychological Association, Los Angeles.

Siegler, I. C., 1975, The terminal drop hypothesis: Fact or artifact?, *Exp. Aging Res.* **1**:169–185.

Terman, L. M., 1916, *The Measurement of Intelligence,* Houghton Mifflin, Boston.

Thorndike, E. L., and Gallup, G. H., 1944, Verbal intelligence of the American adult, *J. Genet. Psychol.* **30**:75–85.

von Verschuer, O. V., and Kober, E., 1956, Tuberkulose und Krebs bei Zwillingen, *Acta Genet. Stat. Med.* **6**:106–113.

Wechsler, D. 1944, *The Measurement of Adult Intelligence,* Williams and Wilkins, Baltimore.

Wechsler, D., 1958, *The Measurement and Appraisal of Adult Intelligence,* 4th Ed., Williams and Wilkins, Baltimore.

Wolstenholme, G. E. W., and O'Connor, C. M. (eds.), 1959, *Ciba Found. Colloq. Ageing,* Vol. 5, *The Lifespan of Animals,* Little, Brown and Co., Boston.

Yen, F. S., Matsuyama, S. S., and Jarvik, L. F., 1976, Survival of octogenarians: Six years after initial chromosome examination, *Exp. Aging Res.* **2**(2):17–26.

Part IV

Genetic Approaches to Aging Research

Chapter 11

Somatic Cell Genetics in the Analysis of in Vitro Senescence

Thomas H. Norwood

1. Introduction

The limited replicative life span, or "senescence," of cultured human diploid somatic cells is now well established (Hayflick and Moorhead, 1961). During the past decade, extensive investigations have resulted in detailed characterization of these cells; the mechanism or mechanisms that regulate their limited proliferative capabilities, however, remain unknown. Moreover, the relevance of such *in vitro* senescence to the aging of proliferating cell populations *in vivo* is controversial. Indeed, the relative contributions of proliferating cell populations and postmitotic cells to the aging process are also unknown. There is no information that clearly favors one or the other of the various hypotheses concerning the mechanism of senescence in the intact organism. Thus, while we are in this state of relative ignorance, it is important to analyze all potentially relevant model systems with a variety of experimental approaches.

The major objective of this chapter is to discuss the current and future status of the use of somatic cell genetics in the study of the mechanism or mechanisms of *in vitro* senescence of proliferating cell populations. To provide an adequate frame of reference, it is necessary to first describe, in general terms, the historical development of the present concepts of the biology of cultivated cells. Since virtually all the somatic cell genetic studies of senescence have utilized *in vitro* systems, the relevance of this

Thomas H. Norwood ● Department of Pathology, University of Washington, Seattle, Washington 98195

model to *in vivo* aging is then analyzed. Promising experimental systems that may be useful in future cellular genetic studies of aging are also discussed.

2. Biology of Cultured Mammalian Cells

2.1. Historical Background

Until approximately two decades ago, it was widely held that while the intact organism has a limited life span, its somatic cells, removed from constraints of the *in vivo* environment, possess unlimited potential for survival and growth. The observations of Carrel (1912), who apparently was able to maintain cells derived from a chick heart in culture for many years, established this concept as a central dogma of cell culture. It is now considered likely that this "immortality" was the result of reintroduction of viable cells present in the chick embryo extract used to feed the cultures (Hayflick, 1970). Moreover, recent investigations of the proliferative capacity of chick cells *in vitro* led to the opposite conclusion (Hay and Strehler, 1967). The notion of immortality of cultured somatic cells persisted unchallenged, however, until the 1950s, primarily on the basis of observations with murine cells (Gey and Gey, 1938). The tendency for cells derived from this species to transform spontaneously into an abnormal cell type was not appreciated at that time (Rothfels *et al.*, 1963).

2.2. The Phenomenon of in Vitro Senescence

Although previous investigators observed that most cultured human cells derived from various tissues ceased to proliferate after variable periods of time (Swim and Parker, 1957), it was generally assumed that growth limitations were due to technical inadequacies of the existing cell culture systems (Puck *et al.*, 1957, 1958). In the early 1960s, however, after extensive experimentation, Hayflick and Moorhead (1961) clearly demonstrated the limited proliferative capacity of cultured human fetal cells. They argued that this was an intrinsic property of these cells. These investigators reported that the outgrowth from all tissue placed in culture was ultimately a fibroblastlike cell, and that although some variation of the proliferative life span of the culture was noted, all cultures ceased growing and died when propagated by subcultivation with trypsin every third or fourth day. Repeated efforts to demonstrate mycoplasma contamination or latent viruses or both were negative. In addition, media in which old cultures failed to grow were found to support growth of young cultures. Chromosome studies revealed a tight diploid mode throughout the life span of the culture, with a small percentage of tetraploid cells present in most cultures.

(It should be emphasized that the authors could not rule out subtle aberrations with the cytogenetic methodologies used at that time.)

These authors divided the growth characteristics of these cultures into three periods—Phase I, outgrowth from tissue fragments; Phase II, active growth *in vitro;* and Phase III, termination of growth with cell degeneration (Fig. 1). Based mainly on the observation that cultures derived from adults displayed a lower growth potential than those derived from fetal tissues, Hayflick (1965) postulated that this phenomenon is a manifestation of cellular senescence and is a relevant model for the study of aging, proliferating cell populations *in vivo*. Although at that time there was little direct evidence to support such an interpretation, it has stimulated extensive investigative effort, as well as controversy as to the relevance of such research to *in vivo* aging.

Although serious objections have been raised to the concept that all cultivated cells are "immortal" as originally postulated by the early workers in cell culture, the fact remains that many cultures derived from diverse species possess apparently unlimited growth potential (Hayflick and Moorhead, 1961). Thus, these authors emphasized that there are two fundamentally distinct types of cultures, which they termed *cell strains* (normal diploid cells of limited growth capacity) and *cell lines* (aneuploid cells of unlimited growth capacity) (Table I). Subsequently, other contrasting terms have been introduced: Krooth *et al.* (1968) proposed the terms *homonu-*

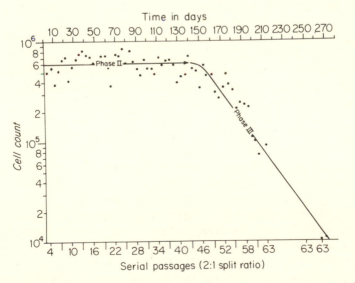

Fig. 1. Growth history of a typical culture of human diploid cells subcultured every 3 days (2:1 split). These results indicate that after intial outgrowth (Phase I), there is a sustained period of growth (Phase II), followed by an exponential decline of proliferative capacity (Phase III). Reproduced from Hayflick (1965), Academic Press, New York, with permission.

Table I.   Comparative Biology of the Basic Cell Types in Cell Culture

Property	Hyperplastoid (cell strains, homonuclear)	Neoplastoid (cell lines, heteronuclear)
Prototype cultures	Human skin fibroblasts	HeLa and mouse L cells
Origin	Normal tissue and stroma of neoplastic tissue	Neoplastic tissue, and in vitro transformation of normal cells
Replicative life span	Finite	Apparently infinite
Karyotype	Same as donor's normal somatic cells	Usually different from donor's normal somatic cells
Tumor assay	Negative	Frequently positive
Saturation density	Comparatively low	Comparatively high

clear (cell strains) and *heteronuclear* (cell lines), and Martin and Sprague (1973) introduced the terms *hyperplastoid* and *neoplastoid* (Table I). It is important to emphasize that any given cell type may not conform to all these criteria. For example, 3T3 cells derived from various strains of mice and subjected to rigid culture conditions display a marked contact inhibition of growth and therefore a low saturation density (Todaro and Green, 1963), yet they have an unlimited growth potential, are aneuploid, and may be tumorigenic in histocompatible hosts (Boone, 1975; Boone *et al.*, 1976). Lymphoblast lines derived from peripheral blood lymphocytes of normal subjects do not enter a senescent phase and may remain apparently diploid for many months. Most if not all of these cultures, however, ultimately become aneuploid (Steel *et al.*, 1971; Povey *et al.*, 1973) and are tumorigenic in appropriate hosts (Deal *et al.*, 1971).

Although this classification of cultured cells has been useful for the interpretation of certain types of experiments, recent developments suggest that reevaluation is needed. It has now been demonstrated that malignant mouse teratocarcinomas, propagated both *in vivo* and *in vitro*, are capable of participating in normal ontogeny following injection into blastocysts, and are capable of contributing cells to most if not all tissues of the adult organism (Mintz and Illmensee, 1975; Papaioannou *et al.*, 1975; Brinster, 1974). These cell lines have been maintained *in vivo* by serial transplantation for long periods of time (Stevens, 1967), and have been converted to an ascites form (Stevens, 1970). Although they appear to have remained diploid *in vivo* (Dunn and Stevens, 1970), there is some evidence of loss of totipotency and chromosomal instability when cultivated *in vitro* (Kahan and Ephrussi, 1970; Lehman *et al.*, 1974; Hogan, 1976; McBurney, 1976). Thus, while these cells appear to possess unique properties, they are considered to be a neoplastoid cell type, because of their capacity to produce malignant tumors. Clearly, further investigations are needed before this cell type can be precisely defined.

2.3. Relevance of in Vitro Senescence to in Vivo Senescence

Since the initial observations of Hayflick and Moorhead, which have been confirmed in many laboratories throughout the world, a number of studies suggest, but by no means prove, that the *in vitro* behavior of human diploid cells is relevant to *in vivo* aging at the cellular level. The inverse correlation between donor age and the *in vitro* proliferative potential first observed by Hayflick has been confirmed in other laboratories (Goldstein *et al.*, 1969; Martin *et al.*, 1970; Hay and Strehler, 1967). The studies of Martin *et al.* (1970) indicated a regression rate of 0.2 ± 0.05 (S.D.) cell doublings per year, based on observation of 100 mass cultures from donors in the first to the ninth decades (Fig. 2). These studies have been criticized because of questionable differences of the proliferative capacity of cells from adult donors between the third and the ninth decades (Kohn, 1975). More recent observations by these investigators show that cultures from donors of this age group display a similar coefficient of regression (Martin *et al.*, 1978).

Another line of evidence often cited as supporting the validity of the *in vitro* model concerns the behavior of cells derived from inherited disorders that display at least a caricature of premature senescence. A dramatic diminution of growth potential was observed in cultures derived from donors with the Werner syndrome (Martin *et al.*, 1970) and progeria (Goldstein, 1969; Danes, 1971), although in the latter disorder, variation between kindreds was observed (Singal and Goldstein, 1973). A variety of other inherited syndromes, including those that result from chromosome

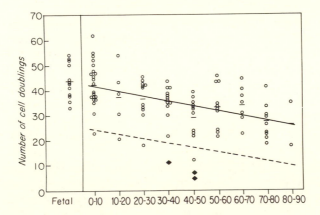

Fig. 2. Proliferative capacity of human diploid cultures as a function of age of the donor. Regression curve of growth potential from donors from the first to the ninth decades of life shows a coefficient of regression of 0.2 population doublings per year, with a correlation coefficient of − 0.50. (---) Lower 95% confidence limit. Reproduced from Martin *et al.* (1970), Williams & Wilkins Co., Baltimore, with permission.

aneuploidy and that also exhibit some aspects of premature aging, display a modest decrease in growth potential, though far less dramatic than the two examples cited above (Kaback and Bernstein, 1970; Schneider and Epstein, 1972; Segal and McCoy, 1974; Kuliev *et al.*, 1974). The most important class of these disorders is diabetes mellitus, a heterogeneous group of metabolic diseases with varying genetic bases (Goldstein *et al.*, 1975). Goldstein *et al.* (1969) showed that the cloning efficiency of cells derived from diabetic and prediabetic donors is reduced throughout most of the life span of the culture. A modest but significant reduction in the replicative life span of such cultures in comparison with that of normal controls was demonstrated by Vracko and Benditt (1975). There are many other inherited disorders in which some aspects of accelerated aging are apparent; there is little or no information, however, concerning the behavior of cultured cells from such donors (Martin, 1977a).

Although age-dependent variation in primary and low-passage cultures is a potentially very important area of study, relatively few investigations of this phenomenon have been reported. A positive correlation between the length of the latent period before cell outgrowth and the age of the donor has been established in cultured tissues from rats (Soukupová *et al.*, 1970), chickens (Lefford, 1964), and the human (Waters and Walford, 1970). The delayed outgrowth could reflect an associated alteration of tissue architecture, such as an increased amount of fibrous connective tissue, rather than an intrinsic alteration in the migrating cell populations. More recently, Schneider and Mitsui (1976) also demonstrated a decreased rate of migration of cells from explanted tissue derived from older human donors. In addition, these investigators showed differences in population doubling time and saturation density in low-passage cultures from old and young donors, suggesting that *in vivo* age-associated alterations occur, at least in those cell populations capable of migration and growth *in vitro*. These differences were not as dramatic, however, as those observed with *in vitro* aging. Rosenbloom *et al.* (1976) recently demonstrated that insulin binding to low-passage cells increases as a function of donor age and genotype (progeria and the Rothmund–Thomson syndrome). This demonstration is the first evidence of an age-related alteration manifested in cultured somatic cells that is of obvious potential functional significance *in vivo*. The relationship of insulin binding to such parameters as cell size and cell cycle stage must be further investigated before the significance of this observation can be evaluated (Thomopoulos *et al.*, 1976).

The relationship between longevity of a species and the *in vitro* replicative capacity of its cultured cells has not been intensively investigated. Sporadic observations have suggested that such a correlation may exist (Hayflick, 1974). As indicated above, human cells survive approximately 50 population doublings (Hayflick and Moorhead, 1961), while cell strains from chickens, which have a life span less than one third that of man, are capable of about 25 population doublings (Hay and Strehler, 1967;

Pontén, 1970; Lima and Macieira-Coelho, 1972). Similar studies with cultured mouse cells indicate a maximum potential of 20 or fewer population doublings; precise analysis in this regard is difficult, however, because of the frequency of spontaneous transformation in these cultures (Rothfels *et al.*, 1963). Cells from the Galapagos tortoise, which probably has a potential life span of more than 150 years, were observed to achieve approximately 100 doublings (Goldstein, 1974), although it is difficult to compare cells derived from a poikilothermic species with those derived from mammals, since culture conditions, such as optimum temperature, have not been precisely defined for the former. More recently, however, in a study of a wide variety of mammalian species including some marsupials, Stanley *et al.* (1975) concluded that no such correlation exists. Indeed, cells derived from the fattailed dunnart (*Sminthopsis crassicaudata*), which has an estimated life span of 3 years, are apparently capable of at least 170 population doublings. Thus, the comparative longevities of cultured cells have provided little support for the validation of the *in vitro* system as an aging model. In any case, one must be cautious in interpreting such experiments, since culture conditions, such as origin of serum and optimum concentrations of other media constituents, have not been precisely defined for each species. Furthermore, there is the possibility that different cell types may be cultivated, especially when comparing widely divergent species.

Critics have questioned both the relevance of this system to the problem of aging and, more basically, the adequacy of present cell culture laboratories for subcultivation. For example, proteolytic agents are used by virtually all cell culture laboratories for subcultivation. Incredibly, there is to date no published study of the effect of these enzymes on the reproductive potential of these cultures. Studies carried out in our laboratory in which portions of the culture were removed by scraping to maintain continual growth of the remaining cells indicated that these cultures senesce even in the absence of exposure to chemical or mechanical passage of the cells (Sprague and Martin, unpublished). Alternative techniques of passage are available (Waters and Walford, 1971), and should be investigated in this regard. It is unlikely, however, that susceptibility to the effects of proteolytic agents is responsible for the difference in the growth potential between hyperplastoid and neoplastoid cells.

Senescence of cultured human cells has been observed in many laboratories and has been established as a reproducible phenomenon. However, it is now clear that certain manipulations can alter the proliferative potential of these human cell cultures. For example, proliferative life span was increased by the addition of cortisone (Macieira-Coelho *et al.*, 1966; Cristofalo, 1970), as well as by alterations of the amino acid composition of the medium (Litwin, 1972). In addition, the stability of human somatic cell cultures is remarkable in that both spontaneous and chemically induced transformation rarely, if ever, occur. It is therefore unlikely that environmental or technical factors are the primary cause of the cessation of cell growth. Recent publications have reported the occurrence of spontaneous transformation in cultures derived from the skin of individuals with carcinoma of the lung (Azzarone *et al.*, 1976), and in cultures from donors with xeroderma pigmentosum after exposure to a chemical mutagen (Shimada *et al.*, 1976). These observations suggest that increased susceptibility to transformation may be associated with certain genotypes or pathological conditions or both.

The relevance of this system to the general problem of aging is an important and controversial issue. It has been pointed out that *in vivo* transplantation studies indicate that proliferating cell populations are capable of survival and growth beyond the life span of the donor. That they are has been demonstrated with serial transplants of marrow erythrocyte stem cells (Harrison, 1973), skin (Krohn, 1966), and mammary tissue (Daniel *et al.*, 1968). Unlike transplantable tumor lines, however, these cells do not survive indefinitely on serial transplantation. Indeed, proliferating populations of human diploid cells can be obtained with ease from biopsies from donors in the eighth and ninth decades of life, indicating that only a modest fraction of the proliferative potential is consumed during a lifetime (Martin *et al.*, 1970). The answer to these arguments remains speculative at this time. Hayflick (1974, 1976) argued that functional alterations occur that are common to both proliferating and postmitotic cell populations, the effects of which are manifested as a loss of division potential in the former. An understanding of the mechanism of *in vitro* senescence (i.e., loss of proliferative capacity) will therefore be relevant to aging in all cell populations *in vivo*. The observations of Rosenbloom *et al.* (1976), indicating an increase of insulin receptors as a function of age, suggest that the alterations may occur *in vivo* before the cessation of mitotic activity. It is certainly conceivable that modest changes in growth capability may have profound effects on reparative and homeostatic responses *in vitro*. Certainly, these questions are worth exploring in the context of aging and senescence. In any case, the elucidation of the mechanism of *in vitro* clonal senescence would be of great relevance to the problem of control of cell replication and neoplasia. Finally, knowledge that would lead to the prolongation of the proliferative life span of human diploid cells in culture would have important applications in the field of human somatic genetics.

3. Phenotype of the Senescent Culture

3.1. Alterations of Proliferative Behavior with Senescence

As indicated above, senescence occurs in cultured cells derived from many species. Human diploid cells (cultured from lung or skin), however, have been the object of the vast majority of experimental studies. This discussion will therefore be confined, for the most part, to studies of these cell types. It should be emphasized that extensive information concerning other species is lacking, and for some purposes, human cells may not provide the optimum model. Also, this discussion will be confined to those areas relevant to somatic cell genetic studies; extensive reviews emphasizing other aspects have been published (Cristofalo, 1972; Hayflick, 1974, 1976).

The early studies of Hayflick (1965) indicated a plateau of constant growth during Phase II, followed by a decline in cell replication during Phase III, and, finally, rapid death of the culture (see Fig. 1). As reviewed by J. W. Littlefield (1976), however, several subsequent observations indicate that alterations in proliferative behavior occur much earlier. Merz and Ross (1969), after dilute plating, located individual cells and determined the percentage of nondividing cells at 4–5 days. They observed that this fraction increased exponentially with passage number throughout the life span of the culture. Subsequent experiments have supported the concept of a progressive loss of division potential. Goldstein *et al.* (1969) observed an almost linear decrease in cloning efficiency during the replicative life of a cell culture. Cristofalo and Sharf (1973) made similar observations concerning the fraction of cells able to incorporate tritiated thymidine ([³H]TdR) under defined conditions (Fig. 3).

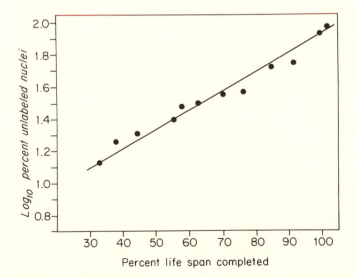

Fig. 3. Percentage of unlabeled nuclei as a function of the *in vitro* age of cultured human diploid cells. A continuous increase of cells not labeled with [³H]TdR is apparent throughout most of the replicative life of the cultures. Reproduced from Cristofalo and Sharf (1973), Academic Press, New York, with permission.

This latter observation has spurred interest in using this thymidine labeling index as a means of estimating the remaining life span of a culture. Good and Smith (1974) challenged this notion on the basis of cloning studies. In our experience, there is considerable variation among strains with respect to the kinetics of the decline of labeling indices. J. R. Smith *et al.* (1977) made preliminary observations indicating that the precentage of clones achieving a minimum number of doublings under certain standard conditions may serve as a more reliable index of proliferative potential.

Other studies of the proliferative behavior of human diploid cells have been directed toward measuring alterations in cell-cycle duration and determination of the point in the cycle at which cells are arrested. Macieira-Coelho *et al.* (1966) concluded from autoradiographic studies of old and young cultures of diploid fetal cells that increasing heterogeneity of cell-cycle time occurred with age mainly due to lengthening of the G_1 and G_2 phases of the cell cycle. More recently, Grove *et al.* (1976), also using autoradiographic methods on the same cell strains, reported that cell-cycle prolongation with advancing *in vitro* age was due almost entirely to changes in G_1. No measurable alterations were observed in the S period, and only slight increments in G_2. These authors also noted a decreased average grain density over [^{3}H]TdR-labeled late-passage cells. They speculated that this decrease could reflect a decreased rate of DNA synthesis, although, as the authors suggested, alterations in transport or pool sizes of thymidine could account for this observation. In an earlier study, Petes *et al.* (1974) observed a decreased rate of DNA synthesis in late-passage cultures as measured by fiber autoradiography. These observations are, at present, difficult to interpret, since the length of the S phase and the distance between initiation points of DNA synthesis appear to be unchanged. They could reflect a change in the temporal sequence of initiation of DNA synthesis in aging cells.

There have been only a few reported studies attempting to determine whether senescent cells cease replicating at a certain point in the cell cycle. Yanishevsky *et al.* (1974) and Grove *et al.* (1976), both using quantitative cytophotometric methods, concluded that the majority of cells are arrested in G_1. The former group noted an accumulation of cells with a DNA content consistent with either a G_2 diploid or G_1 tetraploid state, as well as an increased frequency of intermediate values. Utilizing an alternative approach, Yanishevsky and Carrano (1975) fused senescent cultures to mitotic cells to induce premature chromosome condensation (Rao, P. N., and Johnson, 1972), and observed that the majority of cells revealed a G_1 chromosome configuration (i.e., the prematurely condensed chromosomes were composed of single chromatids). Flow microfluorometric analysis of senescent cell cultures also revealed an increased frequency of G_1-phase cells (Schneider and Fowlkes, 1976). Although there is a striking consensus in these experimental results, it is not clear whether they reflect complete termination of the proliferative functions of these cells in the G_1 phase. Macieira-Coelho (1974) demonstrated that up to 90% of the cells in late-passage cultures could be labeled with [^{3}H]TdR following prolonged exposure periods. Although there are alternative interpretations, this observation is consistent with an elongation, but not complete cessation, of cell-cycle activity.

It is important to stress that with respect to growth behavior, these cultures are extremely heterogeneous, and that they become increasingly so with age. This heterogeneity was revealed by various cloning studies (Smith, J. R., and Hayflick, 1974; Martin *et al.*, 1974), but was revealed most vividly in the time-lapse cinemicrophotometric studies of Absher *et al.* (1974). Yet, alterations in the proliferative behavior of these cultures remain to date, the only marker that has been available for somatic cell genetic studies. Ideally, age-associated markers should involve biochemically defined alterations in a specific gene product or gene products that are of functional significance in the appearance of the senescence phenotype. Recently, several promising observations concerning this problem have been reported. Mayne *et al.* (1976) demonstrated a change in the type of collagen synthesized by aging chick chondrocytes. The loss of a neutral protease was observed with the onset of senescence in at least one strain of human diploid cells (Bosmann *et al.*, 1976). Clearly, the significance of these observations in relation to cell senescence remains to be established; they could be extremely important, however, for future studies.

3.2. Cytogenetic Alterations

Karyotypic stability of cultured human diploid cells has been documented in numerous studies (Chu and Giles, 1959; Hayflick and Moorhead, 1961; Tjio and Puck, 1958). As cells enter the terminal phase of their life span, however, increases in aneuploidy, polyploidy, and aberrant chromosomes have been observed (Yoshida and Makino, 1963; Saksela and Moorhead, 1963; Thompson, K. V. A., and Holliday, 1975), and are generally interpreted to be secondary to cellular senescence. More recently, there have been reports of the emergence of cytogenetically aberrant clones in long-term cultures, some with complex rearrangements (Chen and Ruddle, 1974; Littlefield, L. G., and Mailhes, 1975; Harnden *et al.*, 1976). The donor genotype could certainly be significant in this regard. Hoehn *et al.* (1975*a*) reported a high incidence of abnormal clones in cultures from a donor with the Werner syndrome and from an apparently normal donor. No such aberrations were observed in early and senescent cultures from four other normal donors. Whitaker *et al.* (1974) observed that the frequency of unstable aberrations may be increased by some batches of serum, suggesting that culture conditions may alter the frequency of some anomalies. Although tests for the presence of mycoplasma were carried out in all these studies, occult infections remain a possible cause of chromosomal alterations (Schneider *et al.,* 1974).

Thus, while clonal chromosomal abnormalities may appear in long-term cultures of certain human cell strains under certain conditions, these cultures are in general remarkably stable, and it is unlikely that the changes seen in the terminal phase are a primary cause of senescence. A detailed analysis of the cytogenetic changes with aging is presented in Chapter 2.

3.3. Morphology

During the active growth phase of human cultures, the cells maintain a relatively uniform spindle-shaped morphology, tending to display parallel orientation at confluence. As senescence approaches, there is increasing variation in cell shape, a marked increase in cell volume, and accumulation of extracellular debris. Terminally, dramatic variation in nuclear size and shape ocurs. The increased cell size in late-passage cells was quantitatively documented in several independent studies (Simons, 1967; Cristofalo and Kritchevsky, 1969; Bowman and Daniel, 1975). Recently, Mitsui and Schneider (1976a,b) demonstrated an inverse relationship between growth rate and both nuclear size and cell volume. As with the other age-associated changes described above, no causal relationship between cell volumetric changes and loss of proliferative potential has been established. The experiments of Mitsui and Schneider (1976a) also revealed increases in cell volume following inhibition of growth by both chemical and physical agents, suggesting that alterations in cell volume may be secondary to the inhibition in cell replication seen during Phase III.

Ultrastructural studies have been carried out on aged human fibroblast cultures (Robbins *et al.,* 1970; Lipetz and Cristofalo, 1972) and senescent chick cells (Brock and Hay, 1971). The most striking and consistent change is an increase in the number of lysosomes, many of them transforming into autophagic vacuoles and residual bodies. Such changes were correlated with an increase in the activity of lysosomal enzymes (Cristofalo, 1970). Other observations included a decrease in the number of free and membrane-bound ribosomes, an increase in glycogen, alterations of mitochondrial structure, and increased variation of nuclear shape. Nuclear alterations are striking in light-microscopic preparations of extremely senescent cells. In our experience, binucleation and micronucleation may approach 20% in cells that have been maintained for months after cessation of replication (unpublished). These changes correlate with the karyotypic alterations described above, and suggest that impairment of both nuclear and cytoplasmic division occurs.

3.4. Implication for Genetic Studies

While there is now a large body of descriptive literature characterizing the changes that occur as cells enter the senescent phase, we remain completely ignorant of the basic mechanisms involved. We do not know which, if any, of these observations are manifestations of, or, alternatively, causes of, the loss of proliferative functions. Indeed, as Martin *et al.* (1975) suggested, many of the observed alterations may be epiphenomena. For example, the loss of replicative function may be under genetic control and the subsequent morphological alterations the result of unbalanced growth or accumulation of abnormal molecules or both. On the other hand, one could argue that the observed chromosomal and morphological alterations in nuclei are the result of continued "attempts" to replicate after the onset of molecular alterations within the cell. It must be emphasized, however, that the results of studies with terminally senescent cultures may very well reflect alterations that have occurred after the transition to a nongrowing state.

The heterogeneity present throughout the replicative life span of these cultures obviously increases the complexity of experimental design, as well as interpretation of such experiments. Moreover, in many cases, evaluation of cell-cycle function involves the measurement of incorporation of labeled precursors into DNA. Virtually nothing is known about changes in thymidine transport, pool sizes, or metabolism with increasing age of a culture. In view of this lack of information, the interpretation of many of the experiments discussed below is of necessity very tentative. Clearly, in view of the heterogenous nature of these cell populations, analyses must be carried out at the cellular level (cytological studies) as well as the population level (biochemical studies). Herein lies the value of somatic cell genetic methodology, for, as will be discussed, some of the methods allow the assessment of the behavior of individual cells.

4. Somatic Cell Genetic Studies of in Vitro Cellular Senescence

4.1. Theories of the Mechanism of in Vitro Senescence

Limitations of space preclude a detailed discussion of theories of aging. Virtually all theories pertaining to *in vitro* senescence can be discussed, however, in terms of two broad categories: (1) That random accumulation of abnormal molecules, injurious to the organism, is the primary event leading to senescence. The most prominent example of such theories is the protein error catastrophe hypothesis of Leslie Orgel (1963), which has stimulated extensive research of the aging phenomenon in both *in vitro* and *in vivo* systems. The model predicts that the accumulation of abnormal proteins, resulting from mistakes in transcription or translation or both, is the initial cause of senescence. Since certain classes of proteins are essential for macromolecular synthesis, a variety of other aberrations, such as gene alteration, may occur in the cell or organism during the aging process. Other stochastic models predict such events as somatic gene mutations (Burnet, 1974*a,b*), intracellular free-radical accumulation (Harman, 1956, 1961), or extensive cross-linking of macromolecules (Bjorksten, 1974) as the primary causes of senescence. Genetically controlled corrective systems that affect the rate and character of these processes could be determinants of the longevity of the species. For example, in the case of the protein error theory, scavenger proteolytic enzyme systems (Goldberg, 1972; Capecchi *et al.,* 1974) may be of significance. (2) Genetic control of division potential of proliferating cell population both *in vivo* and *in vitro*. The nonproliferative state, the final result of a series of genetically controlled events, would be a fully differentiated cell that, in the case of cultivated human diploid skin or lung culture, has yet to be defined. A related hypothesis is that of a biological clock that counts cell divisions, with cessation of growth occurring on attainment of a predetermined limit. Such simple clock models of *in vitro* senescence have been virtually ruled out by serial cloning studies (Martin *et al.,* 1974, 1975). Indeed, as the authors suggest, the pattern of loss of growth potential in individual clones appears to be a stochastic process analogous to what has been observed in other differentiating populations *in vitro* (Till *et al.,* 1964). They also speculated that growth regulation may be a function of cell populations rather than individual cells. Many theories of aging have been put forward, all of which emphasize one of the broad concepts discussed here. To date, however, no single hypothesis has gained prominence, nor is one favored by a majority of investigators.

4.2. Scope of Somatic Cell Genetics

The discipline of somatic cell genetics involves the modification and application of classic genetic methods in the analysis of somatic cell behavior. A basic experimental paradigm of genetics is the study of cell structure and function through the isolation and analysis of stable variants or mutants. The major classes of stable variants that thus far have been isolated from somatic cells include: drug resistance, nutritional auxotrophy, conditional lethality, and alterations of gene products with a differentiated function (Siminovitch, 1976). Variants resistant to purine analogues have provided the most widely used selective system in somatic cell genetics. When cell populations are exposed to such analogues as 8-azaguanine, 6-thioguanine, or 6-mercaptopurine, a proportion of the surviving (resistant) clones, depending on the stringency of the selective system (Sharp *et al.,* 1973), will show greatly reduced levels of activity of the enzyme hypoxan-thine-guanine phosphoribosyltransferase (HGPRT), which is essential for the function of the salvage pathway in purine metabolism (Littlefield, J. W., 1976). Cells of this phenotype are then sensitive to anifoliate agents, such as aminopterine, that block endogenous synthesis of purines. A medium containing preformed purines, thymidine, and hypoxanthine, as well as aminopterine (HAT medium), provides a system for the selection of rever-tants (Szybalska and Szybalski, 1962; Littlefield, J. W., 1964). Isolation of clones resistant to ouabain has also been reported (Baker *et al.,* 1974; Mankovitz *et al.,* 1974). The cytoplasmic membrane enzyme Na/K ATPase in these variants displays decreased sensitivity to this compound. In hybrids with wild-type cells, this phenotype is dominant or codominant, which makes it potentially very useful in somatic cell genetics. Although variants have been selected from human diploid cells (Albertini and DeMars, 1973; Cox and Masson, 1974; Mankovitz *et al.,* 1974), their usefulness has been limited because of restricted growth potential *in vitro.*

The most fundamental aspect of characterization of a variant pheno-type is the demonstration of its mutational origin. There has been contro-versy as to the true nature of these variants (Siminovitch, 1976). This controversy stems, for the most part, from experimental evidence that indicates that ploidy does not influence the frequency of recovery of at least some markers (Harris, M., 1971, 1974; Mezger-Freed, 1971, 1972; Prickett *et al.,* 1975). Mezger-Freed (1971, 1972) examined this question using haploid and pseudodiploid lines derived from frog (*Rana pipiens*) embryos. The observed frequency of variants resistant to puromycin and bromode-oxyuridine (BrdU) was independent of the ploidy, and exposure to muta-gens in the case of puromycin resistance in the haploid cells. Based on these results and on studies of the permeability of puromycin in the wild-type and mutant cells, it was suggested that autonomous or "self-determin-ing" units are present in the plasma membrane or other structures of the cell, or in both. These and most studies, however, were carried out on aneuploid lines in which variations due to mitotic recombinations or chro-mosome loss or both cannot be accurately assessed. There is at least one report that suggests that these events may account in part for the observa-tions described above (Chasin and Urlaub, 1975).

There are, however, more stringent criteria for evaluating the genetic basis of variants isolated under selective conditions. Those given by L. H. Thompson and Baker (1972) are as follows: (1) enhancement of the fre-quency of the event by known mutagenic agents; (2) stability in the absence of the selective environment; (3) demonstration of an abnormal gene prod-uct; and (4) genetic mapping of the mutant and demonstration of its Mendelian segregation. Virtually all "mutants" satisfy the first two criteria;

moreover, there are now reports demonstrating altered gene products (Sharp *et al.,* 1973; Thompson, L. H., *et al.,* 1973; Shin, 1974; Beaudet *et al.,* 1973). Although it is now clear that at least some cell culture variants almost certainly result from gene mutation, it is reasonable to expect that epigenetic mechanisms (which are likely to be the usual basis of the heritable variation that occurs during differentiation) may also be operant.

The last criterion cited by Thompson and Baker (1972) is the most stringent, yet the least available to the somatic cell geneticist because somatic cells have no true sexual cycle. This problem can be circumvented, in part (albeit less efficiently), by means of artificially enhanced cell fusion. For the past decade, cell fusion has been accomplished by exposing cells to inactivated Sendai virus, a parainfluenza virus (Harris, H., and Watkins, 1965). More recently, polyethylene glycol has been found to fuse cells efficiently. Because of ease of handling and reproducibility, this chemical will probably replace Sendai virus as the fusigen of choice (Pontecorvo, 1975; Davidson and Gerald, 1976; Davidson *et al.,* 1976; Norwood *et al.,* 1976).

Following exposure to the fusing agent, bi- and multinucleate cells are formed; these cells are termed *heterokaryons* if the parental cells are of different genotypes, *homokaryons* if the genotypes are identical. In a small percentage of binucleate cells, nuclear fusion will occur, forming a *synkaryon*. Some of these synkaryons are capable of proliferation as a hybrid clone. Obviously, hybrid clones can be selected for if the parental cells are carrying selective markers such as drug resistance or nutritional auxotrophy. Depending on the cell type used and the culture conditions, these hybrid clones may be karyotypically stable or may preferentially lose one set of parental chromosomes (Ruddle and Creagan, 1975). The nomenclature for hybrid cells is similar to that of heterokaryons, a *homosynkaryon* being derived from genetically identical parental cells and a *heterosynkaryon* from genetically dissimilar parental cells. The technique of cell fusion has been extensively used in a number of major areas of study: (1) gene mapping, mainly of the human genome (Ruddle and Creagan, 1975); (2) analysis of the mechanism of differentiation (Davis and Adelberg, 1973); (3) analysis of the malignant phenotype *in vivo* and *in vitro* (Weiner *et al.,* 1974); and (4) study of cell-cycle control through fusion of heterophasic cell populations (Rao, P. N., and Johnson, 1970). Only in the last several years have serious attempts been made to analyze the phenomenon of *in vitro* senescence using cell hybridization and other techniques of somatic cell genetics. As mentioned above, the only meaningful "markers" of *in vitro* senescence are those related to cell replication, which are DNA synthesis and cell division (mitosis). These are certainly the result of many complex and, at present, poorly understood events. The use of such poorly defined markers limits the precision of interpretation of genetic studies. They are, however, technically easy to demonstrate and amenable to quantitation.

The major objective of the initial somatic cell genetic studies of *in vitro* senescence has been to attempt to distinguish among the broad theories of aging discussed above. The basic strategy has been to study the complementary behavior of senescent cells with respect to proliferative functions after fusion of these cells with other dividing cell populations. Three basic types of experiments will be discussed below: (1) heterokaryon studies, in which the parental nuclei are separate but in a common cytoplasm; (2) enucleation–fusion studies, also termed *heteroplasmosis* (Wright and Hayflick, 1975*a*) or *cybridization* (Bunn *et al.*, 1974), in which one fusion partner is an anucleate cytoplasm or a nucleus (with a small remnant of cytoplasm and a surrounding cytoplasmic membrane) (Wise and Prescott, 1973); and (3) synkaryon studies, in which nuclear fusion occurs and is followed by proliferation of a hybrid clone.

4.3. Heterokaryon Studies

The first heterokaryon studies involving crosses between late-passage cells and actively proliferating early-passage cells were attempted by Norwood *et al.* (1974, 1975). These authors had previously suggested, on the basis of cloning studies of human diploid cells, that cessation of proliferative activity is the result of terminal differentiation similar or identical to that observed in cell populations of known differentiated function, such as the hematopoietic system (Martin *et al.*, 1974). Although it was suggested that the differentiated cell type may be a type of histiocyte or macrophage, no evidence for a differentiated function or gene product has yet been demonstrated (Martin *et al.*, 1975). The experimental rationale of Norwood *et al.* (1974, 1975) was based on the observations of Professor Henry Harris and his associates, who demonstrated reactivation of nuclei from bona fide terminally differentiated cells when fused to an actively dividing partner (Harris, H., *et al.*, 1966; Harris, H., 1967). The most definitive demonstration was achieved with the introduction of hen erythrocyte nuclei into the cytoplasm of HeLa cells. Reinitiation of RNA and DNA synthesis occurs in the erythrocyte nucleus, and is associated with an increase in nuclear volume. The reappearance of hen specific cell-surface antigens coincided with the formation of a recognizable nucleolus (Harris, H., *et al.*, 1969). Norwood *et al.* (1974) reasoned that if the postmitotic, senescent cells are a differentiated population, then nuclear DNA synthesis should be reinitiated on fusion with a cycling cell. The first crosses were between this human diploid senescent cell type and low-passage, actively dividing cells. Identification of the parental origin of these cells was achieved by isotopic prelabeling of the cytoplasm of the senescent cell with [^{3}H]methionine and of the nucleus of the proliferating young cell with [^{14}C]thymidine. Double-layer autoradiography was used for identification of the prelabeled nucleus (Baserga and Nemeroff, 1962). Following fusion with inactivated Sendai virus, the cultures were challenged with three consecutive 24-hr pulses of [³H]TdR to determine the pattern of nuclear DNA synthesis. Contrary to the expected result, the young cells fused to a senescent cell not only failed to stimulate nuclear thymidine incorporation in the latter, but also were themselves markedly inhibited with respect to this function (Fig. 4). This result was observed in both isologous (intrastrain) and homologous (interstrain) crosses. In heteropolykaryons, there was no apparent dosage effect with varying ratios of parental nuclei. Although these results would appear to be nonsupportive of the differentiation hypothesis, it was noted that, with one possible exception, Harris used cell lines or, neoplastoid cells, not cell strains, or hyperplastoid cells (see Section 2.2). The studies were therefore repeated using the same protocol, except that HeLa cells or Simian-Virus-40 (SV-40)-transformed human cells were used as the actively

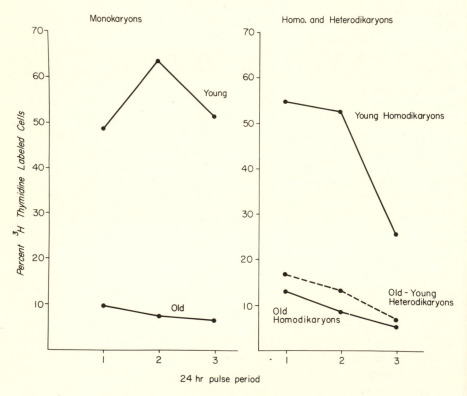

Fig. 4. [³H]TdR labeling indices of human diploid cell mono-, homo-, and heterodikaryons following Sendai-virus-mediated cell fusion between senescent and low-passage, actively dividing human diploid cells of the same strain. The slightly higher labeling indices of the old–young heterodikaryons in comparison with those of old homodikaryons are not significant. Reproduced from Martin *et al.* (1975), Plenum Press, New York, with permission.

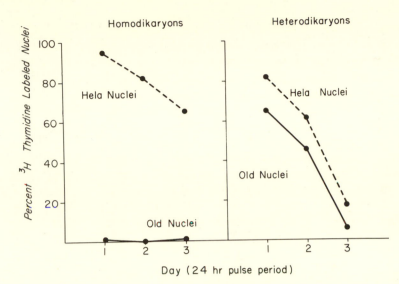

Fig. 5. [³H]TdR labeling indices of nuclei in homodikaryons and heterodikaryons resulting from Sendai-virus-induced fusion between senescent human diploid cells and HeLa cells. In contrast to the previous studies (Fig. 4), individual nuclei in the multinucleate cells were enumerated in these experiments. A decline of labeling indices observed in both nuclei in the heterodikaryons is apparent, and has been observed in multiple experiments. Reproduced from Martin *et al.* (1977), Elsevier–Excerpta Medica–North-Holland, with permission.

dividing partner (Norwood *et al.,* 1975). These experiments yielded quite different results in that marked stimulation of thymidine incorporation was observed in the nuclei of senescent cells (Figs. 5 and 6). Each cell type, however, exhibited a different kinetic pattern; in the case of HeLa cells, the [³H]thymidine labeling indices of both the senescent and the HeLa nuclei declined to less than 20% by the third pulse period. On the other hand, in the crosses with the SV-40-transformed cells, the labeling indices of both parental nuclei remained approximately 60–80 percent throughout all three pulse periods. Analysis of HeLa–old cell heteropolykaryons indicated a positive dose effect: the higher the ratio of HeLa to senescent cell nuclei, the greater the probability of nuclear thymidine incorporation by one or more of the senescence nuclei. These experiments were interpreted by the authors as supporting, but clearly not proving, a differentiation hypothesis. To explain the recessive behavior of low-passage, actively dividing human cells, it was suggested that the senescent cell elaborates a repressor or repressors that specifically inhibit the growth function of diploid cell strains (Norwood *et al.,* 1975).

These observations could also be interpreted within the framework of a stochastic model that predicts the random accumulation of abnormal

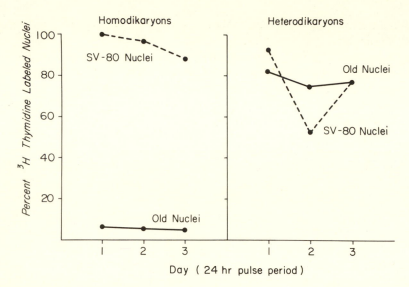

Fig. 6. [³H]TdR labeling indices of nuclei in homo- and heterodikaryons induced by Sendai-virus-induced fusion between senescent human diploid cells and SV-40-transformed human cells (designated SV-80). Unlike the labeling indices observed in the fusions between senescent cells and HeLa cells, those of both parental nuclei in heterodikaryons remain elevated throughout all three labeling periods. Reproduced from Martin *et al.* (1977a), Elsevier–Excerpta Medica–North-Holland, with permission.

molecules. It is certainly possible that immortal cells possess extremely efficient repair mechanisms that are capable of rapidly cleansing the senescent cell of deleterious molecules. The decline in [³H]TdR labeling indices in crosses with HeLa cells would suggest that this effect may be transient. As a positive control to test this notion, the authors exposed low-passage human diploid cells to amino acid analogues that, if incorporated into protein, might be expected to simulate the various types of injury postulated in the protein error catastrophe theory (Orgel, 1963). Concentrations were used that caused a sustained inhibition of growth but were not completely lethal. In the first series of experiments, low-passage, actively dividing human diploid cells were exposed to a combination of amino acid analogues known to be incorporated into proteins of eukaryote cells. This treatment resulted in very low [³H]TdR labeling indices comparable to those observed in late-passage cultures. In separate experiments, these cells were then crossed with untreated young human diploid cells and HeLa cells utilizing the same protocol described above (Norwood *et al.*, 1978a). The results were very similar to those observed in the studies with senescent cells with respect to labeling indices and kinetic pattern. A second series of identical experiments were initiated, except that the nonproliferating parent of low-passage human diploid cells was treated with mitomycin C, a bifunctional alkylating agent known to cross-link DNA and possibly other macromolecules (Iyer and Szybalski, 1963, 1964). This treatment also reduced the [³H]TdR labeling indices to the range seen in late-passage, senescent cultures. Once again, the pattern of nuclear thymidine incorporation was almost indistinguishable from that observed in original studies with senescent cells (Norwood *et al.*, 1978*b*).

Critical to the interpretation of these experiments is how precisely these agents produce a phenocopy of the senescent cell. Among the criteria were (1) the morphology of the treated cells and (2) the extent of reversibility of the injury. With the light microscope, the analogue-treated cells appeared remarkably unchanged over a period of days, while the mitomycin-C-treated cells assumed certain of the morphological features of senescent cells, such as apparent increase in size (by light microscopy) and increase in granular and filamentous structures in the cytoplasm. Clonal outgrowth is apparent after 2 weeks in the analogue-treated cells at the doses and duration of exposure used in these experiments. The recovery of mitomycin-treated cells at doses used by these investigators has not been examined; at lower doses (0.1 as compared with 0.5 μg/ml), however, clonal recovery occurs beginning at 4–6 weeks (Hoehn and Martin, 1972). Thus, the observations to date indicate that treatments of young cells by these agents do not produce an exact phenocopy of *in vitro* senescence.

The most important conclusion to be drawn from these experiments is that the [³H]TdR heterokaryon assay system does not discriminate among various types of cell injury. It is therefore impossible at this time to render any interpretation that supports the differentiation hypothesis. It is conceivable that *in vitro* senescence is multifactorial, and that the phenotype is the result of a variety of injurious events, some of which may be similar to those induced by the agents used in these experiments (the effects of which, it should be emphasized, have not been completely defined). These observations do raise the possibility that acquisition of a highly efficient error-correcting mechanism or mechanisms may be a necessary requisite for *in vitro* immortality of somatic cells.

There have been only a few other attempts to analyze the senescent phenotype by means of heterokaryon studies. Stein and Yanishevsky (1976) fused senescent WI-38 fetal lung fibroblasts to T98G human glioblastoma cells to analyze whether the ability to induce DNA synthesis in a senescent nucleus is correlated with immortality or with the pattern growth regulation. T98G cells were used because they are highly aneuploid and of unlimited proliferative potential, yet they show marked density-dependent inhibition of replication and high serum dependence and are apparently nontumorigenic (Stein, 1976). The results showed that in heterodikaryons, the T98G nucleus incorporated [³H]TdR, while the senescent nucleus did not. This observation suggests that T98G cells are not sensitive to a putative repressor or repressors, or alternatively, aberrant molecules, elaborated by senescent cells; this may be true of all immortal cells. In addition, the failure to the T98G cells to stimulate thymidine incorporation in senescent nuclei suggests that "reactivation" may require another factor or factors that alter growth regulation *in vitro*. This observation indicates that a variety of responses may be elicited, depending on the parental cell types used, a possibility further supported by the different kinetic pattern observed in the crosses with HeLa and SV-40-transformed cells. For example, the 3T3 cell line displays *in vitro* behavior very similar to that of the T98G cells. It would be of interest to determine how these cells behave in the experimental system. Using a slightly different approach, M. V. N. Rao (1975) introduced chicken erythrocyte nuclei, via Sendai virus fusion, into old and young human diploid cells. Reactivation occurred in the heterokaryons with young cells, but not with senescent cells. Although the author suggested that failure to reactivate the chick nucleus reflects the loss of specific nuclear proteins in the senescent cell, these results could also be attributable to the presence of defective proteins in the old cells.

Thus, analyses of the senescent phenotype by means of heterokaryon studies have yielded no evidence strongly supporting any of the hypotheses concerning the mechanism of *in vitro* senescence. There remains, however, a deficiency of information necessary for further interpretation of these experiments, i.e., the nature of the nuclear thymidine incorporation observed in the heterokaryons. To assume that this represents replicative DNA synthesis on the sole basis of autoradiographic observation is at best tenuous. The labeling could be the result of repair-type synthesis, a type of metabolic reutilization of the labeled substrate (Fox and Prusoff, 1965), or, less likely, the passage of labeled, acid-insoluble molecules directly between the two nuclei. To test for the possible induction of a repair-type synthesis, it should be possible to conduct similar experiments in the presence of agents (Wolff, 1972) or a nutritional environment (Stich and San, 1970) that selectively inhibits semiconservative DNA synthesis. It is also important to perform parallel synkaryon experiments in which clonal growth provides unambiguous evidence of cell growth, but, as will be discussed below, the heterogeneity of human diploid cell cultures imposes demands on both the design and the interpretation of such experiments.

4.4. Enucleation–Fusion Studies

Since the observations by Carter (1967) that cytochalasin B, a metabolite isolated from *Helminthosporum dematoideum,* induces nuclear protrusion and, in some cells, spontaneous enucleation, it has been demonstrated that a combination of exposure to cytochalasin B and centrifugation will efficiently enucleate mass populations of a variety of cell types (Prescott and Kirkpatrick, 1973; Wright, 1973). Veomett *et al.* (1976) termed the enucleate cytoplasm, cytoplasts, and the nuclei, with residual cytoplasm and surrounding cytoplasmic membrane, *karyoplasts*. It is of obvious interest to determine whether the capacity to rescue the senescent cell or, conversely, the factor or factors that induce senescence is predominantly a cytoplasmic or a nuclear function or both. The first experiments that attempted to answer this question were carried out by Wright and Hayflick (1975*a*–*d*). Specifically, these authors attempted to determine whether nuclear functions are responsible for loss of growth potential. They exposed low-passage proliferating cells to iodoacetate (a reagent that bonds to sulfhydryl groups) before fusion and to retenone (an inhibitor of oxidative metabolism) after fusion. It was claimed that these agents produced irreversible cytoplasmic injury. The authors reasoned that if nuclear functions were responsible for the onset of senescence, then enucleate cytoplasms from senescing cultures should be able to rescue those injured cells. The cell cultures to be enucleated were exposed to mitomycin C to prevent growth of the residual nonenucleated cells. Apparent rescue with extensive proliferation was demonstrated in the young cytoplast × young cell and the old cytoplast × young cell crosses, but not in the young cytoplast × old cell or old cytoplast × old cell crosses. From these observations, Wright and Hayflick concluded that the regulation of *in vitro* senescence resides in the nucleus. Although this interpretation is certainly reasonable, the experimental design does not exclude other possibilities. Cytoplasmic markers were not available, and the authors did not make use of nuclear markers (chromosome or biochemical), which precludes unambiguous identification of the hybrid nature of the rescued populations. A proportion of the experiments had to be rejected because of growth in the controls, indicating that the selective system is not amenable to precise control. In addition, the authors mention that in separate experiments, they observed rescue of iodoacetate-''killed'' cells, both when cocultivated and when fused to human cells bearing a selective genetic marker (hypoxanthine phosphoribosyltransferase) (Wright and Hayflick, 1975*a*). The rescued populations were diploid, indicating that the recovery was unlikely to have occurred as a result of hybridization. Thus, rescue by another mechanism such as metabolic cross-feeding (Subak-Sharpe, 1965) cannot be excluded.

In experiments concerned with the same question but using different methodology, Muggleton-Harris and Hayflick (1976) harvested the karyoplasts following enucleation of young and old cultures and carried out fusions of the karyoplasts and cytoplasts in the following combinations: young karyoplasts × young cytoplasts, old karyoplasts × young cytoplasts, and young karyoplasts × old cytoplasts. These crosses were accomplished in a nonselective system in which fusions and resultant clones were monitored by direct microscopic observations. The clones deriving from young karyoplast × old cytoplasm reconstructions showed a slightly greater proliferative capacity than the opposite crosses, but far less than what was observed with the young karyoplast × young cytoplast reconstructions. Indeed, the intermediate proliferative capacity of the young karyoplasts × old cytoplasts suggests that cytoplasmic alterations may occur after or in association with cessation of replication. Again, certain technical limitations necessitate conservative interpretations. As indicated above, the karyoplasts are surrounded by a cytoplasmic membrane with some residual cytoplasm. Clearly, potent cytoplasmic regulatory factors could affect the outcome of these experiments. It is also possible that nuclei from senescent cells are more susceptible to trauma and therefore less likely to initiate replicative activity under these conditions, even in a favorable cytoplasmic environment. Lukas *et al.* (1976) reported that karyoplasts from mouse L cells are capable of regenerating cytoplasms, although in the Muggleton-Harris and Hayflick work, direct observations by light microscopy make it unlikely that the observed clones arise by this mechanism or from contaminating whole cells. Nonetheless, nuclear and cytoplasmic selective markers could be very useful in these types of experiments. Cytoplasmic selective markers, such as resistance to chloramphenicol, have been isolated (Spolsky and Eisenstadt, 1972), although the isolation procedure is prolonged and the variants are not as "clean" as variants resulting from nuclear gene mutations.

In an extension of their previous studies, Norwood *et al.* (1978*a*) investigated the capacity of karyoplasts or cytoplasts or both to stimulate or inhibit nuclear thymidine incorporation. The only experiments completed to date are fusions of HeLa cytoplasts to senescent human cells. The HeLa cells were prelabeled with [³H]methionine, a cytoplasmic label, and [¹⁴C]thymidine, a nuclear label, the latter allowing for identification of intact (nonenucleated) HeLa cells. Following the prelabeling procedure, enucleation was accomplished using a modification of a published technique (Croce and Koprowski, 1973) in which cells were cultivated and enucleated in Corex glass centrifuge tubes. The mononuclear senescent cells displaying a cytoplasmic label (i.e., silver grains over the cytoplasm) were interpreted as having fused with HeLa cytoplasms. In several experiments, using either inactivated Sendai virus or polyethylene glycol as the fusigen, the senescent cells with cytoplasmic label displayed a two- to threefold higher labeling index than those without the label, considerably less than with intact HeLa cells, which induce a 10- to 15-fold increase in the senescent nuclei (see Fig. 5). Because of the technical complexity of such experiments, this result is difficult to interpret, and many controls are necessary. In the initial experiments, trypsin was used to remove the cytoplasts from the centrifuge tubes. Since cytoplasts removed by mechanical scraping yielded very similar results, this technical variable seems not to be important. Similarly, the stimulating activity of nucleated HeLa cells was not diminished by exposure to bytochalasin B. The combined effects of cytochalasin B and centrifugation, however, must also be considered.

It is possible that the stimulatory activity resides in a labile cell-cycle-dependent gene product. This possibility could be tested by fusing cytoplasts derived from synchronized populations. An alternative interpretation would be that a stimulatory cytoplasmic environment is due to multiple factors that decay rapidly after removal of the nucleus.

Fusion of pure karyoplast populations to senescent cells is yet to be accomplished. In view of the different kinetic patterns of labeling observed in the heterokaryon experiments, fusion studies with isolated karyoplasts and cytoplasts from SV-40-transformed human cells should be carried out. Initial trials indicate, however, that these cells are less amenable to efficient enucleation (Norwood, unpublished).

4.5. Synkaryon Studies

Successful recovery of clones from senescent human cultures after fusion with cell lines (neoplastoid cells) was reported by Goldstein and Lin (1972), Croce and Koprowski (1974), and Stanbridge (1976). In all experiments, a selective marker [hypoxanthine phosphoribosyltransferase deficiency (HPRT$^-$)] was present in the proliferating parental cell. These experiments are difficult to interpret because of the degree of heterogeneity in senescent cultures; the hybrid cells could have been derived from a residual population of replicating cells. Whether the sustained growth of these clones was due to loss of chromosomes responsible for senescence or to positive control by the heteroploid genome is not clear. Croce and Koprowski (1974), in crosses between SV-40-transformed human cells and senescent human diploid cells, reported that chromosome 7, to which the SV-40 tumor antigen was assigned, was present in all clones, indicating positive control. It was not possible, however, to determine whether concomitant loss of certain chromosomes (determining senescence) from the senescent parent was also occurring. Stanbridge (1976), using two HeLa lines as the proliferating parents, also isolated proliferating hybrid clones. In contrast to those recovered by Croce and Koprowski, however, these hybrid cells did not form tumors when injected into nude and appropriately pretreated mice. Dominance of the benign phenotype in hybrid clones was observed by other investigators (Weiner *et al.,* 1974), and indicates that other factors in addition to the intrinsic regulation of proliferation are involved in determining the malignant potential of a cell. That the SV-40-transformed cells appear to be dominant with respect to tumorigenicity suggests that transformation by at least some oncogenic viruses produces other, as yet unidentified, alterations in the cell. In a slightly different system, Davidson and Ephrussi (1970) recovered clones following fusion of the HPRT⁻ A9 mouse line with slowly growing secondary cultures of euploid mouse embryo cultures. The well-known tendency of cultured mouse cells to transform (Rothfels *et al.*, 1963) obscures interpretation of these experiments. The authors noted and emphasized, however, that the efficiency of recovery of hybrid colonies increased with decreasing number of the "senescent" parental cells.

Rescue of cells from senescent populations by hybridization with young, actively dividing cells has not been reported. J. W. Littlefield (1972) failed to recover clones in crosses with senescent cultures utilizing low-passage cells carrying a selective marker (HPRT⁻, derived from a donor with Lesch–Nyhan syndrome). The senescent culture was pretreated with BrdU in an attempt to cleanse the culture of residual replicating cells. Failure to observe clonal outgrowth again suggests dominance of the senescent phenotype, as was observed in the heterokaryon studies. Caution is warranted, however, because of the obvious difficulties of interpreting negative results.

Isolation of proliferating clones from euploid human cells is of interest not only to the study of *in vitro* aging, but also to human somatic cell genetics. The lack of selective markers has been a major problem, though numerous differentiating genetic markers are available (Harris, H., and Hopkinson, 1972). Genetic complementation of various inborn errors of metabolism have been demonstrated in heterokaryon studies (Nadler *et al.*, 1970; Lyons *et al.*, 1973; Thomas *et al.*, 1974). Two laboratories have reported demonstration of proliferating hybrids (Migeon *et al.*, 1974; Siniscalco *et al.*, 1969); in both cases, however, the presence of contaminating parental cells in the recovered clones prevented unambiguous determination of the proliferative capacity of hybrid cells. Heterokaryosis and metabolic cross-feeding could as well account for the observations (Subak-Sharpe, 1965). Furthermore, evaluation of karyotypic stability was impossible. Recently, Hoehn *et al.*, (1975b), using a nonselective system and glucose-6-phosphate dehydrogenase (G-6-PD) isozymes as a differentiating marker, isolated pure hybrid clones from human diploid cultures. These authors screened for putative hybrid clones by comparing the width of the equatorial plate in metaphase cells of a large number of clones, the width being greater in tetraploid cells (Sprague *et al.*, 1974). The presumptive hybrid clones were then screened for the presence of the G-6-PD heteropolymer and the karyotype of the clones analyzed to determine the fraction of tetraploid cells. Three types of crosses with low-passage, actively dividing cultures were made: (1) G-6-PD A and B strains, both male; (2) the two cell phenotypes from a female strain, mosaic for G-6-PD A and B; and (3) G-6-PD A male strain and G-6-PD B female strain derived from a patient with clinically diagnosed Werner syndrome. In the first two types of crosses,

Table II.   Types of Crosses Carried Out in a Nonselective System and Resultant Number of Pure Tetraploid Clones of Hybrid Origin as Evidenced by Presence of G-6-PD Heteropolymer[a]

Type of fusion	Clones prescreened[b]	Clones isolated and tested[c]	G-6-PD heteropolymer present
G-6-PD A male × G-6-PD B male	3203	102	6
G-6-PD A/B × Self	6944	127	3
G-6-PD A male × Werner G-6-PD B	8160	151	0

[a]From Martin *et al.* (1977).
[b]Visual screening under inverted microscope for tentative ploidy.
[c]G-6-PD electrophoresis and cytogenetics.

approximately 1 clone in 1000 screened proved to be a pure hybrid (Table II). On the other hand, none of the 8000 clones screened from the cross with the Werner syndrome cells has proved to be hybrid. Although suggestive, the data are not extensive enough to conclude that the phenotype of the Werner cells is dominant. Moreover, the Werner syndrome could be a special case, since the clinical presentation is not an exact phenocopy of true senescence (Epstein *et al.,* 1966; Martin, 1978*a*) and, more important, there is evidence of a propensity to chromosomal instability in cultured skin fibroblasts from patients with the Werner syndrome (Hoehn *et al.,* 1975*a*). Hybridization studies with senescent cells from normal donors should also be performed. Table III shows the life histories of pure hybrid and mixoploid clones. Although the number of observations is limited, the pure tetraploid clones display a stable karyotype and a growth potential, in terms of cumulative population doublings, similar to those of diploid controls and to previously reported cloning studies (Smith, J. R., and Hayflick, 1974).

Table III.   Life Histories and Ploidy of Selected Hybrid Clones Showing Both Tetraploid and Mixoploid Karyotypes

Clone No.	Tetraploid cells (%)		Cumulative population doublings
	Initial	Final	
1	100	100	35.3
3	41	10	43.6
4	100	100	46.6
5	95	100	33.9
6	42	15	31.9
7	16	0	46.5
8	100	100	< 25.0

Since the pure tetraploid clones remained stable throughout their life histories, it was concluded that the mixoploid clones resulted from the interclonal contamination that occurred during the initial isolation procedure, and the change in proportion reflects the relative growth advantage of one or the other cell type.

Although some tentative conclusions can be made, synkaryon studies to date have been sporadic and variable in design. For example, in none of the studies using heteroploid cells was there an attempt to rid the culture of residual growing cells (Davidson and Ephrussi, 1970; Goldstein and Lin, 1972; Stanbridge, 1976; Croce and Koprowski, 1974). That there was not, of course, makes any comparison with the observations of J. W. Littlefield (1973) of the young–senescent human diploid cell fusions very tentative, at best. Certainly these types of experiments should be repeated using rigidly controlled conditions with respect to the ratio of parental cells during the fusion (Davidson and Ephrussi, 1970). Pretreatment of senescent cultures should also be performed to remove replicating cells. Ideally, these studies should be designed to yield quantitative as well as qualitative results, which would make comparisons with the heterokaryon studies more meaningful. Recent technical advances in selective techniques against cycling cells will be useful for such experiments (Stetten *et al.*, 1976).

5. Discussion

Table IV summarizes the behavior of senescent cells with respect to proliferative functions in the various types of hybridization experiments reported as of this writing. As indicated above, conclusions drawn from many of these studies are very tentative because of the limited number of supporting observations. It is obvious from Table IV that a number of experiments have yet to be completed. The heterokaryon and synkaryon studies indicate dominance of the senescent cell with respect to their young, actively proliferating counterparts. On the other hand, such cells appear to be recessive to at least some neoplastoid cell lines. The enucleation–hybridization studies, at an even more preliminary stage, suggest that control of proliferation may be regulated by nuclear functions in human diploid cells. There is no evidence to date to indicate whether nuclei from neoplastoid cells with minimal amounts of cyoplasm are capable of rescuing senescent cells. More controls are needed before it can be concluded that HeLa cytoplasms possess minimal capacity to stimulate nuclear thymidine incorporation, as indicated in the first experiments of this type. Indeed, the cytoplasm of an ovum has the capacity to reprogram nuclei of somatic cells to an undifferentiated state capable of directing normal ontogeny (Gurdon and Woodland, 1970).

Table IV. Reproductive Behavior of Senescent Fibroblastlike Cells, Karyoplasts, and Cytoplasts Following Various Fusions

Intact senescent cell fused to:	Result[a]	Ref. No.[b]	Senescent cytoplast fused to:	Result[a]	Ref. No.[b]	Senescent karyoplast fused to:	Result[a]	Ref. No.[b]
A. Hyperplastoid cell			A. Hyperplastoid cell	Recessive[c,d]	6	A. Hyperplastoid cell	NR	—
Heterokaryon studies	Dominant[c,e]	1						
Synkaryon studies	Dominant[c,f]	2						
B. Neoplastoid cell			B. Neoplastoid cell	NR	—	B. Neoplastoid cell	NR	—
Heterokaryon studies	Recessive[c,e,g]	3						
Synkaryon studies	Recessive[c,h]	4						
C. Hyperplastoid karyoplast	NR	—	C. Hyperplastoid karyoplast	Recessive?[c,i]	7			
D. Hyperplastoid cytoplast	NR	—				D. Hyperplastoid cytoplast	Dominant[c,i]	7
E. Neoplastoid karyoplast	NR	—	E. Neoplastoid karyoplast	NR	—			
F. Neoplastoid cytoplast	±[j]	5				F. Neoplastoid cytoplast	NR	—

[a](NR) Not reported.   [b]References: (1) Norwood et al. (1974); (2) Littlefield, J. W. (1973); (3) Norwood et al. (1975); (4) Goldstein and Lin (1972); Croce and Kaprowski (1974), Stanbridge (1976); (5) Norwwod et al. (1977); (6) Wright and Hayflick (1975, a–d); (7) Muggleton-Harris and Hayflick (1976).   [c]Dominant: hybrid cells or heteroplasmons that display the reproductive phenotype of the senescent cell; recessive: hybrid cells or heteroplasmons that display the reproductive phenotype of the proliferating partner.   [d]As measured by the capacity to rescue chemically injured low-passage diploid cells.   [e]Pattern of nuclear [3H]TdR incorporation.   [f]Recovery of proliferating hybrid clones.   [g]May vary with type of neoplastoid cell.   [h]Clones may be derived from residual replicating cells in the senescent population.   [i]Cell reconstruction by nonselective techniques; statistically significant data not reported.   [j]Minimal (2 ×) increase in [3H]TdR labeling index of senescent nuclei.

Have these somatic cell genetic experiments provided any insight into the mechanisms of *in vitro* senescence? At the risk of equivocating, the answer must be a "not yet," due to the very preliminary state of affairs. The results of heterokaryon studies with cells in which replicative functions have been inhibited by exposure to toxic agents indicate that this approach lacks specificity and will not distinguish among the proposed models. As mentioned above, it is possible that acquisition of highly efficient error-correcting systems is a necessary requisite for cellular immortality.

Of the models proposing the accumulation of abnormal molecules to explain the process of aging, the protein error catastrophe theory of Leslie Orgel (1963, 1973) has been extensively tested *in vitro*. Experimental evidence both for (Holliday and Tarrant, 1972; Lewis and Tarrant, 1972; Holliday and Porterfield, 1974; Goldstein and Moerman, 1976) and against (Pendergrass *et al.*, 1976; Holland *et al.*, 1973; Tomkins *et al.*, 1974; Ryan *et al.*, 1974; Pitha *et al.*, 1975) this hypothesis has been reported; the issue is at present very much unresolved. Of interest in this regard is that selective degradation of abnormal proteins has been demonstrated in both prokaryotic (Goldberg, 1972; Prouty and Goldberg, 1972) and eukaryotic cells (Shaeffer, 1973; Capecchi *et al.*, 1974; Hendil, 1976). A recent study showed increased rates of protein degradation in senescent cells, yet some evidence indicated that senescent cells may degrade analogue-containing protein less efficiently than low-passage, dividing cells (Bradley *et al.*, 1976). This result could reflect impairment of an error-correcting system or, on the other hand, merely competition with other abnormal proteins accumulating in the aging cell. These authors found no difference in rates of protein degradation (either normal or analogue-substituted) between Phase II diploid human cells and their SV-40-transformed counterparts. Differences in the regulation of protein degradation were observed, however, with transformation of 3T3 cells (Hershko *et al.*, 1971). Clearly, qualitative as well as quantitative differences in systems responsible for degradation of abnormal proteins could exist. One approach to this problem would be to select for variants possessing scavenger systems with altered efficiencies, the experimental strategy being to select for increased as well as decreased sensitivity to a combination of amino acid analogues. Such variants, if isolated, could be used to study the efficiency of rescue of senescent cells.

Another error-correcting system that has recently received increasing attention in gerontological research is that of DNA repair. As above, conflicting observations have complicated the evaluation system for *in vitro* senescence. With regard to UV-induced repair, most studies have shown a decline in unscheduled DNA synthesis (UDS) after the onset of senescent changes. The authors unanimously concluded that the loss of UV repair capacity was not of causal significance (Goldstein, 1971; Painter *et al.*, 1973; Hart and Setlow, 1976). Studies of DNA repair following ionizing irradiation have yielded conflicting results. One laboratory observed decreased rates of repair in senescing cultures from normal donors (Little, 1976) and patients with progeria (Epstein *et al.*, 1974). Other investigators were not able to demonstrate significant changes with age in cultures from either normal donors (Clarkson and Painter, 1974) or patients with progeria (Regan and Setlow, 1974). Moreover, cultures derived from donors with xeroderma pigmentosum, which is known to result from a genetically determined deficiency of UV-induced repair (Cleaver and Bootsma, 1975), do not display restricted growth potential (Goldstein, 1971). Other genetic syndromes that may result from defective DNA repair or replication, which include the Bloom syndrome (Hand and German, 1975), Fanconi anemia (Sasaki, 1975; Fujiwara and Tatsumi, 1975; Poon *et al.*, 1974), and ataxia–telangiectasia (Taylor *et al.*, 1976; Paterson *et al.*, 1976), show no obvious decrease in growth potential. Subtle alterations may exist, however, as was documented in the latter two syndromes (Elmore and Swift, 1975, 1976).

Although it is apparent that the significance of DNA repair to aging, if any, is far from established, there are some recent observations that may be very important in this regard. Hart and Setlow (1974) showed that the initial rate and extent of UV-induced UDS in cultured cells correlated positively with the longevity of the species from which they are derived (Fig. 7). Clearly, many more studies both *in vivo* and *in vitro* in a wider variety of species are needed to confirm this observation. This is, however, the first study indicating that an error-correcting system may play some role in regulating life span. More recently, Schwartz (1975) reported an inverse correlation between the life span of a species and the ability of its cultured cells to metabolically convert 7,12 dimethylbenz(a)anthracene to a mutagenic form, suggesting that at least some aspects of cell metabolism may play a role in determination of longevity (Fig. 8). These observations could be interpreted as supporting a somatic mutation theory of aging (Burnet, 1974*a,b*). Alternatively, these differences could reflect the number of senescent or possibly differentiated cells that appear at lower passages in cultures from short-lived species. A decline in UV-induced repair synthesis was demonstrated with differentiation in some tissues (Stockdale, 1971; Hahn *et al.*, 1971). In addition, the observations of Hoehn *et al.* (1975*b*) are not supportive of a somatic mutation hypothesis in that tetraploid, hybrid clones do not display complementation in terms of a greater growth potential, indicating that recessive somatic mutations are unlikely to account for *in vitro* senescence. A detailed discussion of the significance of DNA-repair mechanisms is presented in Chapter 3.

Clearly, the present lines of experimentation must be completed and verified before their significance can be evaluated in terms of any contributions to our understanding of *in vitro* senescence. For example, a variety of neoplastoid cell lines with varying *in vitro* behavior should be examined in

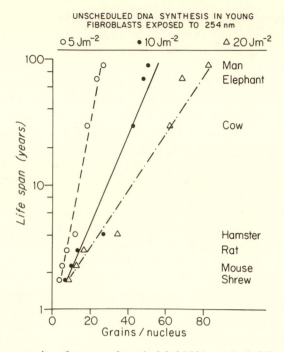

Fig. 7. Graphic presentation of amount of unscheduled DNA synthesis following exposure to UV irradiation (254 nm). A positive correlation between the magnitude of the response and the longevity of the species is evident. Reproduced from Hart and Setlow (1974), The National Academy of Sciences, Washington, D.C., with permission.

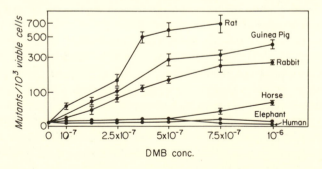

Fig. 8. Mutagenicity of 7,12-dimethylbenz(a)anthracene (DMB) to hamster cells as a function of dose. The test cells were cocultured with X-irradiated cells from various mammalian species to test the efficiency of the metabolic conversion of this compound to a mutagenic product. An inverse relationship to the longevity of the species is apparent. Reproduced from Schwartz (1975), Academic Press, New York, with permission.

both heterokaryon and synkaryon studies. Enucleation–fusion experiments should be continued, employing cytoplasmic and nuclear selective markers. There are, however, other experimental strategies that are relevant for consideration in future studies.

As stated above, one area that has been surprisingly neglected is that of the comparative biology of cultured cells; experimental studies to date are inconclusive (Hayflick, 1974; Stanley *et al.,* 1975). Such studies would certainly provide data pertinent to the relevance of *in vitro* cell behavior to aging and senescence *in vivo.* Ideally, the growth potential of cultured cells from closely related species with widely varying life spans should be analyzed, primate species probably being the best candidates. Such studies should, of course, be carried out under rigidly controlled conditions with coded cultures to maximize objectivity. Optimum *in vitro* growth conditions for each species would have to be defined. In addition, it would be necessary to determine for each species the predominant cell type that migrates and proliferates *in vitro,* utilizing both morphological and biochemical criteria. The major problems with these types of studies would be the cost and time required to adequately complete such an undertaking, both of which would be prohibitive for many laboratories. Other complicating factors include the frequency of spontaneous transformation in cell populations derived from many species, especially rodents (Todaro and Green, 1963), and the activation of latent viruses, especially in primate cultures (Martin and Sprague, 1973; Rogers *et al.,* 1967), which would not only affect survival of the cultures but also, most importantly, could be a potential biohazard for personnel handling them. Clearly, the costs and risks must be considered before such a project can be initiated. If the studies were properly done, however, a wealth of information benefiting not only aging research but also cell biology in general could be forthcoming.

As cited above, except for loss of proliferative function, there are no specific markers associated with senescence. Indeed, the only cell-cycle markers are those relative to DNA content, DNA synthesis, and mitosis. In the past decade, a number of laboratories have successfully isolated temperature-sensitive (Ts) conditional lethal variants (e.g., Thompson, L. H., *et al.,* 1970; Scheffler and Buttin, 1975; Roscoe *et al.,* 1973; Smith, D. B., and Chu, 1973), some of which have been partially characterized at the molecular level (Thompson, L. H., *et al.,* 1973; Toniolo *et al.,* 1973). One class of Ts mutants appears to be inhibited at specific points in the cell cycle. Some variants appear to be inhibited in the G_1 phase (Smith, B. J., and Wigglesworth, 1973; Burstin *et al.,* 1974; Liskay, 1974), while others appear to have defects in cytokinesis or mitosis (Wang, 1974, 1976; Hatzfeld and Buttlin, 1975; Shiomi and Sato, 1976; Thompson, L. H., and Lindl, 1976), and one mutant may have a defect in DNA synthesis (Sheinin, 1976).

This group of mutants may be of particular interest in that, although they are not characterized at the molecular level, they have the potential of providing additional markers of cell-cycle function. It would be of interest to study the complementation pattern of a series of these mutants with the senescent phenotype at the nonpermissive temperature. If a specific pattern of complementation were observed, then further characterizations of the noncomplementing mutants might provide information relevant to the mechanisms of proliferative failure in senescent cells. Failure of all such mutants to complement would best support the concept of accumulation of abnormal, toxic molecules. On the other hand, rescue by all classes of cell-cycle variants would suggest that the reproductive apparatus of the cells was intact, and that genetically mediated mechanisms may be involved in the cessation of proliferation. Since the difference between the permissive and nonpermissive temperatures in these cells is only 5–6°, meticulous attention to details of experimental design must be observed; such experiments are, however, technically feasible.

Another area that must be pursued with greater vigor is the *in vivo* studies of somatic cell behavior. Most of the age-related changes in proliferating cell populations *in vivo* show lengthening of the cell-cycle time with decreased cell-division rate (Lesher and Sacher, 1968; Thrasher and Greulich, 1968; Thrasher, 1971; Cameron, 1972), though not in all studies (Hamilton, 1976). Whether these alterations reflect environmental changes or are intrinsic modifications of the cell populations remains unresolved. It has been shown that BrdU incorporation into DNA can be demonstrated with fluorescent dyes (Latt, 1973) or with a modified Giemsa stain (Perry and Wolff, 1974). These dyes will distinguish between mono- and bifilial chromatid substitution of BrdU. Sister chromatid exchanges (SCEs), which appear to be a very sensitive indicator of DNA damage (Kato, 1974; Latt, 1974; Perry and Evans, 1975), are unambiguously demonstrated by this procedure. More recently, application of these techniques to *in vivo* systems was demonstrated (Allen and Latt, 1976; Vogel and Bauknecht, 1976; Tice *et al.*, 1976). This methodology will be useful not only for the analysis of cell-cycle alterations, but also for evaluation of DNA damage as a function of age. Clearly, emphasis should be placed not only on studies of resident cell populations *in vivo*, but also on transplantation studies to evaluate environmental effects.

The mouse teratocarcinoma system, described above, has the potential of being extremely valuable in gerontological research (Martin, 1977, 1978*a,b*). The teratocarcinoma cells participate in the development of virtually every organ in the chimeric animals (Papaioannou *et al.*, 1975), including the germ cells (Mintz and Illmensee, 1975). The effect of a specific gene locus on longevity could potentially be tested in this system. In addition, it may be feasible to test interspecific gene action or cytoplasmic factors through nuclear–cytoplasmic reconstructions. The technical complexities of these manipulations, however, should not be underestimated.

Thus, while genetic analysis has not elucidated the mechanisms of *in vitro* senescence, there are many experiments yet to be completed. Most certainly, as the discipline of somatic cell genetics evolves, so will the opportunities to apply this approach to the problem of aging. As indicated in the last part of this discussion, techniques are now available to carry out *in vivo* somatic cell genetic studies. Such studies will, it is to be hoped, help establish the relevancy of the *in vitro* model to senescence in the intact animal.

ACKNOWLEDGMENTS

I am grateful to Dr. George M. Martin for his critical review of the manuscript. Portions of the experimental material presented here were supported by NIH grants AG 00257 and AM 04826.

References

Absher, P. M., Absher, R. G., and Barnes, W. D., 1974, Genealogies of clones of diploid fibroblasts, *Exp. Cell Res.* **88:**95–104.

Albertini, R. J., and DeMars, R., 1973, Somatic-cell mutation, detection and quantification of X-ray-induced mutation in cultured, diploid human fibroblasts, *Mutat. Res.* **18:**199–224.

Allen, J. W., and Latt, S. A., 1976, Analysis of sister chromatid exchange formation *in vivo* in mouse spermatogonia as a new test system for environmental mutagens, *Nature (London)* **260:**449–451.

Azzarone, B., Pedulla, D., and Romanzi, C. A., 1976, Spontaneous transformation of human skin fibroblasts derived from neoplastic patients, *Nature (London)* **202:**74–75.

Baker, R. M., Brunette, D., Mankovitz, R., Thompson, L. R., Whitmore, G. F., Siminovitch, L., and Till, J. E., 1974, Ouabain-resistant mutants of mouse and hamster cells in culture, *Cell* **1:**9–21.

Baserga, R., and Nemeroff, K., 1962, Two-emulsion radioautography, *J. Histochem. Cytochem.* **10:**628–635.

Beaudet, A. L., Roufa, D. J., and Caskey, C. T., 1973, Mutations affecting the structure of hydoxanthine:guanine phosphoribosyltransferase in cultured Chinese hamster cells, *Proc. Natl. Acad. Sci. U.S.A.* **70:**320–324.

Bjorksten, J., 1974, Theoretical aspects of aging, in: *Symposium on the Theoretical Aspects of Aging* (M. Rockstein, ed.), pp. 43–59, Academic Press, New York.

Boone, C. W., 1975, Malignant hemangioendotheliomas produced by subcutaneous inoculation of BALB/3T3 cells attached to glass beads, *Science* **188:**68–70.

Boone, C. W., Takeichi, N., Paranjpe, M., and Gilden, R., 1976, Vasoformative sarcomas arising from BALB/3T3 cells attached to solid substrates, *Cancer Res.* **36:**1625–1633.

Bosmann, H. B., Gutheil, R. L., and Case, K. R., 1976, Loss of a critical neutral protease in ageing WI-38 cells, *Nature (London)* **261:**499–501.

Bowman, P. D., and Daniel, C. W., 1975, Characteristics of proliferative cells from young, old, and transformed WI-38 cultures, in: *Cell Impairment in Aging and Development* (V. J. Cristofalo and E. Holečková, eds.), pp. 107–122, Plenum Press, New York.

Bradley, M. O., Hayflick, L., and Schimke, R. T., 1976, Protein degradation in human fibroblasts (WI-38), *J. Biol. Chem.* **251**:3521–3529.

Brinster, R. L., 1974, The effect of cells transferred into the mouse plastocyst on subsequent development, *J. Exp. Med.* **140**:1049–1056.

Brock, M. A., and Hay, R. J., 1971, Comparative ultrastructure of chick fibroblasts *in vitro* at early and late stages during their growth span, *J. Ultrastruct. Res.* **36**:291–311.

Bunn, C. L., Wallace, D. C., and Eisenstadt, J. M., 1974, Cytoplasmic inheritance of chloramphenicol resistance in mouse tissue culture, *Proc. Natl. Acad. Sci. U.S.A.* **71**:1681–1685.

Burnet, F. M., 1974*a*, Intrinsic mutagenesis: A genetic basis of ageing, *Pathology* **6**:1.

Burnet, F. M., 1974*b*, *Intrinsic Mutagenesis: A Genetic Approach to Aging,* John Wiley & Sons, New York.

Burstin, S. J., Meiss, H. K., and Basilico, C., 1974, A temperature-sensitive cell cycle mtuant of the BHK cell line, *J. Cell. Physiol.* **84**:397–408.

Cameron, I. L., 1972, Cell proliferation and renewal in aging mice, *J. Gerontol.* **27**:162–172.

Capecchi, M. R., Capecchi, N. E., Hughes, S. H., and Wahl, G. M., 1974, Selective degradation of abnormal proteins in mammalian tissue culture cells, *Proc. Natl. Acad. Sci. U.S.A.* **71**:4732–4736.

Carrel, A., 1912, On the permanent life of tissues outside of the organism, *J. Exp. Med.* **15**:516–528.

Carter, S. B., 1967, Effects of cytochalasins on mammalian cells, *Nature (London)* **213**:261–264.

Chasin, L. A., and Urlaub, G., 1975, Chromosome-wide event accompanies the expression of recessive mutations in tetraploid cells, *Science* **187**:1091–1092.

Chen, T. R., and Ruddle, F. H., 1974, Chromosome changes revealed by the Q-band staining method during cell senescence, *Proc. Soc. Exp. Biol. Med.* **147**:533–536.

Chu, E. H. Y., and Giles, N. H., 1959, Human chromosome complements in normal somatic cells in culture, *Am. J. Hum. Genet.* **11**:63–79.

Clarkson, J. M., and Painter, R. B., 1974, Repair of X-ray damage in aging WI-38 cells, *Mutat. Res.* **23**:107–112.

Cleaver, J. E., and Bootsma, D., 1975, Xeroderma pigmentosum: Biochemical and genetic characteristics, *Annu. Rev. Genet.* **9**:19–38.

Cox, R., and Masson, W. K., 1974, X-ray dose response for mutation to fructose utilization in cultured diploid human fibroblasts, *Nature (London)* **252**:308–310.

Cristofalo, V. J., 1970, Metabolic aspects of aging in diploid human cells, in: *Aging in Cell and Tissue Culture* (E. Holečková and V. J. Cristofalo, eds.), pp. 83–119, Plenum Press, New York.

Cristofalo, V. J., 1972, Animal cell cultures as a model system for the study of aging, *Adv. Gerontol.* **4**:45–79.

Cristofalo, V. J., and Kritchevsky, D., 1969, Cell size and nucleic acid content in the diploid human cell line WI-38 during aging, *Med. Exp.* (Basel) **19**:313–320.

Cristofalo, V. J., and Sharf, B. B., 1973, Cellular senescence and DNA synthesis, *Exp. Cell Res.* **76**:419–427.

Croce, C. M., and Koprowski, H., 1973, Enucleation of cells made simple and rescue of SV40 by enucleated cells made even simpler, *Virology* **51**:227–229.

Croce, C. M., and Koprowski, H., 1974, Positive control of transformed phenotype in hybrids between SV-40-transformed and normal human cells, *Science* **184**:1288–1289.

Danes, B. S., 1971, Progeria: A cell culture study on aging, *J. Clin. Invest.* **50**:2000–2003.

Daniel, C. W., deOme, K. B., Young, J. R., Blair, P. B., and Faulkin, L. J., 1968, The *in vivo* lifespan of normal and preneoplastic mouse mammary glands: A serial transplantation study, *Proc. Natl. Acad. Sci. U.S.A.* **61**:53–59.

Davidson, R., and Ephrussi, B., 1970, Factors influencing the "effective mating rate" of mammalian cells, *Exp. Cell Res.* **61**:222–226.

Davidson, R. L., and Gerald, P. S., 1976, Improved techniques for the induction of mammalian cell hybridization by polyethylene glycol, *Somat. Cell Genet.* **2**:165–176.

Davidson, R. L., O'Malley, K. A., and Wheeler, T. B., 1976, Polyethylene glycol-induced mammalian cell hybridization: Effect of polyethylene glycol molecular weight and concentration, *Somat. Cell Genet.* **2**:271–280.

Davis, F. M., and Adelberg, E. A., 1973, Use of somatic cell hybrids for analysis of the differentiated state, *Bacteriol. Rev.* **37**:197–214.

Deal, D. R., Gerber, P., and Chisari, F. V., 1971, Heterotransplantation of two human lymphoid cell lines transformed *in vitro* by Epstein–Barr virus, *J. Natl. Cancer Inst.* **47**:771–780.

Dunn, G. R., and Stevens, L. C., 1970, Determination of sex of teratomas derived from early mouse embryos, *J. Natl. Cancer Inst.* **44**:99–105.

Elmore, E., and Swift, M., 1975, Growth of cultured cells from patients with Fanconi anemia, *J. Cell. Physiol.* **87**:229–234.

Elmore, E., and Swift, M., 1976, Growth of cultured cells from patients with ataxia–telangiectasia, *J. Cell. Physiol.* **89**:429–432.

Epstein, C. J., Martin, G. M., Schultz, A. S., and Motulsky, A. G., 1966, Werner's syndrome: A review of its symptomatology, natural history, pathology features, genetics, and relationships to the aging process, *Medicine (Baltimore)* **45**:177–221.

Epstein, C. J., Williams, J. R., and Little, J. B., 1974, Rate of DNA repair in progeric and normal human fibroblasts, *Biochem. Biophys. Res. Commun.* **59**:850–857.

Fox, B. W., and Prusoff, W. H., 1965, The comparative uptake of I^{125}-labeled 5-iodo-2′-deoxyuridine and thymidine-H^3 into tissues of mice bearing hepatoma-129, *Cancer Res.* **25**:234–240.

Fujiwara, Y., and Tatsumi, M., 1975, Repair of mitomycin C damage to DNA in mammalian cells and its impairment in Fanconi's anemia cells, *Biochem. Biophys. Res. Commun.* **66**:592–595.

Gey, G. O., and Gey, M. K., 1938, The maintenance of human normal cells and tumor cells in continuous culture, *Am. J. Cancer* **27**:45–76.

Goldberg, A. L., 1972, Degradation of abnormal proteins in *Escherichia coli*, *Proc. Natl. Acad. Sci. U.S.A.* **69**:422–426.

Goldstein, S., 1969, Lifespan of cultured cells in progeria, *Lancet* **1**:424.

Goldstein, S., 1971, The role of DNA repair in aging of cultured fibroblasts from xeroderma pigmentosum and normals, *Proc. Soc. Exp. Biol. Med.* **137**:730–734.

Goldstein, S., 1974, Aging *in vitro*, growth of cultured cells from the Galapagos tortoise, *Exp. Cell Res.* **83**:297–302.

Goldstein, S., and Lin, C. C., 1972, Rescue of senescent human fibroblasts by hybridization with hamster cells *in vitro*, *Exp. Cell Res.* **70**:436–439.

Goldstein, S., and Moerman, E. J., 1976, Defective proteins in normal and abnormal human fibroblasts during aging *in vitro*, *Interdiscip. Top. Gerontol.* **10**:28–43.

Goldstein, S., Littlefield, J. W., and Soeldner, J. S., 1969, Diabetes mellitus and aging: Diminished plating efficiency of cultured human fibroblasts, *Proc. Natl. Acad. Sci. U.S.A.* **64**:155–160.

Goldstein, S., Niewiarowski, S., and Singal, D. P., 1975, Pathological implications of cell aging *in vitro*, *Fed. Proc. Fed. Am. Soc. Exp. Biol.* **34**:56–63.

Good, P. I., and Smith, J. R., 1974, Age distribution of human diploid fibroblasts, *Biophys. J.* **14:**811–823.

Grove, G. L., Kress, E. D., and Cristofalo, V. J., 1976, The cell cycle and thymidine incorporation during aging *in vitro, J. Cell Biol.* **70:**133a (abstract).

Gurdon, J. P., and Woodland, H. R., 1970, On the long term control of nuclear activity during cell differentiation, *Curr. Top. Dev. Biol.* **5:**39–70.

Hahn, G. M., King, D., and Yang, S., 1971, Quantitative changes in unscheduled DNA synthesis in rat muscle cells after differentiation, *Nature (London)* **230:**242–244.

Hamilton, E., 1976, Aging and the proliferative capacity of mouse colon cells *in vivo, J. Cell Biol.* **70:**27a (abstract).

Hand, R., and German, J., 1975, A retarded rate of DNA chain growth in Bloom's syndrome, *Proc. Natl. Acad. Sci. U.S.A.* **72:**758–762.

Harman, D., 1956, Aging: A theory based on free-radical and radiation chemistry, *J. Gerontol.* **11:**298–300.

Harman, D., 1961, Prolongation of the normal lifespan and inhibition of spontaneous cancer by antioxidants, *J. Gerontol.* **16:**247–254.

Harnden, D. G., Benn, P. A., Oxford, J. M., Taylor, A. M. R., and Webb, T. P., 1976, Cytogenetically marked clones in human fibroblasts cultured from normal subjects *Somat. Cell Genet.* **2:**55–62.

Harris, H., 1967, The reactivation of the red cell nucleus, *J. Cell Sci.* **2:**23–32.

Harris, H., and Hopkinson, D. A., 1972, Average heterozygosity per locus in man: An estimate based on the incidence of enzyme polymorphisms, *Ann. Hum. Genet.* **36:**9–38.

Harris, H., and Watkins, J. F., 1965, Hybrid cells derived from mouse and man: Artificial heterokaryons of mammalian cells from different species, *Nature (London)* **205:**640–646.

Harris, H., Watkins, J. F., and Schoefl, G. I., 1966, Artificial heterokaryons of animal cells from different species, *J. Cell Sci.* **1:**1–30.

Harris, H., Sidebottom, E., Grace, D. M., and Bramwell, M. E., 1969, The expression of genetic information: A study with hybrid animal cells, *J. Cell Sci.* **4:**499–525.

Harris, M., 1971, Mutation rates in cells at different ploidy levels, *J. Cell. Physiol.* **78:**177–184.

Harris, M., 1974, Comparative frequency of dominant and recessive markers for drug resistance in Chinese hamster cells, *J. Natl. Cancer Inst.* **52:**1811–1816.

Harrison, D. E., 1973, Normal production of erythrocytes by mouse marrow continuous for 73 months, *Proc. Natl. Acad. Sci. U.S.A.* **70:**3184–3188.

Hart, R. W., and Setlow, R. B., 1974, Correlation between deoxyribonucleic acid excision-repair and life-span in a number of mammalian species, *Proc. Natl. Acad. Sci. U.S.A.* **71:**2169–2173.

Hart, R. W., and Setlow, R. B., 1976, DNA repair in late-passage human cells, *Mech. Ageing Dev.* **5:**67–77.

Hatzfeld, J., and Buttlin, G., 1975, Temperature-sensitive cell cycle mutants: A Chinese hamster cell line with a reversible block in cytokinesis, *Cell* **5:**123–129.

Hay, R. J., and Strehler, B. L., 1967, The limited growth span of cell strains isolated from the chick embryo, *Exp. Gerontol.* **2:**123–135.

Hayflick, L., 1965, The limited *in vitro* lifetime of human diploid cell strains, *Exp. Cell Res.* **37:**614–636.

Hayflick, L., 1970, Aging under glass, *Exp. Gerontol.* **5:**291.

Hayflick, L., 1974, The longevity of cultured human cells, *J. Am. Geriatr. Soc.* **22:**1–12.

Hayflick, L., 1976, The cell biology of human aging, *N. Engl. J. Med.* **295:**1302–1309.

Hayflick, L., and Moorhead, P. S., 1961, The serial cultivation of human diploid cell strains, *Exp. Cell Res.* **25:**585–621.

Hendil, K. B., 1976, Degradation of abnormal proteins in HeLa cells, *J. Cell. Physiol.* **87:**289–296.

Hershko, A., Mamont, P., Shields, R., and Tomkins, G. M., 1971, Pleiotypic response, *Nature (London) New Biol.* **232**:206–211.

Hoehn, H., and Martin, G. M., 1972, Heritable alteration of human constitutive heterochromatin induced by mitomycin C, *Exp. Cell Res.* **75**:275–278.

Hoehn, H., Bryant, E. M., Au, K., Norwood, T. H., Boman, H., and Martin, G. M., 1975a, Variegated translocation mosaicism in human skin fibroblast cultures, *Cytogenet. Cell Genet.* **15**:282–298.

Hoehn, H., Bryant, E. M., Johnston, P., Norwood, T. H., and Martin, G. M., 1975b, Nonselective isolation, stability and longevity of hybrids between normal human somatic cells, *Nature (London)* **258**.608–610.

Hogan, B. L. M., 1976, Changes in the behavior of teratocarcinoma cells cultivated *in vitro, Nature (London)* **263**:136–137.

Holland, J. J., Kohne, D., and Doyle, M. V., 1973, Analysis of virus replication in ageing human fibroblast cultures, *Nature (London)* **245**:316–319.

Holliday, R., and Porterfield, J. S., 1974, Premature ageing and occurrence of altered enzyme in Werner's syndrome fibroblasts, *Nature (London)* **248**:762–763.

Holliday, R., and Tarrant, G. M., 1972, Altered enzymes in ageing human fibroblasts, *Nature (London)* **238**:26–30.

Iyer, V. N., and Szybalski, W., 1963, A molecular mechanism of mitomycin action: Linking of complementary DNA strands, *Proc. Natl. Acad. Sci. U.S.A.* **50**:355–362.

Iyer, V. N., and Szybalski, W., 1964, Mitomycins and porfiromycin: Chemical mechanism of activation and cross-linking of DNA, *Science* **145**:55–58.

Kaback, M. M., and Bernstein, L. H., 1970, Biologic studies of trisomic cells growing *in vitro, Ann. N. Y. Acad. Sci.* **171**:526–536.

Kahan, B. W., and Ephrussi, B., 1970, Developmental potentialities of clonal *in vitro* cultures of mouse testicular teratoma, *J. Natl. Canc. Inst.* **44**:1015–1029.

Kato, H., 1974, Induction of sister chromatid exchanges by chemical mutagens and its possible relevance to DNA repair, *Exp. Cell Res.* **85**:239–247.

Kohn, R. R., 1975, Aging and cell division, *Science* **188**:203–204.

Krohn, P. L., 1966, Transplantation and aging, in: *Topics in the Biology of Aging* (P. L. Krohn, ed), p. 133, John Wiley & Sons, New York.

Krooth, R. S., Darlington, G. A., and Velazques, I. A. A., 1968, The genetics of cultured mammalian cells, *Annu. Rev. Genet.* **2**:141–164.

Kuliev, A. M., Kukharenko, V. I., Grinberg, K. N., Terskikh, V. V., Tamarkina, A. D., Bogomazov, E. A., Redkin, P. S., and Vasileysky, S. S., 1974, Investigation of a cell strain with trisomy 14 from a spontaneously aborted fetus, *Humangenetik* **21**:1–12.

Latt, S. A., 1973, Microfluorometric detection of deoxyribonucleic acid replication in human metaphase chromosomes, *Proc. Natl. Acad. Sci.* **70**:3395–3399.

Latt, S. A., 1974, Sister chromatid exchanges, indices of human chromosome damage and repair: Detection by fluorescence and induction by mitomycin C, *Proc. Natl. Acad. Sci. U.S.A.* **71**:3162–3166.

Lefford, F., 1964, The effect of donor age on the emigration of cells from chick embryo explants *in vitro, Exp. Cell Res.* **35**:557–571.

Lehman, J. M., Speers, W. C., Swartzendruber, D. E., and Pierce, G. B., 1974, Neoplastic differentiation: Characteristics of cell lines derived from a murine teratocarcinoma, *J. Cell. Physiol.* **84**:13–28.

Lesher, S., and Sacher, G. A., 1968, Effects of age on cell proliferation in mouse duodenal cysts, *Exp. Gerontol.* **3**:211–217.

Lewis, C. H., and Tarrant, G. M., 1972, Error theory and ageing in human diploid fibroblasts, *Nature (London)* **239**:316–318.

Lima, L., and Macieira-Coelho, A., 1972, Parameters of aging in chicken embryo fibroblasts cultivated *in vitro, Exp. Cell Res.* **70:**279–284.

Lipetz, J., and Cristofalo, V. J., 1972, Ultrastructural changes accompanying the aging of human diploid cells in culture, *J. Ultrastruct. Res.* **39:**43–56.

Liskay, M. R., 1974, A mammalian somatic "cell cycle" mutant defective in G_1, *J. Cell. Physiol.* **84:**49–56.

Little, J. B., 1976, Relationship between DNA repair capacity and cellular aging, *Gerontology* **22:**28–55.

Littlefield, J. W., 1964, Selection of hybrids from matings of fibroblasts *in vitro* and their presumed recombinants, *Science* **145:**709–710.

Littlefield, J. W., 1973, Attempted hybridizations with senescent human fibroblasts, *J. Cell. Physiol.* **82:**129–132.

Littlefield, J. W., 1976, *Variation, Senescence, and Neoplasia in Cultured Somatic Cells,* Harvard University Press, Cambridge, Massachusetts.

Littlefield, L. G., and Mailhes, J. B., 1975, Observations of *de novo* clones of cytogenetically aberrant cells in primary fibroblast cell strains from phenotypically normal women, *Am. J. Hum. Genet.* **27:**190–197.

Litwin, J., 1972, Human diploid cell response to variations in relative amino acid concentrations in Eagle medium, *Exp. Cell Res.* **72:**566–568.

Lukas, J. J., Szekely, E., and Kates, J. R., 1976, The regeneration and division of mouse L-cell karyoplasts, *Cell* **7:**115–122.

Lyons, L. B., Cox, R. P., and Dancis, J., 1973, Complementation analysis of maple syrup urine diseases in heterokaryons derived from cultured human fibroblasts, *Nature (London)* **243:**533–535.

Macieira-Coelho, A., 1974, Are non-dividing cells present in ageing cell cultures?, *Nature (London)* **248:**421–422.

Macieira-Coelho, A., Pontén, J., and Philipson, L., 1966, The division cycle and RNA synthesis in diploid human cells at different passages levels *in vitro, Exp. Cell Res.* **42:**673–684.

Mankovitz, R., Buchwald, M., and Baker, R. M., 1974, Isolation of ouabain-resistant human diploid fibroblasts, *Cell* **3:**221–226.

Martin, G. M., 1977, Cellular Aging—Part I. Clonal senescence, Part II. Postreplicative cells, *Am. J. Pathol.* **89:**484–530.

Martin, G. M., 1978a, Genetic syndromes in man with potential relevance to the pathobiology of aging, in: *Genetic Effects on Aging, Birth Defects: Orig. Artic. Ser.* (D. Bergsma and D. E. Harrison, eds.), The National Foundation–March of Dimes, New York (in press).

Martin, G. M., 1978b, Summary discussion, in: *Genetic Effects on Aging, Birth Defects: Orig. Artic. Ser.* (D. Bergsma and D. E. Harrison, eds.), The National Foundation–March of Dimes, New York (in press).

Martin, G. M., and Sprague, C. A., 1973, Symposium on *in vitro* studies related to atherogenesis: Life histories of hyperplastoid cell lines from aorta and skin, *Exp. Mol. Pathol.* **18:**125–141.

Martin, G. M., Sprague, C. A., and Epstein, C. J., 1970, Replicative life-span of cultivated human cells: Effects of donor's age, tissue, and genotype, *Lab. Invest.* **23:**86–92.

Martin, G. M., Sprague, C. A., Norwood, T. H., and Pendergrass, W. R., 1974, Clonal selection, attenuation and differentiation in an *in vitro* model of hyperplasia, *Am. J. Pathol.* **74:**137–154.

Martin, G. M., Sprague, C. A., Norwood, T. H., Pendergrass, W. R., Bornstein, P., Hoehn, H., and Arend, W. P., 1975, Do hyperplastoid cell lines differentiate themselves to death?, *Adv. Exp. Med. Biol.* **53:**67–90.

Martin, G. M., Norwood, T. H., and Hoehn, H., 1977, Somatic cell genetic investigations of clonal senescence, in: *The Molecular Biology of the Mammalian Genetic Apparatus* (P. O. P. Ts'o, ed.), Chapt. 23, pp. 289–302, Elsevier–Exerpta Medica, Holland.

Martin, G. M., Ogburn, C. E., and Sprague, C. A., 1978, Effects of age on cell division capacity, in: Le Vierllissement: Un Défi à la Science et a la Politique Sociale (M. Marois and D. Danor, eds.), Elsevier–Exerpta Medica, Holland.

Mayne, R., Vail. M. S., Mayne, P. M., and Miller, E. J., 1976, Changes in type of collagen synthesized as clones of chick chondrocytes grow and eventually lose division capability, *Proc. Natl. Acad. Sci. U.S.A.* **73:**1674–1678.

McBurney, M. W., 1976, Clonal lines of teratocarcinoma cells *in vitro:* Differentiation and cytogenetic characteristics, *J. Cell. Physiol.* **89:**441–456.

Merz, G. S., and Ross, J. D., 1969, Viability of human diploid cells as a function of *in vitro* age, *J. Cell. Physiol.* **74:**219–222.

Mezger-Freed, L., 1971, Puromycin resistance in haploid and heteroploid frog cells: Gene or membrane determined?, *J. Cell Biol.* **51:**742–751.

Mezger-Freed, L., 1972, Effect of ploidy and mutagens on bromodeoxyuridine resistance in haploid and diploid frogs, *Nature (London) New Biol.* **235:**245–246.

Migeon, B. R., Norum, R. A., and Corsaro, C. M., 1974, Isolation and analysis of somatic hybrids derived from two human diploid cells, *Proc. Natl. Acad. Sci. U.S.A.* **71:**937–941.

Mintz, B., and Illmensee, K., 1975, Normal genetically mosaic mice produced from malignant teratocarcinoma cells, *Proc. Natl. Acad. Sci. U.S.A.* **72:**3585–3589.

Mitsui, Y., and Schneider, E. L., 1976a, Relationship between cell replication and volume in senescent human diploid fibroblasts, *Mech. Ageing Dev.* **5:**45–56.

Mitsui, Y., and Schneider, E. L., 1976b, Increased nuclear sizes in senescent human diploid fibroblast cultures, *Exp. Cell Res.* **100:**147–152.

Muggleton-Harris, A., and Hayflick, L., 1976, Cellular aging studied by the reconstruction of replicating cells from nuclei and cytoplasms isolated from normal human diploid cells, *Exp. Cell Res.* **103:**321–330.

Nadler, H. L., Chacko, C. M., and Rachmeler, M., 1970, Interallelic complementation in hybrid cells derived from human diploid strains deficient in galactose-1-phosphate uridyl transferase activity, *Proc. Natl. Acad. Sci. U.S.A.* **67:**976–982.

Norwood, T. H., Pendergrass, W. R., Sprague, C. A., and Martin, G. M., 1974, Dominance of the senescent phenotype in heterokaryons between replicative and post-replicative human fibroblast-like cells, *Proc. Natl. Acad. Sci. U.S.A.* **71:**223–236.

Norwood, T. H., Pendergrass, W. R., and Martin, G. M., 1975, Reinitiation of DNA synthesis in senescent human fibroblasts upon fusion with cells of unlimited growth potential, *J. Cell Biol.* **64:**551.

Norwood, T. H., Zeigler, C. J., and Martin, G. M., 1976, Dimethyl sulfoxide enhances polyethylene glycol mediated somatic cell fusion, *Somat. Cell Genet.* **2:**263–270.

Norwood, T. H., Hoehn, H., Martinez, A. O., and Martin, G. M., 1978a, Synkaryon and heterokaryon analyses of clonal senescence, in: *Cellular Senescence and Somatic Cell Genetics, Vol 2, Senescence: Dominant or Recessive in Somatic Cell Crosses* (W. Nichols and D. Murphy, eds.), Plenum Press, New York (in press).

Norwood, T. H., Pendergrass, W., Bornstein, P., and Martin, G. M., 1978b, Behavior of chemically injured cells in heterokaryons and its relevance to clonal senescence (in prep.).

Orgel, L. E., 1963, The maintenance of the accuracy of protein synthesis and its relevance to ageing, *Proc. Natl. Acad. Sci. U.S.A.* **49:**517–521.

Orgel, L. E., 1973, Ageing of clones of mammalian cells, *Nature (London)* **243:**441–445.

Painter, R. B., Clarkson, J. M., and Young, B. R., 1973, Ultraviolet-induced repair replication in aging diploid human cells WI-38, *Radiat. Res.* **56:**560–564.

Papaioannou, V. E., McBurney, M. W., Gardner, R. L., and Evans, M. J., 1975,

Fate of teratocarcinoma cells injected into early mouse embryos, *Nature (London)* **258**:70–73.

Paterson, M. C., Smith, B. P., Lohman, P. H. M., Anderson, A. K., and Fishman, L., 1976, Defective excision repair of X-ray-damaged DNA in human (ataxia–telangiectasia) fibroblasts, *Nature (London)* **260**:444–447.

Pendergrass, W. R., Martin, G. M., and Bornstein, P., 1976, Evidence contrary to the protein error hypothesis for *in vitro* senescence, *J. Cell. Physiol.* **87**:3.

Perry, P. E., and Evans, H. J., 1975, Cytological detection of mutagen–carcinogen exposure by sister chromatid exchange, *Nature (London)* **258**:121–125.

Perry, P., and Wolff, S., 1974, New Giemsa method for the differential staining of sister chromatids, *Nature (London)* **251**:156–158.

Petes, T. D., Farber, R. A., Tarrant, G. M., and Holliday, R., 1974, Altered rate of DNA synthesis in aging fibroblast cultures, *Nature (London)* **251**:434–436.

Pitha, J., Stork, E., and Wimmer, E., 1975, Protein synthesis during aging of human cells in culture, *Exp. Cell Res.* **94**:310–314.

Pontecorvo, G., 1975, Production of mammalian somatic cell hybrids by means of polyethylene glycol treatment, *Somat. Cell Genet.* **1**:397–400.

Pontén, J., 1970, The growth capacity of normal and Rous-virus-transformed chicken fibroblasts *in vitro*, *Int. J. Cancer* **6**:323–332.

Poon, P. K., O'Brian, R. L., and Parlear, J. W., 1974, Defective DNA repair in Fanconi's anemia, *Nature (London)* **250**:223–225.

Povey, S., Gardiner, S. E., Watson, B., Mowbray, S., and Harris, H., 1973, Genetic studies on human lymphoblastoid lines: Isozyme analysis on cell lines from forty-one different individuals and on mutants produced following exposure to a chemical mutagen, *Ann. Hum. Genet.* **36**:247–266.

Prescott, D. M., and Kirkpatrick, J. B., 1973, Mass enucleation of cultured animal cells, *Methods Cell Biol.* **7**:189–202.

Prickett, M. S., Coultrip, L., Patterson, M. K., and Morrow, J., 1975, Effect of ploidy on spontaneous mutation rate to asparagine non-requirement in cultured cells, *J. Cell Physiol.* **85**:621–626.

Prouty, W. F., and Goldberg, A. L., 1972, Effects of protease inhibitors on protein breakdown in *Escherichia coli*, *J. Biol. Chem.* **247**:3341–3352.

Puck, T. T., Cieciura, S. J., and Fisher, H. W., 1957, Clonal growth *in vitro* of human cells with fibroblastic morphology: Comparison of growth and genetic characteristics of single epithelioid and fibroblast-like cells from a variety of human organs, *J. Exp. Med.* **106**:145–157.

Puck, T. T., Cieciura, S. J., and Robinson, A., 1958, Genetics of somatic mammalian cells. III. Long-term cultivation of euploid cells from human and animal subjects, *J. Exp. Med.* **108**:945–955.

Rao, M. V. N., 1975, Reactivation of chicken erythrocyte nucleus in young and senescent WI-38 cells, *J. Cell Biol.* **67**:352a (abstract).

Rao, P. N., and Johnson, R. T., 1970, Mammalian cell fusion: Studies on the regulation of DNA synthesis and mitosis, *Nature (London)* **255**:159–164.

Rao, P. N., and Johnson, R. T., 1972, Cell fusion and its application to studies on the regulation of the cell cycle, *Methods Cell Physiol.* **5**:76–122.

Regan, J. D., and Setlow, R. B., 1974, DNA repair in human progeroid cells, *Biochem. Biophys. Res. Commun.* **59**:858–864.

Robbins, E., Levine, E. M., and Eagle, H., 1970, Morphologic changes accompanying senescence of cultured human diploid cells, *J. Exp. Med.* **131**:1211–1221.

Rogers, N. G., Basnight, M., Gibbs, C. J., and Gajdusek, D. C., 1967, Latent viruses in chimpanzees with experimental Kuru, *Nature (London)* **216**:446–449.

Roscoe, D. H., Robinson, H., and Carbonelli, A. W., 1973, DNA synthesis and mitosis in a temperature sensitive Chinese hamster cell line, *J. Cell. Physiol.* **82**:333–338.

Rosenbloom, A. L., Goldstein, S., and Yip, C. C., 1976, Insulin binding to cultured human fibroblasts increases with normal and precocious aging, *Science* **193**:412–414.

Rothfels, K. H., Kupelwieser, E. B., and Parker, R. C., 1963, Effects of X-irradiated feeder layers on mitotic activity and development of aneuploidy in mouse-embryo cells *in vitro*, *Can. Cancer Conf.* **5**:191–223.

Ruddle, F. H., and Creagan, R. P., 1975, Parasexual approaches to the genetics of man, *Annu. Rev. Genet.* **9**:407–486.

Ryan, J. M., Duda, G., and Cristofalo, V. J., 1974, Error accumulation and aging in human diploid cells, *J. Gerontol.* **29**:616–621.

Saksela, E., and Moorhead, P. S., 1963, Aneuploidy in the degenerative phase of serial cultivation of human cell strains, *Proc. Natl. Acad. Sci. U.S.A.* **50**:390–395.

Sasaki, M. S., 1975, Is Fanconi's anaemia defective in a process essential to the repair of DNA crosslinks?, *Nature (London)* **257**:501–503.

Scheffler, I. E., and Buttin, G., 1975, Conditional lethal mutations in Chinese hamster cells: Isolation of a temperature-sensitive line and its investigation by cell cycle studies, *J. Cell. Physiol.* **81**:199–216.

Schneider, E. L., and Epstein, C. J., 1972, Replication rate and lifespan of cultured fibroblasts in Down's syndrome, *Proc. Soc. Exp. Biol. Med.* **141**:1092–1094.

Schneider, E. L., and Fowlkes, B. J., 1976, Measurement of DNA content and cell volume in senescent human fibroblasts utilizing flow multiparameter single cell analysis, *Exp. Cell Res.* **98**:298–302.

Schneider, E. L., and Mitsui, Y. 1976, The relationship between *in vitro* cellular aging and *in vivo* human age, *Proc. Natl. Acad. Sci. U.S.A.* **73**:3584–3588.

Schneider, E. L., Stanbridge, E. J., Epstein, C. J., Golbus, M., Abbo-Halbasch, G., and Rodgers, G., 1974, Mycoplasma contamination of cultured amniotic fluid cells: Potential hazard to prenatal chromosomal diagnosis, *Science* **184**:477–480.

Schwartz, A. G., 1975, Correlation between species lifespan and capacity to activate 7,12-dimethylbenz(a)anthracene to a form mutagenic to a mammalian cell, *Exp. Cell Res.* **94**:445–447.

Segal, D. J., and McCoy, E. E., 1974, Studies on Down's syndrome in tissue culture. 1. Growth rates and protein contents of fibroblast cultures, *J. Cell. Physiol.* **83**:85–90.

Schaeffer, J. R., 1973, Structure and synthesis of the unstable hemoglobin sabine $(\alpha_2\beta_2^{91Leu} \rightarrow {}^{Pro})$, *J. Biol. Chem.* **248**:7473–7480.

Sharp, J. D., Capecchi, N. E., and Capecchi, M. R., 1973, Altered enzymes in drug-resistant variants of mammalian tissue culture cells, *Proc. Natl. Acad. Sci. U.S.A.* **70**:3145–3149.

Sheinin, R., 1976, Preliminary characterization of temperature sensitive defect in DNA separation in the mouse L cell, *Cell* **7**:49–57.

Shimada, H., Shibuta, H., and Yoshikawa, M., 1976, Transformation of tissue-cultured xeroderma pigmentosum fibroblast by treatment with *N*-methyl-*N*-nitro-*N*-nitrosoguanidine, *Nature (London)* **264**:547–548.

Shin, S., 1974, Nature of mutations conferring resistance to 8-azaguanine in mouse cell lines, *J. Cell Sci.* **14**:235–251.

Shiomi, T., and Sato, K., 1976, A temperature-sensitive mutant defective in mitosis and cytokinesis, *Exp. Cell Res.* **100**:297–302.

Siminovitch, L., 1976, On the nature of hereditable variation in cultured somatic cells, *Cell* **7**:1–11.

Simons, J. W. I. M., 1967, The use of frequency distribution of cell diameters to characterize cell populations in tissue culture, *Exp. Cell Res.* **45**:336–350.

Singal, D. P., and Goldstein, S., 1973, Absence of detectable *HL-A* antigens on cultured fibroblasts in progeria, *J. Clin. Invest.* **52**:2259–2263.

Siniscalco, M., Klinger, H. P., Eagle, H., Koprowski, H., Fujimoto, R. Y., and Seegmiller, J. E., 1969, Evidence for intergenic complementation in hybrid cells, derived from two human diploid strains, each carrying an X-linked mutation, *Proc. Natl. Acad. Sci. U.S.A.* **62**:793–799.

Smith, B. J., and Wigglesworth, N. M., 1973, A temperature-sensitive function in a Chinese hamster line affecting DNA synthesis, *J. Cell. Physiol.* **82**:339–348.

Smith, D. B., and Chu, E. H. Y., 1973, Isolation and characterization of temperature-sensitive mutants in a Chinese hamster cell line, *Mutat. Res.* **17**:113–138.

Smith, J. R., and Hayflick, L., 1974, Variation in the life-span of clones drived from human diploid cell strains, *J. Cell Biol.* **62**:48–53.

Smith, J. R., Pereira-Smith, O. M., and Good, P. I., 1977, Colony size distribution as a measure of age in cultured human cells, *Mech. Ageing Dev.* **6**:283–286.

Soukupová, M., Holečková, E., and Hněvkovský, P., 1970, Changes of the latent period of explanted tissues during ontogenesis, in: *Aging in Cell and Tissue Culture* (E. Holečková and V. J. Cristofalo, eds.), pp. 41–56, Plenum Press, New York.

Spolsky, C. M., and Eisenstadt, J. M., 1972, Chloramphenicol-resistant mutants of human HeLa cells, *FEBS Lett.* **25**:319–324.

Sprague, C. A., Hoehn, H., and Martin, G. M., 1974, Ploidy of living clones of human somatic cells determined by mensuration at metaphase, *J. Cell Biol.* **60**:781–784.

Stanbridge, E. J., 1976, Suppression of malignancy in human cells, *Nature (London)* **260**:17–20.

Stanley, J. F., Pye, D., and MacGregor, A., 1975, Comparison of doubling numbers attained by cultured animal cells with life span of species, *Nature (London)* **255**:158–159.

Steel, C. M., McBeath, S., and O'Riordan, M. L., 1971, Human lymphoblastoid cell lines. II. Cytogenetic studies, *J. Natl. Cancer Inst.* **47**:1203–1214.

Stein, G. H., 1976, Characterization of T98: A polyploid human tumor cell line showing normal regulation *in vitro, J. Cell Biol.* **70**:24a.

Stein, G. H., and Yanishevsky, R., 1976 (personal communication).

Stetten, G., Latt, S. A., and Davidson, R. L., 1976, 33258 Hoechst enhancement of the photosensitivity of bromodeoxyuridine-substituted cells, *Somat. Cell Genet.* **2**:285–290.

Stevens, L. C., 1967, The biology of teratomas, *Adv. Morphol.* **6**:1–31.

Stevens, L. C., 1970, The development of transplantable teratocarcinomas from intratesticular grafts of pre- and postimplantation mouse embryos, *Dev. Biol.* **21**:364–382.

Stich, H. F., and San, R. H. C., 1970, DNA repair and chromatid anomalies in mammalian cells exposed to 4-nitroquinoline 1-oxide, *Mutat. Res.* **10**:389.

Stockdale, F. E., 1971, DNA synthesis in differentiating skeletal muscle cells: Initiation by ultraviolet light, *Science* **71**:1145–1147.

Subak-Sharpe, H., 1965, Biochemically marked variants of the Syrian hamster fibroblast cell line: BHK21 and its derivatives, *Exp. Cell Res.* **38**:106–118.

Swim, H. E., and Parker, R. F., 1957, Culture characteristics of human fibroblasts propagated serially, *Am. J. Hyg.* **66**:235–243.

Szybalska, E. H., and Szybalski, W., 1962, Genetics of human cell lines. IV. DNA-mediated heritable transformation of a biochemical trait, *Proc. Natl. Acad. Sci. U.S.A.* **48**:2026–2034.

Taylor, A. M. R., Metcalfe, J. A., Oxford, J. M., and Harden, D. G., 1976, Is chromatid-type damage in ataxia telangiectasia after irradiation at G_0 a consequence of defective repair?, *Nature (London)* **260**:441–443.

Thomas, G. H., Taylor, H. A., Miller, C. S., Axelman, J., and Migeon, B. R., 1974, Genetic complementation after fusion of Tay–Sachs and Sandhoff cells, *Nature (London)* **250**:580–582.

Thomopoulos, P., Roth, J., Lovelace, E., and Pastan, I., 1976, Insulin receptors in normal and transformed fibroblasts: Relationship to growth and transformation, *Cell* **8**:417–423.

Thompson, K. V. A., and Holliday, R., 1975, Chromosome changes during the *in vitro* ageing of MRC-5 human fibroblasts, *Exp. Cell Res.* **96**:1–6.

Thompson, L. H., and Baker, R. M., 1972, Isolation of mutants of cultured mammalian cells, *Methods Cell Biol.* **7**:209–281.

Thompson, L. H., and Lindl, P. A., 1976, A CHO-cell mutant with a defect in cytokinesis, *Somat. Cell Genet.* **2**:387–400.

Thompson, L. H., Mankovitz, R., Baker, R. M., Till, J. E., Siminovitch, L., and Whitmore, G. F., 1970, Isolation of temperature-sensitive mutants of L-cells, *Proc. Natl. Acad. Sci. U.S.A.* **66**:377–384.

Thompson, L. H., Harkins, J. L., and Stanners, C. P., 1973, A mammalian cell mutant with a temperature-sensitive leucyl-transfer RNA synthetase, *Proc. Natl. Acad. Sci. U.S.A.* **70**:3094–3098.

Thrasher, J. D., 1971, Age and the cell cycle of the mouse esophageal epithelium, *Exp. Gerontol.* **6**:19–24.

Thrasher, J. D., and Greulich, R. C., 1968, The duodenal progenitor population. I. Age related increase in the duration of the crystal progenitor cycle, *J. Exp. Zool.* **159**:39–46.

Tice, R., Chaillet, J., and Schneider, E. L., 1976, Demonstration of spontaneous sister chromatid exchanges *in vivo, Exp. Cell Res.* **102**:426–428.

Till, J. E., McCulloch, E. A., and Siminovitch, L., 1964, A stochastic model of stem cell proliferation based on the growth of spleen colony-forming cells, *Proc. Natl. Acad. Sci. U.S.A.* **51**:29–36.

Tjio, J. H., and Puck, T. T., 1958, Genetics of somatic mammalian cells, *J. Exp. Med.* **108**:259–268.

Todaro, G. J., and Green, H., 1963, Quantitative studies of the growth of mouse embryo cells in culture, and their development into established lines, *J. Cell Biol.* **17**:299–313.

Tomkins, G. A., Stanbridge, E. J., and Hayflick, L., 1974, Viral probes of aging in the human diploid cell strain WI-38 (38110), *Proc. Soc. Exp. Biol. Med.* **146**:385–390.

Toniolo, D., Meiss, H. K., and Basilico, C., 1973, A temperature sensitive mutation affecting 28 S ribosomal RNA production in mammalian cells, *Proc. Natl. Acad. Sci. U.S.A.* **70**:1273–1277.

Veomett, G., Shay, J., Hough, P. V. C., and Prescott, D. M., 1976, Large-scale enucleation of mammalian cells, *Methods Cell Biol.* **13**:1–6.

Vogel, W., and Bauknecht, T., 1976, Differential chromatid staining by *in vivo* treatment as a mutagenicity test system, *Nature (London)* **260**:448–449.

Vracko, R., and Benditt, E. P., 1975, Restricted replicative life-span of diabetic fibroblasts *in vitro:* Its relationship to microangiopathy, *Fed. Proc. Fed. Am. Soc. Exp. Biol.* **34**:68–70.

Wang, R. J., 1974, Temperature-sensitive mammalian cell line blocked in mitosis, *Nature (London)* **248**:76–78.

Wang, R. J., 1976, A novel temperature-sensitive defective prophase progression, *Cell* **8**:257–261.

Waters, H., and Walford, R. L., 1970, Latent period for outgrowth of human skin explants as a function of age, *J. Gerontol.* **25**:381–383.

Waters, H., and Walford, R. L., 1971, A non-enzymatic method for subculturing monolayer cell cultures, *Proc. Soc. Exp. Biol. Med.* **137**:523–525.

Weiner, F., Klein, G., and Harris, H., 1974, The analysis of malignancy by cell fusion. V. Further evidence of the ability of normal diploid cells to suppress malignancy, *J. Cell Sci.* **15**:177–183.

Whitaker, A. M., Gould, J., and Smith, E. M., 1974, The effect of repeated subcultivations and of a serum with an unusual property, *Exp. Cell Res.* **87**:55–62.

Wise, G. E., and Prescott, D. M., 1973, Ultrastructure of enucleated mammalian cells in culture, *Exp. Cell Res.* **81**:63–72.

Wolff, S., 1972, The repair of X-ray-induced chromosome aberrations in stimulated and unstimulated human lymphocytes, *Mutat. Res.* **15**:435–444.

Wright, W. E., 1973, The production of mass populations of anucleate cytoplasms, in: *Methods in Cell Biology* (D. M. Prescott, ed.), Vol. 8, Chapt. 10, pp. 203–210, Academic Press, New York.

Wright, W. E., and Hayflick, L., 1975*a*, Use of biochemical lesions for selection of human cells with hybrid cytoplasms, *Proc. Natl. Acad. Sci. U.S.A.* **72**:1812–1816.

Wright, W. E., and Hayflick, L., 1975*b*, The regulation of cellular aging by nuclear events in cultured normal human fibroblasts (WI-38), *Adv. Exp. Med. Biol.* **61**:39–55.

Wright, W. E., and Hayflick, L., 1975*c*, Contributions of cytoplasmic factors to *in vitro* cellular senescence, *Fed. Proc. Fed. Am. Soc. Exp. Biol.* **34**:76–79.

Wright, W. E., and Hayflick, L., 1975*d*, Nuclear control of cellular aging demonstrated by hybridization of anucleate and whole cultured normal human fibroblasts, *Exp. Cell Res.* **96**:113–121.

Yanishevsky, R., and Carrano, A. V., 1975, Prematurely condensed chromosomes of dividing and non-dividing cells in aging human cell cultures, *Exp. Cell Res.* **90**:169–174.

Yanishevsky, R., Mendelsohn, M. L., Mayall, B. H., and Cristofalo, V. J., 1974, Proliferative capacity and DNA content of aging human diploid cells in culture: A cytophotometric and autoradiographic analysis, *J. Cell. Physiol.* **84**:165–170.

Yoshida, M. C., and Makino, S., 1963, A chromosome study of non-treated and an irradiated human *in vitro* cell line, *Jpn. J. Hum. Genet.* **8**:39–45.

Chapter 12

Immunogenetics of Aging

R. L. Walford, G. S. Smith, P. J. Meredith, and K. E. Cheney

1. Introduction*

As recently as the late 1960s, a major drawback to an immunological interpretation of aging seemed to be that animals below the vertebrate level did not possess true immunological systems (Walford, 1969). It has been clearly demonstrated by now, however, that at least in echinoderms, annelids, and coelenterates, specific immunocompetence with components of memory or immunorecognition systems or both, exists (Hildemann, 1978). At the same time, it is known that life span may vary independently of phylogenetic or evolutionary position (Hildemann, 1978), and that animals high on the evolutionary scale may display much longer or shorter life spans than animals relatively low on the scale. Broad-ranging possibilities for immunogenetic investigations of aging are therefore evident. Unfortunately, those invertebrates that have been investigated immunologically have not been much studied genetically, and those for which abundant genetic information is available—arthropods, for example—have not been subjected to refined immunological scrutiny. The one form of immune response that is probably common to all metazoa is the recognition of self

---

*Abbreviations used in this chapter: (CML) cell-mediated lymphocytotoxicity; (DNP) dinitrophenyl; (Ig) immunoglobulin; (*Ir* gene) immune respone gene; (L chain) light chain; (LPS) lipopolysaccharide; (MHC) major histocompatibility complex; (MLR) mixed lymphocyte reaction; (PHA) phytohemagglutinin; (PPD) purified protein derivative; (PWM) pokeweed mitogen; (SRBC) sheep red blood cells.

R. L. Walford, G. S. Smith, P. J. Meredith, and K. E. Cheney • Department of Pathology, University of California, Los Angeles, California 90024

from nonself, demonstrable experimentally by transplant rejection. Immunogenetic information relevant to aging in the usual sense, i.e., variation within the species rather than comparisons between species, derives almost entirely from studies of higher animals subjected to laboratory experimentation or clinical observation, such as the mouse, man, rat, guinea pig, and hamster.

2. Histocompatibility Systems and Immune Responses

All vertebrate species so far investigated, including birds and amphibia as well as mammals, possess a major histocompatibility complex (MHC), e.g., the *H-2* system in the mouse and the *HLA* system in man. Each of these systems occupies a chromosomal region—on the 17th chromosome in the mouse and on the 6th in man—of sufficient size to accommodate several hundred genetic loci, although only 6–12 have been identified. *H-2* and *HLA* are so-called "super-gene" systems or regions, a term that refers to a cluster of genes influencing the same type of functions. Thus, the MHC appears to be the master gene system for controlling or influencing the immune response, particularly as it involves thymus-dependent functions (Shreffler, 1977; Svejgaard *et al.*, 1975*a*; Walford, 1977). That the MHC might be fundamentally involved in aging has been suggested by several workers (Walford, 1970, 1974; Yunis *et al.*, 1973). This view is consistent with Cutler's recent conclusion, based on analysis of the aging rate of hominid ancestral species, that primary aging processes may be determined by a relatively small number of genes or genetic regulatory systems (Cutler, 1975).

The *H-2* system of the mouse is the most completely studied of the MHCs. Within it lie genes for controlling the development of specific suppressor cells; the mixed lymphocyte reaction (MLR); the cell-mediated lymphocytotoxicity (CML) reaction; susceptibility or resistance to a number of leukemia viruses; susceptibility or resistance to a number of spontaneously occurring malignancies; the so-called "immune response," or *Ir*, genes, which determine whether an animal can develop immune responses to certain antigens; the so-called "immune-associated," or Ia, antigens, which may be the gene products of the *Ir* genes; the age-specific maturation rates, peaks, and rates of decline of different immune-response capacities; and several components of the complement system. In addition, the gene products located at the *D* and *K* loci of the *H-2* system may be required for recognition of "self" (Bevan, 1975; Doherty and Zinkernagel, 1975). An outline of the *H-2* and *HLA* systems is given in Fig. 1.

Other genes on other chromosomes might also influence the immune response, and even the development of autoimmunity, but non-MHC loci

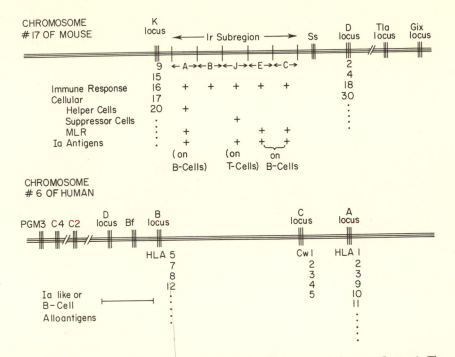

Fig. 1. The *H-2* system of the mouse (top) and the *HLA* system in humans (bottom). The mouse MHC is somewhat dissimilar to that of other species, including man, in that the *Ir* subregion and the locus for the MLR lie between the *K* and *D* loci, whereas in man it lies to the left of the *B* locus (which is homologous to *K* in the mouse.) The specificities shown under the *K, D, B, C,* and *A* loci in the two species are mutually exclusive in that only one can occupy the locus. Over 40 *HLA* specificities are known, counting the *B, C,* and *A* loci only. The different functions thought to be influenced by the *Ir* genes in the mouse are indicated. *Ss,* and *C4* and *C2,* refer to loci that influence complement in mouse and man, respectively.

have been much less studied than MHC because of the difficulty in defining their gene products by serological or cellular immune techniques. Characteristics of some of these, the so-called "minor" histocompatibility systems in the mouse, or *H-1, H-3, H-4* . . . etc., were thoroughly reviewed by Hildemann (1970). The "minor" systems can be demonstrated in the laboratory only by transplantation methods involving either skin or tumor grafts, but at least one of these, the *H-1* system, may influence life span and the type and frequency of spontaneous neoplasms developing in mice (Smith and Walford, 1978). Ultimately, therefore, the term "minor system" may prove to have been misleading. At least 36 and possibly many more histocompatibility systems exist in mice.

While the MHC may influence the maturation rate of thymus-independent as well as thymus-dependent immune functions (Meredith and Walford, 1977), the primary genetic control of responses to at least some thymus-independent antigens, e.g., to bacterial lipopolysaccharide (LPS) in mice (Watson and Riblet, 1974), probably resides elsewhere. Except for studies of proliferative responses to certain mitogens, information about the age-related immune response to thymus-independent antigens, or responses not controlled or influenced by the MHC, is virtually nonexistent.

3. Immune Functional Changes with Age

We shall briefly outline here salient points about what is known regarding immune functional changes with age, chiefly in mice, and later relate these points to specific genetic control where such correlative information is available.

In considering age-specific variation in immune function in any species, e.g., in the mouse, it is important to relate the level of change to the actual life span of the strain. Quite a few otherwise very sophisticated studies purporting to deal with the aging process in mice have employed mice no more than 12–18 months of age as "old" subjects. For a long-lived strain such as C57BL/6, this is merely early middle age, and certain immune responses may not even have reached peak values by that time (Gerbase-DeLima *et al.*, 1975*a*).

A second possible cause of error that is also fairly replete in the literature consists of not relating the level of change to the age-specific peak immune response capacity of the mouse for the particular function being measured. Several pertinent concepts related to peak capacity are illustrated heuristically in Fig. 2. Curve A depicts the response to injected sheep red blood cells (SRBC); curve B, the response to allogeneic cells (the MLR); and curve C, the pokeweed mitogen (PWM) response to LPS. Referring now to curve A, one sees that the peak response capacity occurs at about 20 weeks of age in the illustrative mouse strain. The degree of age-related decline in immune function, as measured by response to SRBC, should therefore be related to this peak. Conceptual errors might arise if one compared the response of a 6-week-old mouse with that of a 1-year-old mouse, and concluded that immune function as measured by this parameter increased with "aging." The second concept illustrated by Fig. 2 is that different immune-response capacities mature, reach peak level, and decline at different rates in the same mouse strain. The overall immune situation of an animal at a particular age should be considered as an "immune slice" of these parameters—many of which, incidentally, are controlled or at least greatly influenced by genes at the MHC.

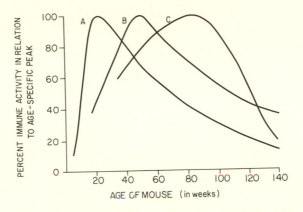

Fig. 2. Heuristic model of maturation rates of different immune response capacities within a single mouse strain. (A) Response to SRBC; (B) MLR; (C) response to PWM.

3.1. T-Dependent Immune Functions

The response of the host lymphoid cells to nonself, altered self, or foreign alloantigens, be they tissue graft, indigenous malignancy, or virus-altered cells, is characterized by a recognition phase during which a sub-population of host cells undergoes blastogenesis. The recognition phase is known as the mixed lymphocyte reaction, and in mice is mediated most strongly by genes at the *Ia* locus of the MHC. Recognition is followed by the development of "killer" cells responsible for a CML reaction in which the foreign or altered cells are lysed. This cytotoxic reaction is not *I*-region-controlled, but is dependent on genetic factors present at the *K* and *D* ends of the *H-2* in the mouse or the *A* and *B* loci of *HLA* in man. Both stimulator and effector aspects of what one may regard as classic transplantation immunity—which to some degree is present in every metazoan animal so far studied in detail—are therefore influenced by the MHC.

With aging, the MLR in mice declines to about a third of its peak youth value (Konen *et al.*, 1973; Gerbase-DeLima *et al.*, 1974). In contrast, the CML reaction corresponding to the effector phase of transplant rejection declines with age to a considerably greater extent (Goodman and Makinodan, 1975).

The humoral immune response involving the manufacture of immunoglobulin (Ig) antibodies, to the extent that it requires T/B-cell cooperation, also declines markedly with age. The most thorough studies of this decline are those of Makinodan *et al.* (1971) and Kishimoto *et al.* (1976).

Certain mitogens, chiefly phytohemagglutinin (PHA) and concanavalin A (Con A), stimulate T-dependent lymphoid cells to undergo blastogenesis and incorporate tritiated thymidine. The response to these mitogens declines markedly with advanced age in mice (Mathies *et al.,* 1973; Meredith and Walford, 1977). It has been shown, however, that the lymphoid cells of an old mouse possess just as many combining sites for PHA as those from a young mouse (Hung *et al.,* 1975). Despite this receptor-site equality, the old lymphoid cell population gives a diminished response, signifying either that many cells respond to a lesser degree or that a lower percentage of cells among the old population respond.

So-called "suppressor cells" are lymphoid cells that suppress another immune reaction or potential reaction. Important in regulatory control of the immune system and in mitigating against autoimmunity, they are coded for by a locus in the *I*-region of the MHC in mice (Shreffler, 1977). There is evidence for the existence of both thymic and splenic suppressor cells that act in different ways (Talal, 1976). Suppressor cells for the MLR and for the response to dinitrophenyl (DNP) hapten increase with normal aging in mice (Gerbase-DeLima *et al.,* 1975*a*; Segre and Segre, 1976). In autoimmune-susceptible NZB mice, on the other hand, suppressor cells were reported to decrease with age (Talal and Steinberg, 1974).

3.2. T-Independent Immune Functions

Much less information is available about age-correlated thymus-independent than thymus-dependent immune functions. There may be a mild functional decline (Gerbase-DeLima *et al.,* 1974), or no change or even some increase with age (Meredith and Walford, 1977; Naor *et al.,* 1976). The area has been poorly explored. None of the "minor" histocompatibility systems has been assessed in relation to aging.

3.3. Autoimmunity

Autoimmune manifestations constitute high-incidence phenomena with age in humans (MacKay, 1972), as well as in most strains of mice (Table I), particularly the age-specific incidence of naturally occurring anti-DNA or anti-DNP antibodies in otherwise normal individuals. This upsurge in autoimmunity is thought to be related to a decline in self/nonself discrimination—in short, to a failure in the homeostatic control of tolerance for self, as originally proposed by us as one possible explanation for the autoimmune features of aging (Walford, 1969). It is quite possible that age-related immune disturbances, including autoimmunity, are due to a failure in active suppressor mechanisms, which normally maintain self-tolerance in younger animals (Cunningham, 1976). Also, old mice have a relatively greater response to "altered-self" antigens than young mice, attributable to failure in regulatory or suppressor T-cell mechanisms for checking the "au-

Table I. Occurrence (%) of Antinuclear Antibodies in Aging
Mice of Various Strains[a]

Strain	7–12 months		13–24 months	
	Strong	Weak	Strong	Weak
NZB	92	8	91	5
A	8	42		
CBA	0	50		
C3H	12	59		
C57BL	4	22	18	45
129/J	0	8	47	24
BALB/C	8	23	62	23

[a]Adapted from Siegal *et al.* (1972).

toimmune'' response to modified-self antigens (Naor *et al.*, 1976). Autoimmunity in aging may take the form of lymphocytes producing autoantibodies such as antinuclear antibodies (Table I), or T-lymphocytes and macrophages infiltrating and destroying target organs. Autoimmune diseases are frequently associated with viral infections or with factors that influence regulation of the immune system. The genetic background of individuals or strains within a species may modify the long-term effects resulting from viral infection, including autoimmune phenomena (Kay, 1978). In a number of instances, viral susceptibility or the course of viral disease is greatly influenced by genes at the MHC. A role for slow viruses in aging was proposed by Gajdusek (1972).

4. Genetic Influences of Immune Function in Aging

4.1. Influence of Sex

Data comparing the immune-response capacities of males and females of various ages to defined antigens are surprisingly scant, although the general impression exists that females respond somewhat better at most ages. There is a higher incidence of autoimmunity in females than in males, at least for humans (MacKay, 1972). The autoimmunity of hybrid NZB/NZW F_1 (B/W) mice is considerably more severe in females than in males (Talal, 1976). If immune dysfunction is involved in aging, one might expect females to display a shorter survival than males, under identical environmental situations. In most instances, this seems to be the case, at least for 50% survival in mice (Smith *et al.*, 1973; Kunstyr and Leuenberger, 1975). Human females enjoy a greater survival in most societies, but the sexes are not under identical environmental conditions. In fact, it is debatable whether sex has any consistent influence on the rate of aging. Simple inspection of survivorship curves in the book by Comfort (1964) suggests that whereas the 50% survival for many animal species may show considerable sex-related differences, longest-lived survivorship is relatively independent of sex, and this is undoubtedly the better estimate of true physiological aging (Sacher, 1959).

4.2. Influence of Strain or Race

Different inbred strains of mice, genetically distinct from one another, may show quite different 50% and even 10th-decile survivals (Storer, 1966; Smith *et al.*, 1973). An appealing interpretation of observed differences in life spans among inbred strains was advanced by Yunis *et al.* (1973), and is illustrated in Fig. 3. Line A represents the normal (immune) functional decline of a long-lived strain. The populations represented by lines B and C reach extinction at the same time, but only B is undergoing accelerated aging. This might be the situation for the autoimmune-susceptible NZB mouse (Yunis *et al.*, 1972), or for diabetes mellitus in man. In C, the strain commences life with a heavy load of genetic defects, but the rate of decline thereafter, and hence the rate of aging, are normal. Persons with ataxia–telangiectasia or progeria, or dwarf mice (Fabris *et al.*, 1972), might fall into this category.

Evaluation of immune functional status in relation to age has been carried out in only a limited number of available mouse strains. Furthermore, the functional status is highly dependent on local husbandry, especially nutrition, and the age-specific peak and rate of decline can be shifted

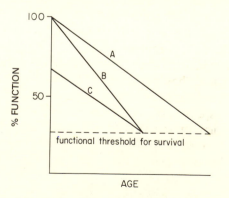

Fig. 3. An interpretation of the relationship among function, aging, and survival. The population becomes extinct by the time the functional threshold for survival is reached. Line A represents the normal (immune) functional decline of a long-lived strain; line B represents accelerated aging. In line C, survival is curtailed by inherited genetic defects or susceptibilities, but the aging rate is not actually accelerated. Adapted from Yunis *et al.* (1973).

either to the right or to the left by nutritional manipulation (Gerbase-DeLima *et al.*, 1975*b*). Meaningful comparisons are therefore relatively few. A study by Kay (1978) of eight strains plus hybrids in which 52 indices were assessed showed age-related strain differences in bone marrow cellularity, and in the onset, magnitude, and rate of decline in PHA responsiveness, as well as other parameters.

The autoimmune-susceptible strains of mice, including A strains and particularly NZB and NZB/NZW F_1 (B/W) mice, have relatively short life spans (Yunis *et al.*, 1972). NZB and B/W mice probably develop premature T-cell maturation, with excessive, early-in-life antibody response to different antigens (Talal, 1976). NZB mice develop an autoimmune hemolytic anemia early, and splenomegaly later in life. Autoimmunity is expressed somewhat differently in B/W mice, which show a high incidence of LE cells, antinuclear factors, and severe immune complex glomerulonephritis.

Genetic, immunological, and virological factors are involved in the pathogenesis of these diseases in the autoimmune-susceptible strains, and it is rather surprising that the formal genetics have not been more thoroughly studied. According to Talal (1976), NZB and B/W mice undergo a relative loss of suppressor T cells beginning at 1–2 months of age. There is an increased proliferative response to allogeneic cells in young NZB mice compared with other strains (Palmer *et al.*, 1976). A detailed comparison of many features of the autoimmune susceptible strains with strains considered nonautoimmune, particularly the CBA mouse, may be found in the comprehensive report by Yunis *et al.* (1972). NZB mice demonstrate nearly all the features of accelerated aging, i.e., line B of Fig. 3, the one possible exception being that suppressor cells may be decreased in NZB mice and are clearly increased in long-lived strains.

NZB mice carry the *H-2^d* allele at the MHC. Other strains of mice with this allele are not necessarily short-lived, nor do they show a high degree of autoimmune susceptibility. The *H-2^d* designation, however, refers to serologically detectable factors representing genes at the *K* and *D* loci, and does not necessarily indicate that other genes in the MHC are precisely the same for different mice having the same *H-2* allele, except in the case of congenic lines. Recent studies suggest that two or more independently segregating genes specify the NZB phenotype and are involved in the genetics of expression of xenotrophic virus and autoimmunity (Datta and Schwartz, 1976). One of these might well be an autoimmune-susceptible, but as yet unidentified, *Ir* gene within the MHC (Talal, 1976).

4.3. Studies in Congenic Mice

Co-isogenic mouse strains are strains that differ from one another only at a single gene locus. Congenic strains, on the other hand, differ from one another at a relatively short chromosomal region. Mice congenic for the H-

2 region can be prepared by selective breeding experiments on any particular background, e.g., on C57BL, C3H, or other backgrounds. A fairly large number of strains congenic for *H-2* and a smaller number congenic for *H-1* or other minor loci are available. A study of 14 strains congenic for *H-2*, and a smaller number for *H-1*, and on C57BL, C3H, and A strain backgrounds led Smith and Walford (1978) to the observation that for mean life span and for mean ages of the 10th decile of survivorship, the variation was as great as that observed in inbred but noncongenic strains. One might have expected greater uniformity of life spans within a congenic set unless the *H-2* region itself exerts a significant effect on aging. The strain background provides a general pattern for the congenic life span, but once this pattern is set, considerable variation exists among life spans of congenic lines. Data for three groups of three lines, each on a different background and for which immune functional data are also available, are given in Table II. The *H-2* alleles are also indicated. Although genetically identical except for the short *H-2* region on the 17th chromosome, the mice within each group demonstrated considerable variation of mean and 10th-decile survivorship. Evidence of a complex interplay between the particular *H-2* allele and the overall genetic backgrounds was provided by the observation that *H-2^b* might promote either longer or shorter life span, depending on the several backgrounds (Table II). The allele *H-2^n* on a C57BL background correlates with greatly shortened survival, premature graying of hair, and other evidence interpretable as accelerated aging (Popp, 1978).

The particular *H-2* allele also has a striking influence on the incidence of different tumors within the background of the congenic lines, although there is no consistent relationship between the overall tumor incidence and life span (Table II). Strain A/WySn, for example, showed the highest tumor incidence among the A lines, but clearly the longest survival by both mean and 10th-decile criteria.

Some insight into the relationship between age-related immune function and life span in these same strains of congenic mice can be garnered from the data presented in Fig. 4, which shows the age-related response of the strains to PHA, purified protein derivative (PPD), and PWM. PHA is known to be a T-cell-specific mitogen, PPD a B-cell-specific mitogen, and PWM to stimulate B cells and cortisone-resistant T cells. For the C3H strains, there was no consistent relationship between the mortality data given in Table I and the age-specific response to several mitogens. For the C57BL strains, however, the longest-lived line, namely, B10.RIII(71NS)/Sn, displayed the highest PHA response throughout most of life, and the shortest-lived line, namely, B10.AKM/Sn, the lowest. The survival patterns of the A strain mice also correlated with the age-specific PHA response, with the longer-lived A/WySn line showing a higher PHA response throughout life than its partners. The response to the thymus-

Table II. Survival Data and Incidences of the Most Common Tumors for Groups of Male Mice Congenic at the H-2 Histocompatibility Region on Three Separate Backgrounds[a]

Strain	H-2 allele	Mean survival (weeks)	Mean of 10th decile (weeks)	Tumor incidence (%)		
				Lymphoma	Hepatoma	Lung tumors
B10.AKM/Sn	m	99	139	53	5	0
C57BL/10Sn	b	134	155	29	2	3
B10.RIII (7INS)/Sn	r	141	170	23	0	10
C3H.JKSn	j	112	136	3	50	14
C3H/HeDiSn	k	98	138	5	51	10
C3H.SW/Sn	b	108	150	3	38	0
A.BY/Sn	b	85	114	10	2	10
A.CA/Sn	f	85	127	0	14	28
A/WySn	a	97	134	13	15	26

[a]Adapted from Smith and Walford (1978). B10.AKM/Sn mice have statistically significantly shorter mean and 10th decile survivorships ($P <$ 0.05, generally much less) than both congenic partners, and C57BL/10Sn a significantly shorter 10th-decile survivorship than B10.RIII (7INS)/Sn mice. On the C3H background, C3H.JKSn mean survival is significantly different from that of C3H/HeDiSn, but not from that of C3H.SW/Sn. C3H.SW/Sn has a significantly longer 10th decile than its partners. On the A strain background, all strains differ significantly from one another at 10th decile, and A/WySn differs from its two partners for mean survival.

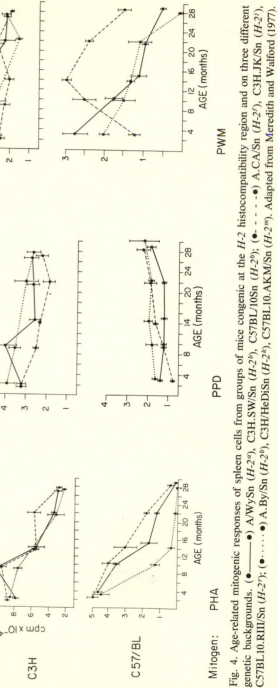

Fig. 4. Age-related mitogenic responses of spleen cells from groups of mice congenic at the *H-2* histocompatibility region and on three different genetic backgrounds. (●———●) A/WySn (*H-2ᵃ*), C3H.SW/Sn (*H-2ᵇ*), C57BL/10Sn (*H-2ᵇ*); (●- - - -●) A.CA/Sn (*H-2ᶠ*), C3H.JK/Sn (*H-2ᶠ*), C57BL10.RIII/Sn (*H-2ʳ*); (●·······●) A.By/Sn (*H-2ᵇ*), C3H/HeDiSn (*H-2ᵏ*), C57BL10.AKM/Sn (*H-2ᵐ*). Adapted from Meredith and Walford (1977).

independent mitogen. PPD, did not correlate with strain-specific life span, although differences on the basis of the *H-2* type were noted. With regard to PWM mitogen, the very long-lived B10.RIII(71NS)/Sn mouse clearly displayed higher responses than its congenic partners. No significant differences were noted for A or C3H strains for this mitogen.

The studies cited above indicate that given any particular genetic background, the MHC in mice exerts a significant influence on life span as determined by mean or 10th-decile survival statistics, and that this influence might be mediated at least in part by preservation of the functional integrity of the immune system by genes within the MHC. Since the MHC may well be the master genetic control region for a wide variety of immune functions, particularly the thymus-dependent functions, negative results would have been strong evidence against an immunological interpretation of the aging process.

4.4. The Major Histocompatibility Complex (HLA System) in Humans in Relation to Aging

A striking disequilibrium exists between the frequency of certain gene products of the *HLA* system and a wide variety of autoimmune and immunological diseases in humans (Svejgaard *et al.*, 1975*b*). The most common *HLA* specificity with a frequency that is significantly increased in various autoimmune diseases is HLA-B8, which suggests that this gene, or more probably a closely linked gene, could be regarded as an autoimmune-susceptibility gene. Interestingly enough, it was recently noted by Yunis and Greenburg (1978) that the frequency of HLA-B8 is decreased in older cohorts of human females, suggesting the possibility of an increased mortality rate in females carrying this marker.

Diabetes mellitus presents many features of accelerated aging, including a shift in the incidence of severe arteriosclerosis to a younger age; an increased frequency of autoantibodies to gastric, thyroid, and nuclear antigens (Whittingham *et al.*, 1971); amyloidosis, especially of the islets of Langerhans (Blumenthal and Berns, 1964); and a sharply decreased replicative potential of fibroblasts in tissue culture (Vracko and Benditt, 1975). Juvenile diabetes, at least, is clearly influenced by the genetic makeup of the MHC, although the precise relationship has not yet been determined. A number of studies report an increased frequency of HLA-B8, as well as of certain MLR determinants, in juvenile diabetes (Thomsen *et al.*, 1975). An increased frequency of recombination or of homozygosity at the *HLA* region was also claimed (Rubenstein *et al.*, 1976), and increased mortality was observed in those older diabetics who demonstrate autoantibodies (Whittingham *et al.*, 1971). L. Greenburg and E. Yunis (personal communication) observed that in maturity-onset familial diabetes, inheritance of diabetes may segregate with one of the *HLA* haplotypes. A rather strong case can therefore be made for the role of immunogenetic factors in diabetes, one of the most characteristic "diseases of aging."

The *HLA* studies in man may be interpreted to lend support to conclusions derived from the congenic mouse data cited above, namely, that the MHC influences aging rates. The situation in humans is simply less clear due to the genetic heterogeneity of the human species, so that the *HLA* types cannot be compared against a common background. By way of illustration, Mittal (1976) found no deviation in *HLA* phenotypes among Caucasians with renal failure, but in Negroes, the specificity HLA-Bw17 was twice that of a normal racially matched population. Racial matching is, of course, still a long way from background genetic homogeneity, but the point is clear. Probably *HLA* typing among family members, and determining that certain traits tend to segregate with *HLA* haplotypes, will prove to be a more fruitful approach than population studies. It should also be noted that the Down syndrome (trisomy 21), which may indeed show more features of accelerated aging than any other human malady (Martin, 1978), shows significant immunological abnormalities as well.

5. Immunogenetic Diseases and Aging

The most ubiquitous disease of aging in vertebrate populations is senile amyloidosis (Walford and Sjaarda, 1964; Walford, 1969). Amyloid is a hyaline material deposited intercellularly and characterized by specific staining reactions with Congo red, thioflavine-T, or other dyes. Electron microscopy reveals its fibrillar composition. Nevertheless, "amyloid" is not a single chemical substance. Most forms fall into one of three types. In primary amyloidosis seen in multiple myeloma, the amyloid consists largely of the light (L) chains of Ig's (Franklin and Zucker-Franklin, 1972). In secondary amyloidosis—such as that occurring after prolonged chronic infections, and probably after all experimental amyloidogenic procedures—the deposited material consists chiefly of a so-called "A" protein, a 76-amino-acid-residue peptide with no relation to L chains or any other known protein. The chemical makeup of senile amyloid is essentially unknown.

It is generally agreed that immune dysfunction plays a major role in the genesis of primary and secondary amyloidosis, but such a role in senile amyloidosis can only be inferred. Evidence based on experimental production of amyloid by hyperimmunization with casein suggests that a decreased T-cell function and a slightly increased B-cell function may potentiate the laying down of amyloid. Such a situation does obtain in normal aging. It is also true that different strains of mice show striking differences in incidence, degree, and organ distribution of senile amyloidosi (Walford, 1969). On the whole, it seems reasonable to regard senile amyloidosis as an immunological disease with strong genetic overtones.

Several human immunodeficiency diseases having a genetic basis show features of accelerated aging. Hereditary ataxia–telangiectasia is transmitted recessively. Ataxia is first noted during infancy, and the telangiectasias usually appear at about 6 years of age or later. Most patients lack both serum and secretory IgA, and often IgE. The thymus is abnormal and cellular-immunity defective. There is a 10–15% incidence of cancer, including all forms, but with lymphomas predominating. Also, premature graying or loss of hair and hypogonadism are characteristic.

In the so-called "primary acquired hypogammaglobulinemia" or "common variable immunodeficiency disease," there is no clear-cut evidence for genetic influence in many instances, but multiple cases in families have also been reported showing both dominant and autosomal recessive inheritance. This disorder may represent a spectrum of diseases. Patients demonstrate enchanced susceptibility to infection, a decreased response of these lymphoid cells to T-dependent mitogens, and frequent occurrence of sprue like syndromes and absorption abnormalities, and many patients develop pernicious anemia relatively early in life, in comparison with the general age-related incidence of this autoimmune disease. Autoantibodies are found in those patients with pernicious anemia. There is a late development of lymphoid malignancies as well as cancers of the GI tract. Other possible relationships between genetically influenced immunodeficiency diseases and aging invite study (Good and Yunis, 1974), but pertinent information is lacking.

6. Summary

Most of our knowledge of immunogenetics as it relates to aging derives from data on higher animals. Central to the understanding of immunogenetics is the concept of the main histocompatibility complex (MHC)—e.g., the *H-2* system in the mouse and the *HLA* system in man—which appears to be the master gene system for controlling or influencing the immune response, particularly thymus-dependent functions. Thymus-dependent immunity declines, whereas autoimmunity increases, with age.

That genetically distinct inbred mouse strains may have quite different ages for their 50% and 10th-decile survivorship attests to the importance of strain differences in influencing the rate of aging. Autoimmune-susceptible strains, such as NZB, have relatively short life spans and demonstrate many features of accelerated aging. Possibly an autoimmune-susceptible immune response gene within the MHC contributes to the pathogenesis of disease in the NZB. Strains of congenic mice, each having identical genetic backgrounds but differing only in the *H-2* regional complex, exhibit considerable variation in mean and 10th-decile survivorship. This significant influence on lifespan by the MHC may be mediated at least in part by preservation of the functional integrity of the immune system by genes within the MHC.

In humans, there is a significant increase in the frequency of the specificity HLA-B8 in a variety of autoimmune and immunological diseases, suggesting that it or a closely linked gene could be an autoimmune-susceptibility gene. Immunogenetic factors may be present in diabetes mellitus, which shows many features of accelerated aging. Senile amyloidosis, the most ubiquitous disease of aging, appears to be an immunological disease with strong genetic overtones. Also, several human immunodeficiency diseases having a genetic basis, including ataxia–telangiectasia and primary acquired hypogammaglobulinemia, manifest features of accelerated aging. The immunogenetic picture in humans is less clear than in the mouse because of the genetic heterogeneity involved. A useful approach may be to determine whether certain traits tend to segregate with *HLA* haplotypes within families.

ACKNOWLEDGMENT

These studies were supported by USPHS Research Grants AI-10088 and AG-00424.

References

Bevan, M. J., 1975, Interaction antigens detected by cytotoxic T-cells with the major histocompatibility complex as modifier, *Nature (London)* **256:**419.

Blumenthal, H. T., and Berns, A. W., 1964, Autoimmunity and aging, *Adv. Gerontol. Res.* **1:**289.

Comfort, A., 1964, *Ageing: The Biology of Senescence,* Holt, Rinehart & Winston, New York.

Cunningham, A. J., 1976, Self-tolerance maintained by active suppressor mechanisms, *Transplant. Rev.* **31:**23.

Cutler, R. G., 1975, Evolution of human longevity and the genetic complexity governing aging rate, *Proc. Natl. Acad. Sci. U.S.A.* **72:**4664.

Datta, S. K., and Schwartz, R. S., 1976, Genetics of expression of xenotropic virus and autoimmunity in NZB mice, *Nature (London)* **263:**412.

Doherty, P. C., and Zinkernagel, R. M., 1975, A biological role for the major histocompatibility antigens, **2:**1406.

Fabris, N., Pierpaoli, W., and Sorkin, E., 1972, Lymphocytes, hormones, and aging, *Nature (London)* **240:**557.

Franklin, E. C., and Zucker-Franklin, D., 1972, Current concepts of amyloid, *Adv. Immunol.* **15:**249.

Gajdusek, D. C., 1972, Slow virus infection and activation of latent infections in aging, *Adv. Gerontol. Res.* **4**:201.

Gerbase-DeLima, M., Wilkinson, J., Smith, G. S., and Walford, R. L., 1974, Age-related decline in thymic-independent immune function of a long-lived mouse strain, *J. Gerontol.* **29**:261.

Gerbase-DeLima, M., Meredith, P., and Walford, R. L., 1975[a], Age-related changes including synergy and suppression in the mixed lymphocyte reaction in long-lived mice, *Fed. Proc. Fed. Am. Soc. Exp. Biol.* **34**:159.

Gerbase-DeLima, M., Liu, R. K., Cheney, K. E., Mickey, R., and Walford, R. L., 1975[b], Immune function and survival in a long-lived mouse strain subjected to undernutrition, *Gerontologia* **21**:184.

Good, R. A., and Yunis, E., 1974, Association of autoimmunity, immunodeficiency and aging in man, rabbits, and mice, *Fed. Proc. Fed. Am. Soc. Exp. Biol.* **33**:2040.

Goodman, S. A., and Makinodan, T., 1975, Effect of age on cell-mediated immunity in long-lived mice, *Clin. Exp. Immunol.* **19**:533.

Hildemann, W. H., 1970, Components and concepts of antigenic strength, *Transplant Rev.* **3**:5.

Hildemann, W. H., 1978, Phylogenetic and immunogenetic aspects of aging, in: *Genetic Effects on Aging, Birth Defects: Orig. Artic. Ser.* (D. Bergsma and D. E. Harrison, eds.), The National Foundation–March of Dimes, New York (in press).

Hung, C., Perkins, E. H., and Yang, W., 1975, Age-related refractoriness of PHA-induced lymphocyte transformation. II. ^{125}I-PHA-binding to spleen cells from young and old mice, *Mech. Ageing Dev.* **4**:103.

Kay, M. M. B., 1978, Immunological aging patterns: Effect of parainfluenza type 1 virus infection on aging mice of 8 strains and hybrids, in: *Genetic Effects on Aging, Birth Defects: Orig. Artic. Ser.* (D. Bergsma and D. E. Harrison, eds.), The National Foundation–March of Dimes, New York (in press).

Kishimoto, S., Takahama, T., and Mizumachi, H., 1976, *In vitro* immune response to the 2,4,6-trinitrophenyl determinant in aged C57Bl/6J mice: Changes in the humoral immune response to and avidity for the TNP determinant and responsiveness to LPS effect with aging, *J. Immunol.* **116**:294.

Konen, T. G., Smith, G. S., and Walford, R. L., 1973, Decline in mixed lymphocyte reactivity of spleen cells from aged mice of a long-lived strain, *J. Immunol.* **110**:1216.

Kunstyr, I., and Leuenberger, H. W., 1975, Gerontological data of C57BL/6J mice. I. Sex differences in survival curves, *J. Gerontol.* **30**:157.

MacKay, I. R., 1972, Ageing and immunological function in man, *Gerontologia* **18**:239.

Makinodan, T., Perkins, E. H., and Chen, M. G., 1971, Immunological activity of the aged, *Adv. Gerontol. Res.* **3**:171.

Martin, G. M., 1978, Genetic syndromes in man with potential relevance to the pathobiology of aging, in: *Genetic Effects on Aging, Birth Defects: Orig. Artic. Ser.* (D. Bergsma and D. E. Harrison, eds.), The National Foundation–March of Dimes, New York (in press).

Mathies, M., Lipps, L., Smith, G. S., and Walford, R. L., 1973, Age-related decline in response to phytohemagglutinin and pokeweed mitogen by spleen cells from hamsters and long-lived mouse strain, *J. Gerontol.* **28**:425.

Meredith, P., and Walford, R. L., 1977, Effect of age on response to T and B cell mitogens in mice congenic at the *H-2* region, *Immunogenetics* **5**:109.

Mittal, K. K., 1976, The *HLA* polymorphism and susceptibility to disease, *Vox Sang.* **31**:161.

Naor, D., Bonavida, B., and Walford, R. L., 1976, Autoimmunity and aging: The age-related response of mice of a long-lived strain to trinitrophenylated syngeneic mouse red blood cells, *J. Immunol.* **117**:2204.

Palmer, D. W., Dauphinee, M. J., Murphy, E., and Talal, N., 1976, Hyperactive T cell function in young NZB mice: Increased proliferative response to allogeneic cells, *Clin. Exp. Immunol.* **23**:578.

Popp, D. M., 1978, Use of congenic mice to study the genetic basis of degenerative disease, in: *Genetic Effects on Aging, Birth Defects: Orig. Artic. Ser.* (D. Bergsma and D. E. Harrison, eds.), The National Foundation–March of Dimes, New York (in press).

Rubenstein, P., Suciu-Foca, N., Nicholson, J. F., Fotino, M., Molinaro, A., Harisiadis, L., Hardy, M. A., Reemtsma, K., and Allan, F. H., Jr., 1976, The *HLA* system in the families of patients with juvenile diabetes mellitus, *J. Exp. Med.* **143**:1277.

Sacher, G. A., 1959, Relation of lifespan to brain weight and body weight in mammals, *Ciba Found. Colloq. Ageing* **5**:115.

Segre, D., and Segre, M., 1976, Humoral immunity in aged mice. II. Increased suppressor T cell activity in immunologically deficient old mice, *J. Immunol.* **116**:735.

Shreffler, D. C., 1977, The *H-2* model: Genetic control of immune functions, in: *HLA and Disease* (J. Dausset and A. Svejgaard, eds.), Munksgaard, Copenhagen.

Siegal, B. V., Braun, M., and Morton, J. I., 1972, Detection of antinuclear antibodies in NZB and other mouse strains, *Immunology* **22**:457.

Smith, G. S., and Walford, R. L., 1978, Influence of the *H-2* and *H-1* histocompatibility systems upon lifespan and spontaneous cancer incidences in congenic mice, in: *Genetic Effects on Aging, Birth Defects: Orig. Artic. Ser.* (D. Bergsma and D. E. Harrison, eds.), The National Foundation–March of Dimes, New York (in press).

Smith, G. S., Walford, R. L., and Mickey, M. R., 1973, Lifespan and incidence of cancer and other diseases in selected long-lived inbred mice and their F_1-hybrids, *J. Natl. Cancer Inst.* **50**:1195.

Storer, J. B., 1966, Longevity and gross pathology at death in 22 inbred mouse strains, *J. Gerontol.* **21**:404.

Svejgaard, A., Hange, M., Jersild, C., Platz, P., Ryder, L. P., Nielsen, L. S., and Thomsen, M., 1975a, The HLA system: An introductory survey, *Mongr. Hum. Genet.*, No. 7.

Svejgaard, A., Platz, P., Ryder, L. P., Nielsen, L. S., and Thomsen, M., 1975b, *HLA* and disease associations—A survey, *Transplant. Rev.* **22**:3.

Talal, N., 1976, Disordered immunologic regulation and autoimmunity, *Transplant. Rev.* **31**:240.

Talal, N., and Steinberg, A. D., 1974, The pathogenesis of autoimmunity in New Zealand black mice, in: *Current Topics in Microbiology and Immunology,* p. 79, Springer-Verlag, New York.

Thomsen, M., Platz, P., Anderson, O. C., Christy, M., Lyngsoe, J., Nerup, J., Rasmussen, K., Ryder, L. P., Nielsen, L. S., and Svejgaard, A., 1975, MLC typing in juvenile diabetes mellitus and idiopathic Addison's disease, *Transplant. Rev.* **22**:125.

Vracko, R., and Benditt, E. P., 1975, Restricted replicative lifespan of diabetic fibroblasts *in vitro:* Its relation to microangiopathy, *Fed. Proc. Fed. Am. Soc. Exp. Biol.* **34**:68.

Walford, R. L., 1969, *The Immunologic Theory of Aging,* Munksgaard, Copenhagen.

Walford, R. L., 1970, Antibody diversity, histocompatibility systems, disease states, and aging, *Lancet* **2**:1226.

Walford, R. L., 1974, The immunologic theory of aging: Current status, *Fed. Proc. Fed. Am. Soc. Exp. Biol.* **33**:2020.

Walford, R. L., 1977, Human B-cell alloantigens: Their medical and biological significance, in: *HLA System: New Aspects,* (G. B. Ferrara, ed.), pp. 105–127, Elsevier–North-Holland Publishing Co., Amsterdam.

Walford, R. L., and Sjaarda, J. R., 1964, Increase of thioflavine-T-staining material (amyloid) in human tissues with age, *J. Gerontol.* **19**:57.

Watson, J., and Riblet, R., 1974, Genetic control of response to bacterial lipopolysaccharide in mice, *J. Exp. Med.* **140**:1147.

Whittingham, S., Mathews, J. D., MacKay, I. R., Stocks, A. E., Ungar, B., and Martin, F. I. R., 1971, Diabetes mellitus, autoimmunity and ageing, *Lancet* **1**:763.

Yunis, E. J., and Greenberg, L. J., 1978, Genetic control of autoimmune disease and aging immune responses, in: *Genetic Effects on Aging, Birth Defects: Orig. Artic. Ser.* (D. Bergsma and D. E. Harrison, eds.), The National Foundation–March of Dimes, New York.

Yunis, E. J., Fernandes, G., Teague, P. O., Stutman, O., and Good, R. A., 1972, The thymus, autoimmunity and the involution of the lymphoid system, in: *Tolerance, Autoimmunity, and Aging* (M. M., Sigel, ed.), pp. 62–119, Charles C. Thomas,

Yunis, E. J., Fernandes, G., and Greenberg, W. J., 1973, Immune deficiency, autoimmunity and aging, in: *Immunodeficiency Workshop, Birth Defects: Orig. Artic. Ser.*, No. 11, p. 85, Plenum Press, New York.

Chapter 13

Behavior Genetics and Aging

Charles L. Goodrick

1. Introduction

In their classic textbook entitled *Behavior Genetics,* Fuller and Thompson (1960) summarized most of the behavioral information concerning the relationship of genetics and behavior available at that time. Age as a factor affecting behavior was not considered in animal studies of behavior genetics, and in general has not been seriously examined in animal behavioral research. There have been exceptions, including the early age-related research studies of rats by Slonaker (1912), Richter (1922), and Stone (1929). These studies, however, were not continued or followed by additional research by the original investigators or by their students or colleagues. That they were not may be due to factors such as the great length of time needed, the amount of support required, the complications of disease or accidental deaths in the animal colony, and the experimental error that can plague long-term research.

According to Lindzey and Thiessen (1970, p. IX): "*Mus musculus* is, and probably will remain, the principal mammalian species for investigating fundamental relations between genes and behavior." Their ease of maintenance, small size, and short life span have resulted in the selection of *Mus musculus* as the appropriate animal for the study of the effects of heredity, age, training, and environment on behavior (Goodrick, 1973*a*). In addition to these advantages, a vast amount of information is available concerning the genetics of *Mus musculus,* much of which is summarized in *Biology of the Laboratory Mouse* (Green, 1966).

Charles L. Goodrick • Laboratory of Behavioral Science, Gerontology Research Center, National Institute on Aging, National Institutes of Health, Public Health Service, U.S. Department of Health, Education and Welfare, Baltimore, Maryland 21224

To plan behavioral research programs concerned with genetics and aging, it is necessary to know a great deal about both the duration of life and the behavioral characteristics of the population or populations studied. This chapter will be concerned with what is known at present about life span and age differences in behavioral characteristics of inbred mice, hybrid mice, and mutant mice.

2. Life Span

2.1. Inbred Mice

In an earlier report, Russell (1966) summarized the literature on the longevity of inbred mice up to 1964. She indicated that the 44 months of age attained by a male of the NS strain was probably the longest recorded life span for the laboratory mouse (Roberts, 1961). Life span had been measured on inbred mice maintained during different time periods from 1948 to 1962. Average longevity ranged from 9 months for AKR/J virgin female mice to an average longevity of 23 months for LP/J virgin female mice (Russell, 1966, p. 512, Table 26.1). A major finding of this report was the marked reduction in longevity for breeder female mice in comparison with virgin female mice. Most of the inbred lines had an average longevity of 15–20 months, while C57BL/6J inbred mice have an average survival of slightly longer than 20 months. Storer (1966) presented data on longevity (from the same laboratory as Russell) for groups of male and female inbred mice that could be compared with Russell's data (Table I). The inbred virgin mice of Storer, maintained under conditions similar to the inbred mice of Russell, generally lived longer than Russell's inbred mice. Russell (1966, p. 514) had pointed out that following improvement in quarters in

Table I.   Mean Longevity in Days (Where Comparable Groups of Unmated Males and Females Were Available) for Mouse Strains Examined by Russell (1966) and Storer (1966)

| Strain | Male | | Female | | |
	Russell	Storer	Russell	Storer	Average
A/J	503 ± 11	490 ± 18	481 ± 8	590 ± 19	516
AKR/J	272 ± 5	326 ± 16	256 ± 3	276 ± 9	283
BALB/cJ	485 ± 9	539 ± 33	532 ± 15	575 ± 15	533
C57BL/6J	539 ± 7	676 ± 20	653 ± 13	692 ± 16	640
C57BR/CdJ	475 ± 13	703 ± 17	588 ± 14	694 ± 20	615
DBA/1J	438 ± 9	433 ± 31	582 ± 11	750 ± 20	551
DBA/2J	415 ± 9	707 ± 22	547 ± 9	714 ± 21	596

1959, significant increased life spans were observed for seven groups of inbred female breeders. This improvement in living conditions might explain the difference in longevity obtained in these two studies.

According to the averages of the data of Russell and Storer in Table I, the A/J and BALB/cJ strains may be classified as short-lived, the DBA strain as intermediate in life span, and the C57 lines as relatively long-lived. Death is due to a variety of causes for these inbred lines, although the AKR/J very short-lived mice generally die from leukemia. There are specific illnesses that may characterize a given strain, such as mammary tumors for DBA females, lung tumors for A/J and BALB/cJ mice, reticular neoplasia and kidney lesions for C57BL/6J mice, and papillonephritis for A/J mice (Russell, 1966, pp. 514–516). As conditions changed at the Jackson laboratories, however, such specific conditions declined in frequency. For example, in 1960–1962, female DBA/2J mice had a much lower incidence of mammary tumors than previously reported. Moreover, Storer (1966), in a pathology study, found that A/J, BALB/cJ, C57BL/6J, and DBA/2J mice died largely from nonspecific causes.

At the National Institute on Aging, Goodrick (1975a) maintained A/J, BALB/cJ, C57BL/6J, and DBA/2J male and female mice, and the six possible F_1 hybrid crosses, to collect mortality data, to examine sex differences in longevity, and to examine the genetics of longevity. For inbred male and female mice, the results of this study and comparisons with previous data are given in Table II. In general, the C57BL/6J strain is longest-lived, followed by the DBA/2J. The A/J and BALB/cJ mice were relatively short-lived, with the exception of BALB/cJ female mice, the mean life span of which approximated that obtained by C57BL/6J. Systematic study of A/J mice, for which sex differences in longevity were not obtained, and BALB/cJ mice, for which sex differences in longevity were obtained, may yield information concerning causal factors in mammalian sex differences in longevity.

The most consistent differences in longevity are found between A/J and C57BL/6J mice (Table II). If Storer (1966) is correct that these strains die of general rather than specific effects, the A/J and C57BL/6J mice may be used to study the genetics of behavioral changes at different stages of the life span. For A/J mice, the maximal age for behavioral study would be 22–23 months of age, while for C57BL/6J mice, it would be 26–27 months of age (senescence, 50% point of mortality).

2.2. Hybrid Mice

Chai (1959) studied the life span of inbred and hybrid mice in order to study the effects of hybridization (or heterozygosity) on longevity. His conclusions were that hybridization increased mean life span in comparison

Table II. Mean Longevity (Days) and Standard Error of the Mean Obtained in Experimental Studies of Longevity for A/J, BALB/cJ, C57BL/6J, and DBA/2J Inbred Strains of Mice[a]

Reference	A/J Male	A/J Female	BALB/cJ Male	BALB/cJ Female	C57BL/6J[b] Male	C57BL/6J[b] Female	DBA/2J[b] Male	DBA/2J[b] Female
Goodrick (1975a) (1)	662 ± 20.4	688 ± 21.6	648 ± 20.6[c]	816 ± 32.4	827 ± 34.2	818 ± 21.0	722 ± 30.0	683 ± 26.4
(2)	(650	(664) ± 9.4			(805	819) ± 5.1		
Goodrick (1974)					815 ± 14.4			
Grahn (1972)			(460	(609) ± 13.9	(815	874) ± 13.8		
Storer (1966)	490 ± 18.4	590 ± 18.8	539 ± 33.0[c]	575 ± 14.9	676 ± 20.3	692 ± 15.7	707 ± 22.4	714 ± 21.4
Russell (1966)		481 ± 8		532 ± 15		653 ± 13		547 ± 9
Curtis et al. (1966)						750 NA		
Hrubant (1964)					870 ± 4.8	919 ± 6.9		
Silberberg et al. (1962)		522 NA				671 NA		
Silberberg and Silberberg (1954)								631 NA
Russell (1966)					653 NA	586 NA	474 NA	
Retired Breeders								
1948–1956	503 ± 11	405 ± 7	485 ± 9	462 ± 7	539 ± 7	561 ± 8	415 ± 9	407 ± 6
1960–1962		512 ± 9				695 ± 9		661 ± 11
Russell (1972)								
Retired breeders								
1948–1952	488 ± 10.8	438 ± 8.3	468 ± 9.2	473 ±7.6	519 ± 7.3	576 ± 7.7	407 ± 8.7	432 ± 7.0

[a]From Goodrick (1975a).
[b](NA) Standard error not available.
[c]Singly caged due to fighting.
( ) Male and female groups combined in standard error computation.

with inbred lines due to fewer early deaths for hybrid mice than for inbred mice. Chai's inbred mice obtained the same maximal longevity as his hybrid mice.

Russell (1966), however, presented data for hybrid groups that clearly showed both greatly increased mean longevity and maximal longevity in comparison with inbred parental groups (Fig. 26-4, p. 515). The data of Goodrick (1975*a*) are given in Fig. 1, and are clearly in agreement with the data of Russell (1966). All six hybrid groups had increased mean longevity and greater maximal longevity in comparison with parental inbred groups. Moreover, the hybrid life spans are considerably greater than those obtained by Russell (1966). The maximal age for behavioral study of hybrid mice, based on the data of Fig. 1, would be 29–30 months. A second part of the study by Goodrick (1975*a*) obtained life spans similar to those obtained in the first study for groups of A/J, C57BL/6J, and F_1 hybrid mice; i.e., the mean longevities did not differ significantly from the first study. This finding suggests stability in life span for these groups under the conditions of maintenance within that laboratory.

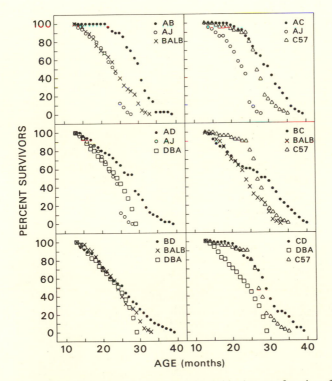

Fig. 1. Percentage of survivors for inbred and hybrid mice as a function of age.

In the study of Goodrick (1975a), the inclusion of an F_2 hybrid group allowed determinations of the number of genetic loci and the coefficient of genetic determination, that portion of the total phenotypic variation attributable to any genetic cause. The minimum number of loci that determine life span was found to be one, and estimates of the coefficient of genetic determination for the two groups were 0.787 and 0.48. The estimates of genetic determination obtained by Storer (1966) were 0.36 for female mice and 0.21 for male mice. Storer's estimates may be low due to the large number of mouse strains used with a similar longevity. On a purely mathematical basis, it can be estimated that half the variance associated with longevity is due to genetic factors.

2.3. Mutant Mice

Estimates of longevity of mutant mice were obtained by Goodrick (1977a) for groups of mutants (on the C57BL/6J background) that differ in maximal body weight. In this study, four groups of male mutant mice and one nonmutant male control group were studied. Two of the mutant groups consisted of obese yellow and black mice (C57BL/6J–A^Y and C57BL/6J–ob), and the other two mutant groups consisted of the nonobese albino and beige mice (C57BL/6J–c^J and C57BL/6J–bg). The average longevity of the control group was 27.9 months, significantly greater than the longevity of any of the four mutant groups: beige, 23.4 months; albino, 24.4 months; yellow, 22.2 months, and obese, 13.0 months. The average longevity of the control group was similar to that obtained earlier (Goodrick, 1975a), and previous studies have given life-span data for the obese mutation (obese, 15 months; control, 25 months: Lane and Dickie, 1958), the yellow mutation (yellow, 26 months; controls, 29 months: Hrubant, 1964), and the albino mutation (albino, 23.2 months; control, 27 months: Goodrick, 1974), with values for longevity consistent with those obtained by Goodrick (1977a). On the basis of these data, the maximal age for behavioral studies would be about 22–23 months for albino, beige, or yellow mutations, and 14–15 months for the obese mutation.

2.4. Body-Weight Increment and Longevity

McCay *et al.* (1935) showed that by restricting body weight increment, in rats it was possible to increase longevity. Inbred, hybrid, or mutant mice, which may differ in peak body weight, growth rate, and food intake patterns, are excellent genetically homogeneous populations for the study of how these factors may affect longevity. One such study (Goodrick, 1977a) used mutant mice on the C57BL/6J background, as well as normal C57BL/6J inbred mice, as subjects. Mutant mice with excessive food intake patterns, obese (*ob*) and yellow (A^Y), as well as mutant mice not known to

Table III.   Mean and Standard Error of the Mean for Measures of Longevity, Peak Body Weight, Body Weight at Last Month of the Life Span, and Month of Peak Body Weight (Growth Duration) for Mutant and Control Mice[a]

Strain	L (months)	BW-P (g)	Bw-LM (g)	GD (month)
Beige (*bg*)	23.4 ± 1.08	30.4 ± 0.18	27.6 ± 0.47	17.4 ± 1.09
Albino (*c*[J])	24.4 ± 1.52	32.5 ± 0.31	32.0 ± 0.40	22.3 ± 1.67
Control (C57BL/6J)	27.9 ± 0.93	35.3 ± 0.42	30.6 ± 0.34	21.3 ± 1.60
Yellow (A[Y])	22.2 ± 0.84	53.7 ± 1.61	35.5 ± 5.01	16.3 ± 0.47
Obese (*ob*)	13.0 ± 1.89	55.2 ± 5.76	27.3 ± 6.56	7.6 ± 0.62

[a]From Goodrick (1977*a*). Abbreviations: (L) longevity; (BW-P) peak body weight; (BW-LM) body weight at last month of the life span; (GD) growth duration.

become obese, albino (*c*[J]) and beige (*bg*), were used. Some of the results are given in Table III. For the control group of C57BL/6J mice and beige, yellow, and obese mutations, the duration of body-weight increment was positively related to mean longevity; i.e., the greater the duration of body-weight increment, the greater the life span. Within groups, correlations of "duration of body weight increment" and "longevity" were all high and positive, with four of the five correlations being statistically significant. Correlations of "longevity" and "growth rate" were all negative, with three of five statistically significant: the slower the growth rate, the greater the longevity.

An additional study (Goodrick, 1977*b*) used inbred A/J and C57BL/6J mice and hybrid F_1 mice fed low dietary protein or normal dietary protein. For individual mice within subgroups, growth rate was negatively related to longevity; i.e., the slower the rate of growth, the greater the life span. Among subgroups, the longer was the mean duration of body-weight increment, the longer was the mean life span, and significant positive relationships were also obtained within subgroups. These results are important, because they were obtained for genetically identical groups that were previously found to differ in mean body weight and mean food intake (Goodrick, 1973*b*). The duration and rate of body-weight increment therefore appear to be more important predictors of longevity than mean body weight or food intake.

3. Behavior

3.1. Exploration and Open-Field Activity

Open-field activity of aged female C57BL/6J mice was about 50% lower than that observed with young female C57BL/6J mice (Goodrick,

1967*a*).* Over a series of four 15-min trials, the young mice maintained much higher levels of open-field activity on all trials. Sprott and Eleftheriou (1974) tested C57BL/6J and DBA/2J male mice cross-sectionally in an open field at different ages using a single 10-min test trial. For both groups, open-field activity decreased with increasing age, with C57BL/6J mice more active than DBA/2J mice at all ages. Another study using the same strains (C57BL/6J and DBA/2J), with a single 5-min test trial, found that open-field activity and exploration decreased with increasing age for C57BL/6J mice, but were very low for DBA/2J mice at all ages (Elias *et al.*, 1975). Goodrick (1975*b*) obtained a similar finding using C57BL/6J and A/J mice. C57BL/6J young mice were more active and explored more than aged C57BL/6J mice, but activity and exploration of young and aged A/J mice was at a low level, with age differences being very small (Goodrick, 1975*b*).

3.2. Wheel Activity

Voluntary wheel-exercise patterns were studied by Wax (1975) for C57BL/6J inbred mice. Aged mice were less active than young mice, and in general, the old mice spent less time in wheel activity. Both aged and young mice had shorter mean periodicities under conditions of constant dark, and longer mean periodicities under conditions of constant light, as predicted by Aschoff (1965).

Goodrick (1975*b*) obtained wheel-activity data for young and senescent A/J and C57BL/6J mice for 7 days. In general, wheel activity increased with time, was greater for C57BL/6J mice than for A/J mice, and was less for senescent than for young mice.

Another study (Wax, 1977) obtained similar results for C57BL/6J and A/J mice over a 30-day time interval, and included an additional group of F_1 hybrid (A/J × C57BL/6J) mice. For all groups, young mice were more active than aged mice. Inbred C57BL/6J mice were reliably more active than inbred A/J mice, with young F_1 mice more active than either parental group and aged F_1 mice as active as aged C57BL/6J mice. In general, genetic differences were found to be reduced for aged groups in comparison with young groups. In all groups, at least 7 full days of activity are needed to obtain maximal activity records with wheel-running.

3.3. Responsiveness to Light Onset

Animals are generally highly responsive to light onset and offset within experimental environments (Lockard, 1963). C57BL/6J and A/J mice were

*For the studies of Goodrick and Wax referred to throughout the remainder of the chapter, young mice were 4–6 months old, aged A/J mice were 23 or more months old, aged C57BL/6J mice were 26 or more months old, and aged hybrid mice were 29 or more months old.

allowed to turn an environmental light on for 2-sec intervals during 30-min daily tests to study acquisition and retention of a learned response (Goodrick, 1967*b*). The two strains did not differ in acquisition or retention, but did differ in level of activity during the test procedures, with A/J mice inactive in comparison with C57BL/6J mice. No differences were found between young and aged C57BL/6J mice in frequency of response to obtain 2-sec bursts of lights during these four daily 1-hr periods (Goodrick 1967*a*). Subsequent experiments examined learning and retention of the light-contingent response for young and aged mice of the A/J and C57BL/6J strains (Goodrick 1975*b*). These studies revealed that aged mice learned the operant task as well, but extinguished more slowly.

Another approach to the study of age differences in responsiveness to light is to allow animals direct control of environmental lighting for long periods of time. Wax and Goodrick (1975) placed young or aged mice of the A/J and C57BL/6J strains into environments in which the mice could control lighting by pressing switches (one switch turned the light on, another turned it off). The major finding of this experiment was that aged mice spent more time in the light than young mice. This difference could be due to age differences in level of activity; i.e., because mice are active in the dark, a greater daily period of light may be preferred by inactive mice than by active mice. A second experiment (Wax, 1977) obtained a similar result for A/J, C57BL/6J, and hybrid mice allowed access to activity wheels during light self-selection procedures. Aged mice spent more time in the light daily than young mice, and during periods of wheel activity, aged mice spent less time wheel-running in the light than young mice. Although unrelated to age, an important finding of the Wax (1977) study was that 52 of 120 mice maintained circadian schedules of light and dark.

3.4. Sucrose Discrimination and Fluid Intake

The ability of an animal to detect the higher of two sucrose concentrations represents a reliable test that may be used as a model in the study of sensory discrimination. Goodrick (1967*a*) used young (4-month-old) and aged (26-month-old) mice of the C57BL/6J strain to determine age differences in the ability to detect sucrose (S) vs. water, as well as to examine the discrimination between the two sucrose solutions. Where differences between the two solutions were large (e.g., 3 vs. 1 g S/dl), young and aged mice did equally well in selecting the sucrose solution of higher concentration, but when differences between the two solutions were small (e.g., 1.125 vs. 1 g S/dl), young mice drank a significantly greater percentage of the higher-concentration sucrose solution than did aged mice. Young mice of this strain therefore have greater taste acuity for sucrose than aged mice, and may therefore have greater sensory acuity than aged mice with respect to taste. This test may be useful in the study of factors that may affect the sensory acuity of aged animals.

Comparisons of age differences for A/J and C57BL/6J strains were made in a further sucrose-discrimination study (Goodrick, 1975b). In this study, age differences for the C57BL/6J groups were similar to the preceding findings obtained by Goodrick (1967a), but age differences in sucrose discrimination were not obtained for A/J mice.

During tests of sucrose discrimination, fluid intake was consistently higher for aged than for young animals in both experiments (Goodrick, (1967a, b). Exceptions occurred where highly palatable sucrose concentrations (1–3 g S/dl) were available. For these sucrose concentrations, young mice increased fluid intake to a greater degree than did aged mice. Thus, two major findings were obtained with respect to age differences in fluid intake: (1) aged inbred mice reliably drank more fluid than young mice and (2) young mice increased their fluid intake more than did aged mice when very palatable solutions were available.

3.5. Alcohol Preference

It has been found that there are large strain differences in the preference of ethanol by mice. McClearn and Rodgers (1961) found that C57BL/6J mice greatly prefer ethanol solutions to water, while the A strain and other strains of mice greatly prefer water to ethanol solutions. Age differences were obtained for C57BL/6J mice (Goodrick, 1967a), with young mice drinking a much greater proportion of 10% ethanol solution (in comparison with water) than aged mice. A further study (Goodrick, 1975b) examined high- and low-ethanol-preference strains, C57BL/6J and A/J, respectively, with young and aged groups of both strains. Over the range of 4–16% ethanol, aged C57BL/6J mice drank a lower percentage of ethanol than did young C57BL/6J mice. Young and aged A/J mice drank less ethanol solution than did C57BL/6J mice, and for A/J mice, age differences were small, with a general avoidance of ethanol by both age groups.

A recent study used A/J and C57BL/6J inbred mice and F_1 and F_2 hybrid mice to examine the effect of age on the genetic determination of ethanol preference of mice (Goodrick, 1977c). Mice were tested cross-sectionally at 5, 14, and 23 months of age. In addition to ethanol preference at different ages, it was possible to obtain information with respect to differences in the genetic system as a function of age. At 5 months of age, C57BL/6J mice preferred ethanol, A/J mice avoided ethanol, and F_1 and F_2 mice were intermediate in ethanol preference. Ethanol preference decreased at 14 months of age, and this decrease was substantial for the C57BL/6J and the F_1 groups. Then, at 23 months of age, there was a large increment in ethanol preference. These age differences are shown in Fig. 2.

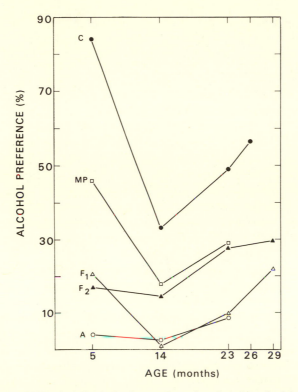

Fig. 2. Percentage of 10% alcohol solution ingested as a function of age for inbred and hybrid mice. (C) C57BL/6J; (A) A/J; (MP) midparent.

The ethanol preference of 5-month-old F_1 hybrids was below the midparental value, but significantly higher than the lower A/J parental value at all three ethanol concentrations. Values normally obtained for this hybrid are at about the midparental value or intermediate in mode of inheritance (e.g., McClearn and Rodgers, 1961). At 14 and 23 months of age, however, the F_1 values for ethanol preference were not significantly different from the A/J parental ethanol-preference value. These data provide ample evidence of systematic age and genetic differences in ethanol preference.

4. Summary

This chapter summarizes a number of research studies that represent a sampling of experimental studies of behavior genetics and aging. It is important to accrue knowledge of behavioral differences and similarities as aging progresses if we are to know how and when to intervene to prolong the period of maximal behavioral vigor during the life span. Since genetic factors and environmental factors interact to determine the behavioral vigor and life span of individual animals within a group, it is necessary to systematically study the effects of different environmental factors on behavioral vigor and life span, utilizing well-defined genetic groups.

References

Aschoff, J., 1965, *Circadian Clocks,* North-Holland, Amsterdam.

Chai, C., 1959, Life span in inbred and hybrid mice, *J. Hered.* **50**:203.

Curtis, H., Tilley, J., Crowley, C., and Fuller, M., 1966, The role of genetic factors in the aging process, *J. Geront.* **21**:365.

Elias, P., Elias, M., and Eleftheriou, B., 1975, Emotionality, exploratory behavior, and locomotion in aging inbred strains of mice, *Gerontologia* **21**:46.

Fuller, J., and Thompson, R., 1960, *Behavior Genetics,* John Wiley & Sons, New York.

Goodrick, C., 1967*a,* Behavioral characteristics of young and senescent inbred female mice of the C57BL/6J strain, *J. Gerontol.* **22**:459.

Goodrick, C., 1967*b,* Learning and retention of a light-contingent bar press response for three inbred strains of mice, *J. Psychol.* **67**:191.

Goodrick, C., 1973*a,* Exploration activity and emotionality of albino and pigmented mice, *J. Comp. Physiol. Psychol.* **84**:73.

Goodrick, C., 1973*b,* The effects of dietary protein upon growth of inbred and hybrid mice, *Growth* **37**:355.

Goodrick, C., 1974, The effects of exercise on longevity and behavior of hybrid mice which differ in coat color, *J. Gerontol.* **29**:129.

Goodrick, C., 1975*a,* Life-span and the inheritance of longevity of inbred mice, *J. Gerontol.* **30**:257.

Goodrick, C., 1975*b,* Behavioral differences in young and aged mice: Strain differences for activity measures, operant learning, sensory discrimination, and alcohol preference, *Exp. Aging Res.* **1**:191.

Goodrick, C., 1977*a,* Body weight change over the life span and longevity for C57BL/6J mice and mutations which differ in maximal body weight, *Gerontology* **23**:405.

Goodrick, C., 1977*b,* Body weight increment and length of life II. The effect of genetic constitution and dietary protein, *J. of Gerontol.* (in press).

Goodrick, C., 1977*c,* Ethanol preference of inbred mice: Mode of inheritance and the effect of age on the genetic system, *J. of Stud. Alcohol* (in press).

Grahn, D., 1972, Data collection and genetic analysis in the selection and study of rodent model systems in aging, in: *Development of the Rodent as a Model System of Aging* (D. Gibson, ed.), pp. 55–65, Department of Health, Education and Welfare, Bethesda, Maryland.

Green, E., (ed.), 1966, *Biology of the Laboratory Mouse,* McGraw-Hill, New York.

Hrubant, H., 1964, Specific genetic control of life span, *J. Gerontol.* **19**:451.

Lane, P., and Dickie, M., 1958, The effect of restricted food intake on the life span of genetically obese mice, *J. Nutr.* **64**:549.

Lindzey, G., and Thiessen, D., 1970, *Contributions to Behavior-Genetic Analysis: The Mouse as a Prototype,* Appleton-Century-Crofts, New York.

Lockard, R., 1963, Some effects of light upon the behavior of rodents, *Psychol. Bull.* **60**:509.

McCay, C., Crowell, M., and Maynard, L., 1935, The effect of retarded growth upon the length of the life span and upon the ultimate body size, *J. Nutr.* **10**:63.

McClearn, G., and Rodgers, D., 1961, Genetic factors in alcohol preference of laboratory mice, *J. Comp. Physiol. Psychol.* **54**:116.

Richter, C., 1922, A behavioristic study of the activity of the rat, *Comp. Psychol. Monogr.* **1**:1.

Roberts, R., 1961, The lifetime growth and reproduction of selected strains of mice, *Heredity* **16**:369.

Russell, E., 1966, Lifespan and aging patterns, in: *Biology of the Laboratory Mouse* (E. Green, ed.), pp. 511–519, McGraw-Hill, New York.

Russell, E., 1972, Genetic considerations in the selection of rodent species and strains for research in aging, in: *Development of the Rodent as a Model System of Aging* (D. Gibson, ed.), pp. 33–53, Department of Health, Education and Welfare, Bethesda, Maryland.

Silberberg, M., and Silberberg, R., 1954, Factors modifying the lifespan of mice, *Am. J. Physiol.* **177**:23.

Silberberg, R., Jarrett, S., and Silberberg, M., 1962, Longevity of female mice kept on various dietary regiments during growth, *J. Gerontol.* **17**:239.

Slonaker, J., 1912, Normal activity of the albino rat from birth to natural death, rate of growth, and duration of life, *J. Anim. Behav.* **2**:20.

Sprott, R., and Eleftheriou, B., 1974, Open-field behavior in aging inbred mice, *Gerontologia* **20**:155.

Stone, C., 1929, The age factor in animal learning. I. Rats in the problem box and the maze, *Genet. Psychol. Monogr.* **5**:1.

Storer, J., 1966, Longevity and gross pathology at death in 22 inbred mouse strains, *J. Gerontol.* **21**:404.

Wax, T., 1975, Runwheel activity patterns in mature-young and senescent mice: The effect of constant lighting conditions *J. Gerontol.* **30**:22.

Wax, T., 1977, Effects of age, strain, and illumination intensity on activity and self-selection of light–dark schedules in mice, *J. Comp. Physiol. Psychol.* **91**:51.

Wax, T., and Goodrick, C., 1975, Voluntary exposure to light by young and aged albino and pigmented inbred mice as a function of light intensity, *Dev. Psychobiol.* **8**:297.

Index